Endocrine
Physiology

Look for these other *Mosby Physiology Monograph Series* titles:

Endocrine Physiology

THIRD EDITION

SUSAN P. PORTERFIELD, PhD

Professor of Physiology, Emeritus and
Associate Dean for Curriculum, Emeritus,
Medical College of Georgia
Augusta, Georgia

BRUCE A. WHITE, PhD

Professor
Department of Cell Biology
University of Connecticut Health Center
Farmington, Connecticut

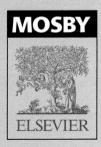

MOSBY

ELSEVIER

MOSBY
ELSEVIER

1600 John F. Kennedy Blvd.
Ste 1800
Philadelphia, PA 19103-2899

ENDOCRINE PHYSIOLOGY

ISBN-13: 978-0-323-03666-5

Copyright © 2007 by Mosby, Inc., an affiliate of Elsevier Inc.

ISBN-10: 0-323-03666-x

Library of Congress Cataloging-in-Publication Data
Porterfield, Susan P.
  Endocrine physiology / Susan P. Porterfield, Bruce A. White. – 3rd ed.
    p. ; cm. – (Mosby physiology monograph series)
  Includes bibliographical references and index.
  ISBN 0-323-03666-x
  1. Endocrine glands—Physiology.   I. White, Bruce Alan. II. Title.
III. Series.
    [DNLM: 1. Endocrine Glands—physiology.   WK 102 P849e 2007]
QP187.P657 2007
612.4—dc22   2006033342

Acquisitions Editor: William Schmitt
Editorial Assistant: Kristin Saunders
Publishing Services Manager: Linda Van Pelt
Project Manager: Priscilla Crater
Design Direction: Lou Forgione
Cover Designer: Lou Forgione

Printed in China
Last digit is the print number: 9 8 7 6 5 4 3 2 1

PREFACE

Endocrinology and reproductive endocrinology are usually taught at the end of a standard physiology course, because the endocrine system regulates all the other organ systems. In this respect, learning about the endocrine system has the added challenge of integrating our knowledge of hormones and their actions with the general function of a specific organ system. The student is encouraged to review previous material on the nervous system, cardiovascular system, GI system, renal-urinary system, and pulmonary system, which are covered in other volumes of the Mosby Monograph Series.

Endocrinology requires some appreciation for the anatomy and histology of each organ (called glands), the hormone(s) secreted (i.e., function) of each organ, the regulation of each organ, and the actions and metabolism of the secreted hormones. It is our hope that the student will gain some understanding of all of these aspects of endocrine function at the molecular, cellular, and organismal levels.

Reproductive endocrinology brings its own challenges, because the reproductive systems are both endocrine systems with glands secreting hormones, and organ systems involved in the production of gametes, copulation, fertilization, placentation, embryogenesis and fetal development, pregnancy, birth and lactation. Reproductive endocrinology is further complicated by sexual dimorphism, and the waxing and waning of reproductive activity during different periods of a human life. In this issue, the endocrinology of reproduction is emphasized, but it is hoped that enough reproductive biology is offered to allow the student to gain some understanding of the many functions of the male and female reproductive systems.

The endocrine system is similar to the nervous and immune systems, and in many instances, these three informational systems interact to promote normal development, maintain homeostatic balance, and allow for sexual reproduction in humans. In fact, some hormones are identical to, or strongly resemble neurotransmitters, while others resemble cytokines. We have tried to emphasize some of these interactions in the third edition of Endocrine Physiology.

The endocrine system, perhaps more than any other organ system, has been defined by its dysfunction. The clinical pictures from hypersecretion and hyposecretion of hormones, and hormone insensitivity inform us about the important roles that hormones play in people. Moreover, many cancers (e.g., breast, prostate, ovarian, uterine, cervical, pituitary, thyroid, testicular) are derived from the endocrine or reproductive systems. Thus, Endocrine Physiology describes both normal physiology of an endocrine gland, and examples of pathophysiology, which often reflect on the normal function of the gland.

As before, this book is designed for preclinical education of medical and dental students, as well as for graduate, nursing, pharmacology, and other allied health students. Susan and I hope that the third edition of Endocrine Physiology will allow the student to gain a foundation of knowledge about the endocrine system that can be built upon in later training, and perhaps invoke a sense of wonder and encourage enthusiastic inquiry about this important and complex organ system.

Bruce A. White

ACKNOWLEDGMENTS

I would like to acknowledge Dr. Ruth-Marie Fincher for her encouragement and direction during the original production of this book. Drs. Janis Work, Tom Wiedmeier, Chester Hendrich, Tom Weidman, Tom Abney and Tom Mills provided invaluable assistance in manuscript review for the original edition. Dr. Clarence Joe graciously provided multiple radiographs included in all editions of the textbook and Dr. Dale Sickles and Mr. Gregory Oblak provided assistance with the histologic sections. I would like to thank my family for the encouragement and support they have provided me during my entire career. In addition, I would like to thank Dr. Robert C. Little, whose teaching and guidance over many years inspired me to write the first edition of the book.

Susan Porterfield

Many colleagues at UConn Health Center helped with the third edition. Dr. Lisa Mehlmann (Department of Cell Biology) made substantive contributions to Chapter 10, especially related to fertilization and IVF. The following individuals provided constructive criticism of various chapters: Alison Nicholes (Dental Class of 2007) and Becky Eleck (Medical Class of 2007), Dr. Margaret (Sam) Pace (currently at Baylor College of Medicine, Houston, TX), Dr. Andrea DiLuigi (Department of Ob/Gyn, UCHC), and Dr. Perry Smith (currently at Yale School of Medicine). Lorri Goldsmith provided excellent administrative assistance.

I also want to acknowledge my wife, Carol, whose understanding and patience allowed me to work on this edition on weekends, vacations, family holidays, etc. At last, we can spend more time together!

Bruce A. White

CONTENTS

CHAPTER 1

INTRODUCTION TO THE ENDOCRINE SYSTEM 1

Objectives   1

Chemical Nature of Hormones   2

Proteins/Peptides   2

Catecholamines   4

Steroid Hormones   4

Thyroid Hormones   7

Eicosanoids   8

Transport of Hormones in the Circulation   8

Cellular Responses to Hormones   9

Signalling from Membrane Receptors   13

Signalling from Intracellular Receptors   18

Hormonal Rhythms   21

Summary   22

Key Words and Concepts   22

Self-Study Problems   23

Appendix: Different Modes of Chemical Signaling   24

CHAPTER 2

THE ENDOCRINE FUNCTION OF THE GASTROINTESTINAL TRACT 25

Objectives   25

Enteroendocrine Hormone Families and Their Receptors   27

The Regulation of Gastric Function   29

Overview of Regulation of Gastric Secretion and Motility   29

Gastrin and the Stimulation of Gastric Function   30

Inhibition of Gastric Function   32

Enteroendocrine Regulation of the Exocrine Pancreas and Gall Bladder   33

Secretin   34

Cholecystokinin   35

Motilin and Stimulation of Gastric and Small Intestinal Contractions During the Interdigestive Period   36

The Insulinotropic Actions of GI Peptides (Incretin Action)   37

Gastric Inhibitory Peptide/ Glucose-dependent Insulinotropic Peptide   38

Glucagon-like Peptide-1   38

The Enterotropic Actions of GI
    Hormones   39
        Gastrin   39
        Secretin and CCK   39
        GLP-1   39
        GLP-2   39
    Summary   40
    Key Words and Concepts   41
    Self-Study Problems   41

CHAPTER 3

ENERGY METABOLISM 43

    Objectives   43
    Overview of Energy Metabolism   43
        Cells Must Make ATP to
            Function and Stay Viable   43
        Making ATP   44
        Storage Forms of Energy   47
        Partial Digestion of VLDL Generates
            Cholesterol-Rich Low-Density
            Lipoprotein   50
        Release of TGs in Adipose Cells   51
        Protein   51
        Gluconeogenesis – Making Glucose
            from Glycerol, Lactate and Amino
            Acids   51
        Summary of Key Metabolic
            Pathways   51
    Key Hormones Involved in Metabolic
        Homeostasis   52
        The Endocrine Pancreas   52
        Insulin   53
        Glucagon   57
        Epinephrine and Norepinephrine   58
    Metabolic Homeostasis – The Integrated
        Outcome of Hormonal and
        Substrate/Product Regulation
        of Metabolic Pathways   58

    The Fasting-to-Fed State Transition
        Involves Anabolic Pathways that
        Store Energy   58
    Release of Energy During the
        Interdigestive Period or an
        Extended Fast   63
    Diabetes Mellitus   65
        Symptoms of Diabetes Mellitus   68
        Acute Complications of Diabetes
            Mellitus   69
        Long-Term Sequelae of Diabetes
            Mellitus   70
        Problems Associated with Diabetes
            Management   72
    Emerging Concepts in Energy
        Homeostasis: Adipose Tissue
        as an Endocrine Organ   73
        Leptin   74
        Adiponectin   75
        Tumor Necrosis Factor-α (TNF-α)   75
    Summary   76
    Key Words and Concepts   77
    Self-Study Problems   79

CHAPTER 4

CALCIUM AND PHOSPHATE
HOMEOSTASIS 81

    Objectives   81
    Calcium and Phosphorus are Important
        Dietary Elements that Play Many
        Crucial Roles in Cellular Physiology   81
    Physiological Regulation of Calcium
        and Phosphate: Parathyroid
        Hormone (PTH) and 1,25-
        dihydroxyvitamin D   82
        Parathyroid Hormone   82
        The Parathyroid Glands   82
        Vitamin D   85

The Small Intestine, Bone, and Kidney
Determine Ca²⁺ and Pi Levels 88

    *Handling of Ca²⁺ and Pi by the
    Small Intestine 88*

    Handling of Ca²⁺ and Pi by Bone 90

    The Histophysiology of Adult Bone 90

    *Handling of Ca²⁺ and Pi by the
    Kidneys 93*

    *Integrated Physiologic
    Regulation of Ca²⁺/Pi
    Metabolism: Response of PTH
    and 1,25-dihydroxyvitamin D
    to a Hypocalcemic Challenge 93*

    *Pharmacologic Hormonal Regulation
    of Calcium and Phosphate:
    Calcitonin 95*

    *Hormonal Regulation of Calcium
    and Phosphate: Regulators
    Overexpressed by Cancers 96*

    *Regulation of Ca²⁺/Pi Metabolism
    by Immune/Inflammatory Cells 97*

    *Regulation of Ca²⁺/Pi Metabolism
    by Gonadal and Adrenal Steroid
    Hormones 97*

Pathologic Disorders of Calcium and
Phosphate Balance 97

    Hyperparathyroidism (Primary) 97

    Pseudohypoparathyroidism 99

    Hypoparathyroidism 99

    Vitamin D Deficiency 101

    Paget's Disease 101

    *Bone Problems of Renal Failure
    (Renal Osteodystrophy) 101*

Summary 102

Key Words and Concepts 103

Self-Study Problems 104

CHAPTER **5**

THE HYPOTHALAMUS-PITUITARY COMPLEX 107

Objectives 107

Embryology and Anatomy 107

The Neurohypophysis 109

    *Synthesis of ADH (Vasopressin)
    and Oxytocin 110*

    Antidiuretic Hormone 112

    Oxytocin 116

The Adenohypophysis 117

    The Endocrine Axes 117

    *The Endocrine Function of the
    Adenohypophysis 121*

    The Corticotrope 121

    The Thyrotrope 124

    The Gonadotrope 125

    The Somatotrope 127

    *Direct Versus Indirect Actions
    of GH 129*

    *Role of Growth Hormone, Insulin-
    like Growth Factor, and Insulin
    in Starvation 131*

    *Pathologic Conditions Involving
    Growth Hormone 131*

    The Lactotrope 133

    *Pathologic Conditions Involving
    Prolactin 135*

    Hypopituitarism 135

    Growth 136

Summary 137

Key Words and Concepts 138

Self-Study Problems 139

CHAPTER **6**

THE THYROID GLAND 141

Objectives   141

Anatomy and Histology of the Thyroid   141

Thyroid Hormones   141

Synthesis of Thyroid Hormones   142

Thyroid Hormone Secretion   145

*Compounds Altering Thyroid
Hormone Synthesis   146*

Thyroid Hormone Transport   146

Metabolism of Thyroid Hormones   147

Control of Thyroid Function   148

Control Mechanisms   148

Perturbations of Control System   149

Mechanisms of Hormone Action   150

Thyroid Hormone Receptors   150

*Thyroid-Stimulating Hormone
Receptor   150*

Actions of Thyroid Hormones   151

*Maturational and Differentational
Effects   151*

Neurologic Effects   151

Effects on Growth   152

Metabolic Actions   152

*Actions Mimicking Sympathetic
Nervous System Activity   153*

Actions on Skeletal Muscle   154

Actions on Cardiovascular System   154

Pathologic Conditions Involving the
Thyroid   154

Hypothyroidism   154

Hyperthyroidism   157

Thyroiditis   159

Summary   159

Key Words and Concepts   160

Self-Study Problems   160

Appendix: Laboratory Data on Thyroid
Function   161

CHAPTER **7**

THE ADRENAL GLAND 163

Objectives   163

Anatomy   163

Adrenal Medulla   164

Synthesis of Epinephrine   164

*Mechanism of Action
of Catecholamines   166*

*Physiological Actions of
Adrenomedullary
Catecholamines   167*

Metabolism of Catecholamines   168

*Pathologic Conditions Involving the
Adrenal Medulla   170*

Adrenal Cortex   170

Zona Fasciculata   170

*The Zona Fasciculata Makes
Cortisol   170*

*Transport and Metabolism of
Cortisol   175*

Mechanism of Action of Cortisol   175

Physiologic Actions of Cortisol   175

Regulation of Cortisol Production   178

Zona Reticularis   179

*The Zona Reticularis Makes
Adrenal Androgens   179*

*Metabolism and Fate DHEAS and
DHEA   180*

*Physiologic Actions of Adrenal
Androgens   180*

*Regulation of Zona Reticularis
Function   182*

Zona Glomerulosa   182

*The Zona Glomerulosa Makes
Aldosterone   182*

*Transport and Metabolism of
Aldosterone   183*

*Mechanism of Aldosterone
Action   183*

Physiologic Actions of Aldosterone   183

Regulation of Aldosterone Secretion   187

Pathologic Conditions Involving the Adrenal Cortex   188

Adrenocortical Insufficiency   188

Adrenocortical Excess   188

Summary   191

Key Words and Concepts   192

Self-Study Problems   194

CHAPTER 8

THE MALE REPRODUCTIVE SYSTEM 197

Objectives   197

Histophysiology of the Testis   198

The Intratubular Compartment   199

The Peritubular Compartment   204

Fates and Actions of Androgens   204

Intratesticular Androgen   204

Peripheral Conversion to Estrogen   204

Peripheral Conversion to DHT   204

Peripheral Testosterone Actions   206

Mechanism of Androgen Action   206

Transport and Metabolism of Androgens   207

Hypothalamus-Pituitary-Testis Axis   207

Regulation of Leydig Cell Function   207

Regulation of Sertoli Cell Function   207

The Male Reproductive Tract   208

Development of the Male Reproductive System   211

Puberty and Senescence   214

Disorders Involving the Male Reproductive System   217

Summary   219

Key Words and Concepts   220

Self-Study Problems   222

CHAPTER 9

THE FEMALE REPRODUCTIVE SYSTEM 223

Objectives   223

Anatomy and Histology of the Ovary   225

Growth, Development, and Function of the Ovarian Follicle   226

Resting Primordial Follicle   226

Growing Preantral Follicles   228

Growing Antral Follicles   228

Dominant Follicle   230

The Dominant Follicle During the Periovulatory Period   231

The Corpus Luteum   234

Follicular Atresia   236

Follicular Development and the Monthly Menstrual Cycle   236

Regulation of Late Follicular Development, Ovulation, and Luteinization: The Human Menstrual Cycle   236

The Female Reproductive Tract   239

The Oviduct   239

The Uterus   241

The Cervix   245

The Vagina   246

The External Genitalia   246

Biology of Estradiol-17β and Progesterone   247

Mechanisms of Estrogen and Progesterone Hormone Action   247

Biological Effects of Estrogen and Progesterone   248

Transport and Metabolism of Ovarian Steroids   248

The Ontogeny of the Female Reproductive System   249

Development of the Female Reproductive Tract   249

Puberty   249

Menopause   250

Ovarian Pathophysiology   251

   Turner Syndrome   251

   Polycystic Ovarian Syndrome   251

Summary   253

Key Words and Concepts   254

Self-Study Problems   256

CHAPTER 10

FERTILIZATION AND PREGNANCY 259

Objectives   259

Fertilization, Early Embryogenesis, Implantation & Placentation   259

   Synchronization with Maternal Ovarian and Reproductive Tract Function   259

   Fertilization   261

   Early Embryogenesis and Implantation   264

   Structure of Mature Placenta   266

   The Endocrine Function of the Placenta   271

   Human Chorionic Gonadotropin   272

   Progesterone   272

   Estrogen   274

   Human Placental Lactogen   274

   Other Placental Hormones   276

Placental Transport   276

The Fetal Endocrine System   277

   Pancreas   277

   Parathyroid Gland   277

   Pituitary Gland   277

   Thyroid Gland   277

   Adrenal Gland   278

   Testes and Ovaries   278

Maternal Endocrine Changes During Pregnancy   278

   Pituitary Gland   278

   Thyroid Gland   279

   Adrenal Gland   279

Maternal Physiologic Changes During Pregnancy   279

   Cardiovascular Changes   279

   Respiratory Changes   280

   Renal Changes   280

   Gastrointestinal Changes   281

   Diabetogenicity of Pregnancy   281

Parturition   281

   Placental Corticotropin-Releasing Hormone and the Fetal Adrenal Axis   281

   Estrogen and Progesterone Secretion   282

   Oxytocin   282

   Prostaglandins   282

   Uterine Size   282

Mammogenesis and Lactation   282

   Structure of the Mammary Gland   282

   Hormonal Regulation of Mammary Gland Development   283

Contraception   285

   Behavioral and Mechanical Approaches   285

   Oral Contraceptives   285

   Hormonal Treatment for Emergency Contraception and Abortion   286

In Vitro Fertilization   286

Summary   287

Key Words and Concepts   288

Self-Study Problems   290

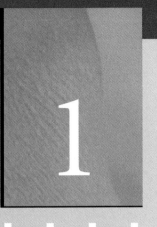

1

INTRODUCTION TO THE ENDOCRINE SYSTEM

OBJECTIVES

1. Identify the chemical nature of the major hormones.
2. Describe how the chemical nature influences hormone synthesis, storage, secretion, transport, clearance, mechanism of action, and appropriate route of exogenous hormone administration.
3. Explain the significance of hormone binding to plasma proteins.
4. Describe the major signal transduction pathways for different classes of hormones and provide a specific example of each.
5. Explain the impact of hormonal rhythms on endocrine function.

Glands are organs that secrete substances in response to stimuli. The secretions of **exocrine glands,** such as the salivary glands, are typically composed of salts, water, immunoglobulins and enzymes, and are conveyed to a major lumen (e.g., the oral cavity) via a duct. In contrast, **endocrine glands** are ductless and secrete chemical messengers, called **hormones,** into the extracellular fluid. Secreted hormones gain access to the circulation, often via fenestrated capillaries, and, in most cases, reach all the cells of the body. In order to function, hormones must bind to specific **receptors** expressed by specific **target cell** types within **target organs**. Hormones are also referred to as **ligands,** in the context of ligand-receptor binding. Hormones are also referred to as **agonists,** in that their binding to the receptor is transduced into a cellular response. Receptor **antagonists** typically bind to a receptor and lock it in an inactive state, unable to induce a cellular response. Loss or inactivation of a receptor leads to **hormonal resistance.** Constitutive activation of a receptor leads to unregulated, hormone-independent activation of cellular processes.

The widespread delivery of hormones in the blood makes the **endocrine system** ideal for the functional coordination of multiple organs and cell types in the following context:

1. Allowing normal development and growth of the organism
2. Maintenance of internal homeostasis
3. Regulating the onset of reproductive maturity at puberty and the function of the reproductive system in the adult

In the adult, endocrine organs produce and secrete their hormones in response to finely regulated feedback control systems that are tuned to **set-points.** These set-points are genetically determined, but may be altered by age, circadian rhythms (24-hour cycles or diurnal rhythms), seasonal cycles, the environment, stress, inflammation, and other influences.

The material in this chapter covers generalizations common to all hormones or to specific groups of hormones. The chemical nature of the hormones and their mechanisms of action are discussed. This presentation provides the generalized information necessary to categorize the hormones and to make predictions about the most likely characteristics of a given hormone. Some of the exceptions to these generalizations are discussed later.

CHEMICAL NATURE OF HORMONES

Hormones are classified biochemically as **proteins/ peptides, catecholamines, steroid hormones,** and **iodothyronines.** The chemical nature of a hormone determines (1) how it is synthesized, stored and released; (2) how it is carried in the blood; (3) its biological half-life ($t_{1/2}$) and mode of clearance; and (4) its cellular mechanism of action.

Proteins/Peptides

The protein and peptide hormones can be grouped into structurally related molecules that are encoded by gene families. Protein/peptide hormones gain their specificity from their primary amino acid sequence, which confers specific higher order structures, and from post-translational modifications, especially glycosylation.

Because protein/peptide hormones are destined for secretion outside the cell, they are synthesized and processed differently than proteins destined to remain within the cell or to be continuously added to the membrane (Box 1-1). The hormones are synthesized on the polyribosome as larger preprohormones or prehormones (Figure 1-1). The nascent peptides have at their N-terminal a group of 15 to 30 amino acids called the **signal peptide.** A **signal recognition complex**

(a complex of six proteins and a ribonucleic acid [RNA]) binds to the N-terminal of the nascent peptide after about 70 amino acids have been polymerized. This stops further translation until the signal recognition complex binds to a **docking protein** located on the cytosolic face of the endoplasmic reticulum. This binding releases the translational block. The growing polypeptide is directed through the endoplasmic reticular membrane into the cisternae. It is released from the signal peptide by a **signal peptidase** located on the cisternal surface of the endoplasmic reticular membrane. The polypeptide is then transported from the cisternae to the Golgi apparatus, where it is packaged into a membrane-bound secretory vesicle and released into the cytoplasm. The carbohydrate moiety of glycoproteins is added in the Golgi apparatus.

The original gene transcript is called either a **prehormone** or a **preprohormone** (Figure 1-2). Removing the signal peptide produces either the prohormone or the hormone. A prohormone is a polypeptide that requires further cleavage before the mature hormone is produced. Often this final cleavage occurs while the prohormone is within the Golgi apparatus or the secretory granule. For example, insulin is produced as preproinsulin, cleaved to proinsulin in the endoplasmic reticulum, and packaged in secretory vesicles as proinsulin. While in the secretory vesicle, a portion of the center of the single chain (connecting [C] peptide) is cleaved to produce the insulin molecule, which contains two peptide chains. The mature secretory vesicle contains equimolar amounts of insulin and C peptide. Sometimes prohormones contain the sequence of multiple hormones. For example, the protein, pro-opiomelanocortin (POMC), contains the amino acid sequences of adrenocorticotropic hormone (ACTH) and α-melanocyte-stimulating hormone (α-MSH). However, ACTH and α-MSH are produced by different cell types. This occurs because different cell types express specific **prohormone** (also called **proprotein**) **convertases,** resulting in cell-specific processing of the prohormone.

Protein/peptide hormones are stored in the gland as membrane-bound secretory granules and are released by **exocytosis** through the **regulated secretory pathway.** This means that hormones are not continually secreted, but rather that they are secreted in response to a stimulus, through a mechanism of **stimulus-secretion coupling.** Regulated exocytosis requires energy, Ca^{2+}, an

---

BOX 1-1
PROTEIN/PEPTIDE HORMONES

- Are synthesized as prehormones or preprohormones
- Are stored in membrane-bound granules
- Are relatively polar
- Often circulate in blood unbound
- Usually cannot be administered orally
- Usually have cell membrane receptors

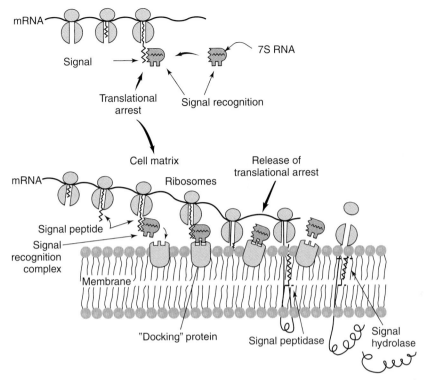

FIGURE 1-1 ■ Synthesis of protein and peptide hormones. *(Redrawn from Wilson JD, Foster DW, Kronenberg HM, Larsen PR, editors: Williams' textbook of endocrinology, ed 10, Philadelphia, 2003, Saunders.)*

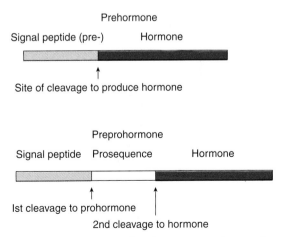

FIGURE 1-2 ■ Structure of prehormones and preprohormones.

intact cytoskeleton (microtubules, microfilaments), and the presence of coat proteins that specifically sort the secretory vesicles to the cell membrane.

Protein/peptide hormones are soluble in aqueous solvents and, with the notable exceptions of the insulin-like growth factors (IGFs) and growth hormone (GH), circulate in the blood predominantly in an unbound form and therefore tend to have short biological half-lives ($t_{1/2}$). Protein hormones are removed by endocytosis and lysosomal turnover of hormone-receptor complexes (see later) or by enzymatic degradation. Many of these protein hormones are small enough to appear in the urine in a physiologically active form. For example, follicle-stimulating hormone (FSH) and luteinizing hormone (LH) are present in urine. Urine of postmenopausal women is an excellent source of gonadotropins because postmenopausal serum gonadotropin levels are high. Pregnancy tests using human urine are based on the urinary presence of the placental hormone human chorionic gonadotropin (hCG).

Proteins/peptides are readily digested if administered orally. Hence, they must be administered by injection or, in the case of small peptides, through a mucous membrane (sublingually or intranasally). Because proteins/peptides do not cross cell membranes readily, they signal through membrane receptors. The **second-messenger hypothesis** was proposed to link membrane receptor binding and intracellular effects.

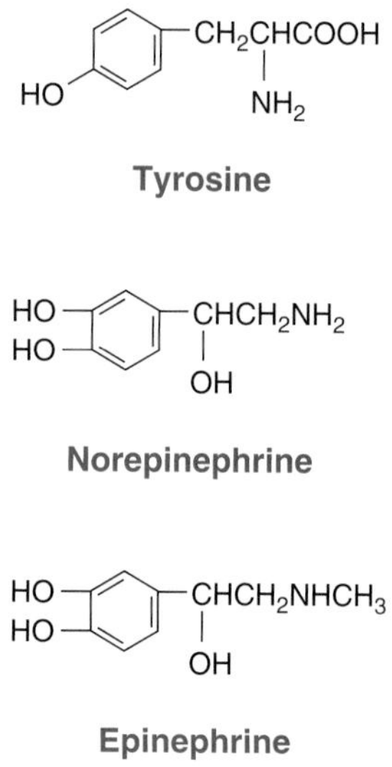

Catecholamines

Catecholamines are synthesized by the adrenal medulla and neurons, and include norepinephrine, epinephrine, and dopamine (Box 1-2). The primary hormonal product of the adrenal medulla is **epinephrine,** and to a lesser extent, **norepinephrine** (Figure 1-3). Catecholamines gain their specificity through enzymatic modifications of the amino acid, tyrosine. Catecholamines are ultimately stored into secretory vesicles that are part of the regulated secretory pathway. Catecholamines are soluble in blood and circulate either unbound or loosely bound to albumin. Catecholamines are similar to protein/peptide hormones in that they do not cross cell membranes readily and hence produce their actions though membrane receptors. They have short biological half-lives ($t_{1/2} = 1$ to 2 minutes), and are primarily cleared by cell uptake and enzymatic modification.

Steroid Hormones

Steroid hormones are made by the **adrenal cortex, ovaries, testes,** and **placenta** (Box 1-3). Steroid hormones from these glands fall into five categories: **progestins, mineralocorticoids, glucocorticoids,**

FIGURE 1-3 ■ Structure of the catecholamines, norepinephrine and epinephrine, and their precursor, tyrosine.

androgens, and **estrogens** (Table 1-1). Progestins and the corticoids are 21-carbon steroids, whereas androgens are 19-carbon steroids and estrogens are 18-carbon steroids. Steroid hormones also include the active metabolite of **vitamin D,** which is a secosteroid (see Chapter 4).

Steroid hormones are synthesized by a series of enzymatic modifications of cholesterol and have the **cyclopentanoperhydrophenanthrene ring** (or a derivative thereof) as their core (Figure 1-4). The enzymatic modifications of cholesterol are of three general types: hydroxylations, dehydrogenations/reductions and lyases. The purpose of these modifications is to produce

---

BOX 1-2
CATECHOLAMINES

- Are derived from tyrosine
- Do not cross cell membranes readily
- Have cell surface receptors
- Are transported in blood free or only loosely associated with proteins
- Are stored in membrane-bound granules
- Could be administered orally but in their native form their half-life is too short to be effective

---

BOX 1-3
STEROID HORMONES

- Are derived from the cyclopentanoperhydrohenanthrene ring
- Have intracellular receptors
- Are nonpolar
- Usually circulate protein-bound in blood
- Are not stored in the endocrine gland
- Can often be administered orally

		TABLE 1-1		
		Steroid Hormones		
FAMILY	NUMBER OF CARBONS	SPECIFIC HORMONE	PRIMARY SITE OF SYNTHESIS	PRIMARY RECEPTOR
Progestin	21	Progesterone	Ovary, placenta	Progesterone receptor (PR)
Glucocorticoid	21	Cortisol, Corticosterone	Adrenal cortex	Glucocorticoid receptor (GR)
Mineralocorticoid	21	Aldosterone, 11-Deoxycorticosterone	Adrenal cortex	Mineralocorticoid receptor (MR)
Androgen	19	Testosterone, Dihydrotestosterone	Testis	Androgen receptor (AR)
Estrogen	18	Estradiol-17β, Estriol	Ovary, placenta	Estrogen receptor (ER)

a cholesterol derivative that is sufficiently unique to be recognized by a specific receptor. Thus, progestins bind to the **progesterone receptor (PR),** mineralocorticoids bind to the **mineralocorticoid receptor (MR)**, glucocorticoids bind to the **glucocorticoid receptor (GR),** androgens bind to the **androgen receptor (AR)**, estrogens bind to the **estrogen receptor (ER)**, and the active vitamin D metabolite binds to the **vitamin D receptor (VDR).** Complexity of steroid hormone action is increased by the expression of multiple forms of each receptor. Additionally, there is some degree of non-specificity between steroid hormones and the receptors they bind to. For example, glucocorticoids bind to the MR with high affinity, and progestins, glucocorticoids, and androgens can all interact with the PR, GR, and AR to some degree. An appreciation of this "cross-talk" is important to the physician who is prescribing synthetic steroids. For example, medroxyprogesterone acetate (a synthetic progesterone given for hormone replacement therapy in postmenopausal women) binds well to the AR, as well as the PR. As discussed subsequently, steroid hormones are hydrophobic and pass through cell membranes easily. Accordingly, classical steroid hormone receptors are localized intracellularly and act by regulating gene expression. Evidence is mounting for the presence of additional membrane and juxtamembrane steroid hormone receptors that mediate rapid, nongenomic actions of steroid hormones.

Steroidogenic cell types are defined as cells that can convert cholesterol to pregnenolone, which is the first reaction common to all steroidogenic pathways. Steroidogenic cells have some capacity for cholesterol synthesis, but often obtain cholesterol from cholesterol-rich lipoproteins (low-density lipoproteins and high-density lipoproteins; see Chapter 3). Pregnenolone is then further modified by six or fewer enzymatic reactions. Because of their hydrophobic nature, steroid hormones and precursors can leave the steroidogenic cell easily, and so are not stored. Thus, steroidogenesis is regulated at the level of uptake, storage and mobilization of cholesterol, and at the level of steroidogenic enzyme gene expression and activity. Steroids are *not* regulated at the level of secretion of the preformed hormone. A clinical implication of this mode of secretion is that high levels of steroid hormone precursors are easily released into the blood when a steroidogenic enzyme within a given pathway is inactive or absent.

An important feature of steroidogenesis is that steroid hormones often undergo further modifications (apart from those involved in deactivation and excretion) after their release from the original steroidogenic cell. For example, estrogen synthesis by the ovary and placenta requires at least two cell types to complete the pathway of cholesterol to estrogen (see Chapters 9 and 10). This means that one cell secretes a precursor, and a second cell converts the precursor to estrogen. There is also considerable peripheral conversion of active steroid hormones. For example, the testis

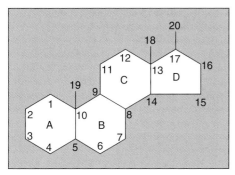

FIGURE 1-4 ■ Cyclopentanoperhydrophenanthrene ring, the backbone of steroid hormones.

secretes sparingly little estrogen. However, adipose, muscle, and other tissues express the enzyme for converting testosterone (a potent androgen) to estradiol-17β (a potent estrogen). Thus, the overall production of a "steroid hormone X" is equivalent to the sum of the secretion of "steroid hormone X" from a steroidogenic cell type, and the **peripheral conversion** of other steroids to "steroid hormone X" (Figure 1-5). Peripheral conversion can produce (1) a more active, but same class, of hormone (e.g., conversion of 25-hydroxyvitamin D to 1,25-dihydroxyvitamin D); (2) a less active hormone that can be reversibly activated by another tissue (e.g., conversion of cortisol to cortisone in kidney, followed by conversion of cortisone to cortisol in abdominal adipose tissue); or (3) a different class of hormone (e.g., conversion of testosterone into estrogen). Peripheral conversion of steroids plays an important role in several endocrine disorders.

Because of their nonpolar nature, steroid hormones are not readily soluble in blood. Therefore, steroid hormones circulate bound to **transport proteins.**

These include albumin, but also the specific transport protein, **sex hormone–binding globulin (SHBG)** and **corticosteroid-binding globulin (CBG)** (see later). Excretion of hormones typically involves inactivating modifications followed by **glucuronide** or **sulfate conjugation** in the liver. These modifications increase the water solubility of the steroid and decrease its affinity for transport proteins, allowing the inactivated steroid hormone to be excreted by the kidney. Steroid compounds are absorbed fairly readily in the gastrointestinal tract and therefore often may be administered orally.

Figure 1-6 compares the ultrastructure of a protein hormone-producing cell to that of a steroidogenic cell. Protein hormone-producing cells store the product in secretory granules and have extensive rough endoplasmic reticulum. In contrast, steroidogenic cells store precursor (cholesterol esters) in the form of lipid droplets, but do not store product. Steroidogenic enzymes are localized to smooth endoplasmic reticulum membrane and within mitochondria, and these two organelles are numerous in steroidogenic cells.

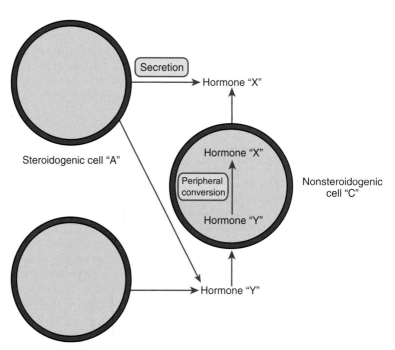

FIGURE 1-5 ■ Peripheral conversion of steroid hormone.

Steroidogenic cell "A"

Secretion

Hormone "X"

Hormone "X"

Peripheral conversion

Hormone "Y"

Nonsteroidogenic cell "C"

Steroidogenic cell "B"

Hormone "Y"

Total production of hormone "X" =
Secretion of hormone "X" + peripheral conversion of hormone "Y" into hormone "X"

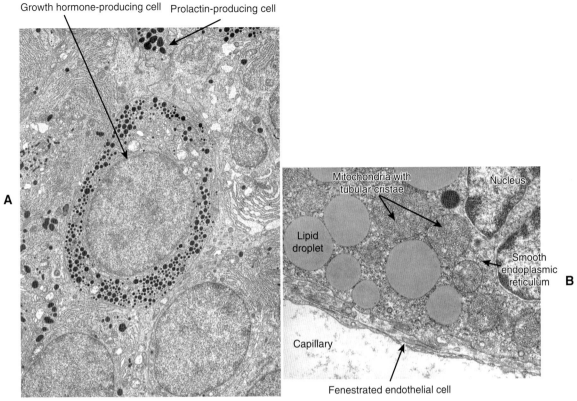

Growth hormone-producing cell   Prolactin-producing cell

A

Mitochondria with tubular cristae

Nucleus

Lipid droplet

Smooth endoplasmic reticulum

B

Capillary

Fenestrated endothelial cell

FIGURE 1-6 ■ Ultrastructure of a protein hormone-producing cell (**A**) and a steroidogenic cell (**B**). Note the presence of secretory granules and rough endoplasmic reticulum in the protein hormone-secreting cell, and the presence of lipid droplets, large mitochondria, and smooth endoplasmic reticulum in the steroidogenic cell. *(From Kierszenbaum AL: Histology and cell biology, Philadelphia, 2002, Mosby.)*

Thyroid Hormones

Thyroid hormones (Box 1-4) are iodothyronines (Figure 1-7) that are made by the coupling of iodinated tyrosine residues through an ether linkage (see Chapter 6). Their specificity is determined by the thyronine structure, but also by exactly where the thyronine is iodinated. Thyroid hormones cross cell membranes by both diffusion and transport systems. They are stored extracellularly in the thyroid as an integral part of the glycoprotein molecule thyroglobulin (see Chapter 6). Thyroid hormones are sparingly soluble in blood and aqueous fluids and are transported in blood bound (>99%) to serum-binding proteins. A major transport protein is **thyroid hormone–binding globulin (TBG).** They have long

BOX 1-4
THYROID HORMONES

- Are derived from tyrosine
- Cross cell membranes
- Are transported in blood bound to proteins
- Have intracellular receptors
- Are stored in the follicle
- Can be administered orally

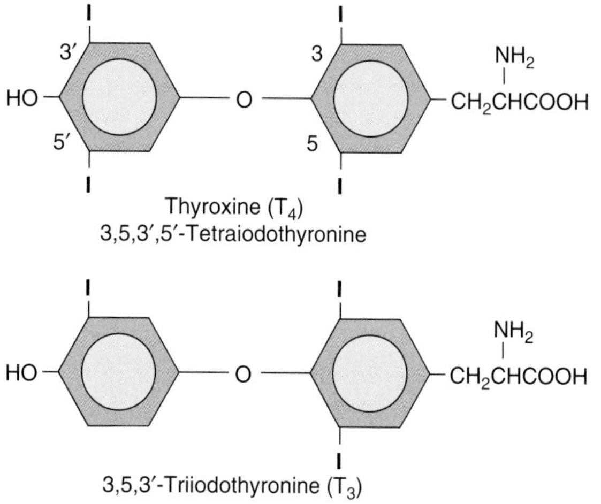

Thyroxine (T_4)
3,5,3′,5′-Tetraiodothyronine

3,5,3′-Triiodothyronine (T_3)

FIGURE 1-7 ■ Structure of thyroid hormones, which are iodinated thyronines.

half-lives (thyroxine [T_4] = 7 days; triiodothyronine [T_3] = 24 hours). Thyroid hormones are similar to steroid hormones in that the **thyroid hormone receptor (TR)** is intracellular and acts as a transcription factor. In fact, the TR belongs to the same gene family that includes steroid hormone receptors and vitamin D receptors.

Thyroid hormones can be administered orally and sufficient hormone is absorbed intact to make this an effective mode of therapy.

Eicosanoids

Eicosanoids are short-lived compounds that are formed from polyunsaturated fatty acids with 18, 20, and 22 carbons. Arachidonic acid is the most important precursor of this group of compounds. This group includes **prostaglandins, leukotrienes, thromboxanes,** and **prostacyclin.** These compounds are not typically considered hormones and are thus not listed in Box 1-5. They are synthesized throughout the body, and their primary actions are autocrine or paracrine. Hormones often regulate the synthesis of these compounds. Whereas most eicosanoids, such as catecholamines and protein/peptide hormones, act by means of cell surface receptors, a few act through intracellular receptors.

TRANSPORT OF HORMONES IN THE CIRCULATION

A significant amount of steroid and thyroid hormones is transported in the blood bound to plasma proteins

---

BOX 1-5

CLASSES OF HORMONES BASED ON STRUCTURE

Glycoproteins	Polypeptides	Steroids	Catecholamines
Follicle-stimulating hormone (FSH)	Adrenocorticotropic hormone (ACTH)	Aldosterone	Epinephrine
Thyroid-stimulating hormone (TSH)	Angiotensin	Cortisol	Norepinephrine **Iodothyronines**
Luteinizing hormone (LH)	Calcitonin, parathyroid hormone (PTH)	Estradiol	Thyroxine (T_4)
Human chorionic gonadotropin (hCG)	Cholecystokinin (CCK)	Progesterone	Triiodothyronine (T_3)
	Melanocyte-stimulating hormone (MSH)	Testosterone	
	Nerve growth factor (NGF), insulin-like growth factor (IGF), epidermal growth factor (EGF)	Vitamin D	
	Oxytocin, antidiuretic hormone (ADH)		
	Relaxin, secretin		
	Somatostatin		
	Releasing hormones		
	Prolactin, growth hormone (GH)		

that are produced in a regulated manner by the liver. Protein and polypeptide hormones are generally transported free in the blood. There is an equilibrium between the concentrations of bound hormone (HP), free hormone (H), and plasma transport protein (P); if free hormone levels drop, hormone will be released from the transport proteins. This relationship may be expressed as

$$[H] \times [P] = [HP] \; or \; K = [H] \times [P]/[HP]$$

where K = the dissociation constant.

The free hormone is the biologically active form for target organ action, feedback control and clearance by uptake and metabolism. Consequently, in evaluating hormonal status, one must sometimes determine free hormone levels rather than total hormone levels alone. This is particularly important because hormone transport proteins themselves are regulated by altered endocrine and disease states.

Protein binding serves several purposes. It prolongs the circulating $t_{1/2}$ of the hormone. Many of these hormones cross cell membranes readily and would either enter the cells or be lost through the kidney were they not protein bound. The bound hormone represents a "reservoir" of hormone and as such can serve to "buffer" acute changes in hormone secretion. Some hormones, such as steroids, are sparingly soluble in blood and protein binding facilitates their transport.

CELLULAR RESPONSES TO HORMONES

Hormones regulate essentially every major aspect of cellular function in every organ system. Hormones control the growth of cells, ultimately determining their size and competency for cell division. Hormones regulate the differentiation of cells and their ability to survive or undergo programmed cell death. Hormones influence cellular metabolism, ionic composition, and transmembrane potential. Hormones orchestrate several complex cytoskeletal-associated events, including cell shape, migration, division, exocytosis, recycling/endocytosis, and cell-cell and cell-matrix adhesion. Hormones regulate the expression and function of cytosolic and membrane proteins, and a specific hormone may determine the level of its own receptor, and/or the receptors for other hormones.

Although hormones can exert coordinated, pleiotropic control on multiple aspects of cell function, any given hormone does not regulate every function in every cell type. Rather, a single hormone controls a subset of cellular functions in only the cell types that express receptors for that hormone. Thus, selective receptor expression determines which cells will respond to a given hormone. Moreover, the differentiated state of a specific cell will determine how it will respond to a hormone. Thus, the specificity of hormonal responses resides in the structure of the hormone itself, the receptor for the hormone, and the cell type in which the receptor is expressed. Serum hormone concentrations are extremely low (10^{-11} to 10^{-9} M). Therefore, a receptor must have a **high affinity,** as well as specificity, for its cognate hormone.

How does hormone-receptor binding get transduced into a cellular response? Hormone binding to a receptor induces conformational changes in the receptor. This is referred to as a **signal.** The signal is **transduced** into the activation of one or more **intracellular messengers.** Messenger molecules then bind to **effector proteins,** which, in turn, modify specific cellular functions. The combination of hormone/receptor binding (signal), activation of messengers (transduction), and the regulation of one or more effector proteins is referred to as a **signal transduction pathway** (also called simply a **signaling pathway**), and the final outcome is referred to as the **cellular response.** Signaling pathways are usually characterized by the following:

1. Multiple, hierarchical steps in which "downstream" effector proteins are dependent on and driven by "upstream" receptors, transducers, and effector proteins. This means that loss or inactivation of one or more component within the pathway leads to a general resistance to the hormone, whereas constitutive activation or overexpression of components can drive a pathway in an unregulated manner.

2. Amplification of the initial hormone-receptor binding. Amplification can be so great that maximal response to a hormone is achieved on hormone binding to a small percentage of receptors.

3. Activation of multiple pathways, or at least regulation of multiple cell functions, from one hormone-receptor binding event. For example, binding of

insulin to its receptor activates three separate signaling pathways. Even in fairly simple pathways (e.g., glucagon activation of adenylyl cyclase), divergent downstream events allow for the regulation of multiple functions (e.g., posttranslational activation of glycogen phosphorylase and increased phosphoenolpyruvate carboxykinase [PEPCK] gene transcription).

4. Antagonism by constitutive and regulated negative feedback reactions. This means that a signal is dampened and/or terminated by opposing reactions, and that loss or gain of function of opposing components can cause hormone-independent activation of a specific pathway or hormone resistance.

In addition, signaling pathways use several common modes of informational transduction and transfer (i.e., intracellular messengers and signaling events). These include the following:

1. **Covalent phosphorylation of proteins and lipids** (Figure 1-8). Signaling components that phosphorylate proteins or lipids are called **kinases,** whereas those that catalyze dephosphorylation are called **phosphatases.** Phosphorylation can activate or deactivate a substrate, and proteins often have multiple sites of phosphorylation that induce quantitative and/or qualitative changes in the protein's activity. Protein kinases and phosphatases can be classified as either **tyrosine-specific** kinases and phosphatases, or **serine/threonine-specific** kinases and phosphatases. There are also **"mixed function"** kinases and phosphatases that are recognize all three residues. An important lipid kinase is phosphatidylinositol-3-kinase (PI3K; see later).

2. **Noncovalent guanosine nucleotide triphosphate (GTP) binding to GTP-binding proteins (G proteins).** G proteins represent a large family of molecular switches, which are latent and inactive when bound to GDP, and active when bound to GTP (Figure 1-9). G proteins are activated by **guanine nucleotide exchange factors (GEFs),** which promote the dissociation of GDP and binding of GTP. G proteins have **intrinsic GTPase activity.** GTP is normally hydrolyzed to GDP within seconds by the G protein, thereby terminating the transducing activity of the G protein. Another G protein termination mechanism (which represents a target for drug development to treat certain endocrine diseases), is the family of proteins called **"regulators of G-protein signaling" (RGS proteins),** which bind to active G proteins and increase their intrinsic GTPase activity.

3. **Noncovalent binding of cyclic nucleotide monophosphates** to their specific effector kinases and ion channels (Figure 1-10). **Cyclic AMP** is generated from ATP by **adenylyl cyclase,** which is primarily a membrane protein. Adenylyl cyclase is activated and inhibited by specific G proteins. Cyclic AMP binds to the **regulatory subunit** of **protein kinase A (PKA; also called cAMP-dependent**

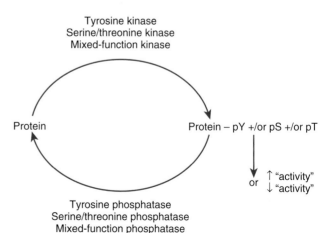

FIGURE 1-8 ■ Phosphorylation/dephosphorylation in signal transduction pathways. pY, phosphorylated tyrosine; pS, phosphorylated serine; pT, phosphorylated threonine.

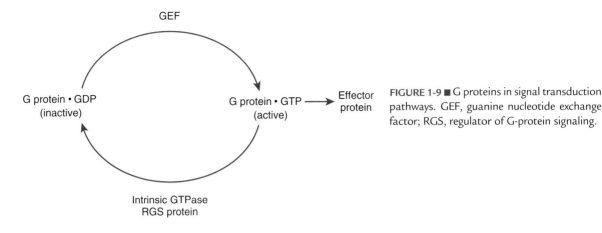

FIGURE 1-9 ■ G proteins in signal transduction pathways. GEF, guanine nucleotide exchange factor; RGS, regulator of G-protein signaling.

protein kinase), causing regulatory subunit-catalytic subunit dissociation and activation of the **PKA catalytic subunit.** PKA phosphorylates numerous proteins on serine and threonine residues. Cyclic AMP also binds to cAMP-gated ion channels, but these are less important to hormonal transduction than PKA. Cyclic AMP is degraded to AMP by **cAMP phosphodiesterases.** The cAMP phosphopdiesterases are inhibited by caffeine and other methylxanthines. **Cyclic GMP** is produced

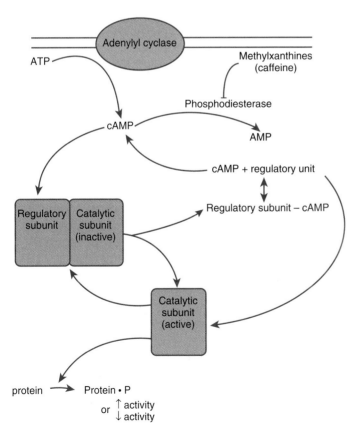

FIGURE 1-10 ■ Cyclic AMP/PKA in signal transduction pathways.

from GTP by **guanylyl cyclase,** which exists in both soluble and membrane forms. The soluble form of guanylyl cyclase is activated by another messenger, **nitric oxide (NO).** Cyclic GMP activates **protein kinase G (PKG),** and lowers cytoplasmic Ca^{2+} levels (possibly through cGMP-gated Ca^{2+} channels). Cyclic GMP is degraded to GMP by cGMP phosphodiesterase. One form of cGMP phosphodiesterase is inhibited by sildenafil (Viagra).

4. **Noncovalent Ca^{2+} binding and activation of proteins** (Figure 1-11). Cytosolic levels of Ca^{2+} are maintained at very low levels (i.e., 10^{-8} M), by either active transport of Ca^{2+} out of the cell, or into intracellular compartments (e.g., endoplasmic reticulum). Some signals are transduced by an increase in the flow of Ca^{2+} through **Ca^{2+} channels** into the cell or into the cytoplasm from intracellular compartments. This leads to an increase in Ca^{2+} binding directly to numerous specific effector proteins, which leads to a change in their activities. Additionally, Ca^{2+} regulates several effector proteins indirectly, through binding to the messenger protein, **calmodulin.** The Ca^{2+}-calmodulin complex then binds to and regulates effector proteins. The Ca^{2+}-dependent message is terminated by the lowering of cytosolic Ca^{2+} by cell membrane and endoplasmic reticular **Ca^{2+} ATPases** (Ca^{2+} pumps).

5. **Generation of lipid informational molecules,** which act as intracellular messengers. These include **diacylglycerol (DAG)** and **inositol 1,4,5-triphosphate (IP_3),** which are cleaved from phosphatidylinositol 4,5-bisphosphate (PIP_2) by phospholipase. DAG activates protein kinase C isoforms (Figure 1-12). IP_3 binds to the IP_3 receptor, which is a large complex including a Ca^{2+} channel, on the endoplasmic reticulum membrane, and promotes Ca^{2+} efflux from the endoplasmic reticulum into the cytoplasm (see Figure 1-12). IP_3 is rapidly metabolized, primarily by dephosphorylation.

Another lipid messenger relevant to hormone signaling is the cell membrane phospholipid, **phosphatidylinositol 3,4,5-triphosphate (PIP_3**—not to be confused with the diffusible lipid molecule, IP_3!). PIP_3 is made from PIP_2 by the enzyme, **phophaditidylinositol-3-kinase (PI3K).** As discussed subsequently, PI3K

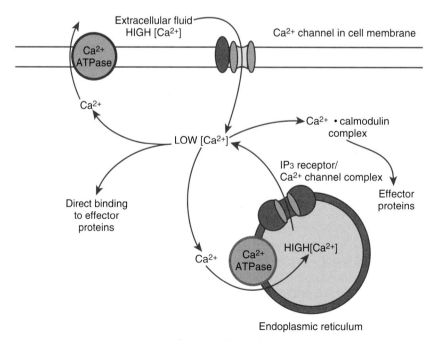

FIGURE 1-11 ■ Ca^{2+} in signal transduction pathways.

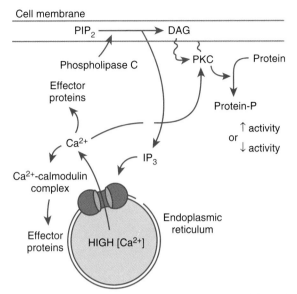

Cell membrane

FIGURE 1-12 ■ Lipid messengers, IP$_3$ and diacylglycerol (DAG) in signal transduction pathways.

Signaling from Membrane Receptors

Receptors Using G Proteins The largest family of hormone receptors belongs to the **G-protein–coupled receptor** (**GPCR**) family. These receptors span the cell membrane 7 times, and are referred to as **7-helix transmembrane receptors.** The G proteins that directly interact with GPCRs are termed **heterotrimeric G proteins** and are composed of an **α subunit (Gα),** and a **β/γ subunit dimer (Gβ/γ).** The Gα binds GTP/GDP and functions as the primary signal transducer. **G-protein–coupled receptors** (**GPCRs**) are, in fact, **ligand-activated GEFs.** This means that on hormone binding, the conformation of the receptor shifts to the active state. Once active, the GPCR induces the exchange of GDP for GTP, thereby activating Gα. One hormone-bound receptor activates 100 or more G proteins. GTP-bound Gα then dissociates from Gβ/γ, and binds to and activates one or more effector proteins (Figure 1-14).

How do G proteins link specific hormone-receptor binding events with specific downstream effector proteins? There are at least 16 Gα proteins that show specificity with respect to cell type expression, GPCR binding, and effector protein activation. A rather ubiquitous Gα protein is called **Gs-α,** which stimulates the membrane enzyme, adenylyl cyclase. As discussed earlier, adenylyl cyclase increases the levels of another messenger, cAMP. Some GPCRs couple to **Gi-α,** which inhibits adenylyl cyclase. A third major hormonal signaling pathway is through **Gq-α,** which activates **phospholipase C.** Phospholipase C generates two lipid messengers, DAG and IP$_3$ from PIP$_2$ (see earlier

is activated by several hormone and growth factor receptors. PIP$_3$ acts in a manner similar to pY residues, in that the specific structure of PIP$_3$ binds tightly to specific proteins, thereby recruiting proteins to the cell membrane. One such protein is **protein kinase B** (**PKB**; also called **Akt**). Recruitment of PKB to the cell membrane brings it close to other PIP$_3$-dependent kinases, which phosphorylate and activate PKB. PKB then phosphorylates effector proteins to produce a specific cellular response (Figure 1-13).

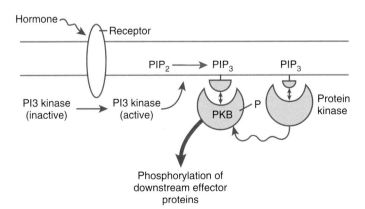

FIGURE 1-13 ■ PI3 kinase-PIP$_3$-PKB signal transduction pathway.

and Figure 1-12). Defects in G protein structure and expression are linked to endocrine diseases such as pseudohypoparathyroidism (loss of Gs activity) or pituitary tumors (loss of intrinsic GTPase activity in Gs, thereby extending its time in the active state).

GPCR-dependent signaling pathways regulate a broad range of cellular responses. For example, the pancreatic hormone, glucagon, regulates numerous aspects of hepatic metabolism (see Chapter 3). The glucagon receptor is linked to the Gs-cAMP-PKA pathway, which diverges to regulate enzyme activity at both posttranslational and transcriptional levels. PKA phosphorylates and thereby activates phosphorylase kinase. Phosphorylase kinase phosphorylates and activates glycogen phosphorylase, which catalyzes the release of glucose molecules from glycogen. In other cases, PKA phosphorylates and inactivates enzymes (e.g., pyruvate kinase). Catalytic subunits of PKA also enter the nucleus, where they phosphorylate and activate the transcription factor, **cAMP response element–binding protein (CREB protein).** Phospho-CREB then increases the transcriptional rate of genes encoding specific enzymes (e.g., phosphoenolpyruvate carboxykinase). In summary, signaling from one GPCR can regulate a number of targets in different cellular compartments (Figure 1-15).

As mentioned, G protein signaling is terminated by intrinsic GTPase activity. Another termination mechanism involves desensitization and endocytosis of the GPCR (Figure 1-16). Hormone binding to the receptor increases the ability of **GPCR kinases (GRKs)** to phosphorylate the intracellular domain of GPCRs. This phosphorylation recruits proteins called **β-arrestins.** GRK-induced phosphorylation and β-arrestin binding inactivate the receptor, and β-arrestin couples the receptor to clathrin-mediated endocytotic machinery. Some GPCRs are dephosphorylated and rapidly recycled back to the cell membrane, whereas others are degraded in lysosomes. GRK/β-arrestin–dependent inactivation and endocytosis is an important mechanism for **hormonal desensitization** of a cell after exposure to excessive hormone.

Receptor Tyrosine Kinases (RTKs) RTKs can be classified into two groups: the first acting as receptors for several growth factors (e.g., epidermal growth factor,

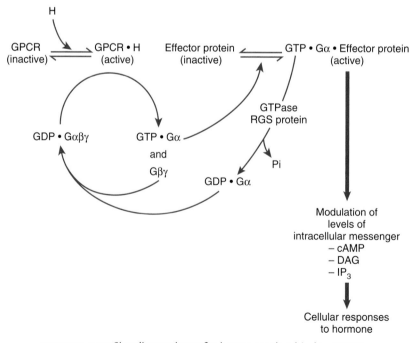

FIGURE 1-14 ■ Signaling pathway for hormones that bind to GPCRs.

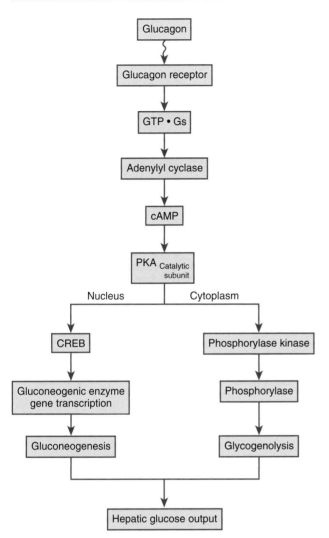

FIGURE 1-15 ■ Coordinated regulation of cytoplasmic and nuclear events by PKA to produce a general cellular response.

platelet-derived growth factor), and the second group for insulin and insulin-like growth factors (IGFs). The former group of RTKs comprises membrane glycoproteins containing three domains: an extracellular domain containing the hormone-binding site, and single transmembrane domain, and an intracellular domain containing intrinsic tyrosine kinase activity. Growth factor binding induces dimerization of the RTK, followed by transphosphorylation of tyrosine residues, generating **phosphotyrosine (pY).** The phosphotyrosines function to recruit proteins that specifically recognize pYs. One recruited protein

is phospholipase C, which is then activated by phosphorylation and generates the messengers, DAG and IP_3 from PIP_2 (see earlier). A second critically important protein that is recruited to pY residues is the adapter protein, **Grb2,** which is complexed with a GEF named **SOS.** Recruitment of SOS to the membrane allows it to activate a small, membrane-bound monomeric G protein called **Ras.** Ras then binds to its effector protein, **Raf.** Raf is a serine-specific kinase that phosphorylates and activates the dual-function kinase, **MEK.** MEK then phosphorylates and activates a **mitogen-activated protein kinase (MAP kinase,**

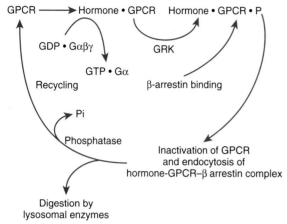

FIGURE 1-16 ■ GPCR inactivation and endocytosis to lysosomes (desensitization) and/or recycling back to the cell membrane in a dephosphorylated form (resensitization).

also called **ERKs).** Activated MAP kinases then enter the nucleus, and phosphorylate and activate several transcription factors. This signaling pathway is referred to as the MAP kinase cascade, and it transduces and amplifies a growth factor-RTK signal into a cellular

response involving a change in the expression of genes encoding proteins involved in proliferation and survival.

The **insulin receptor (IR)** is also an RTK and extremely relevant to health care (see Chapter 3). However, the IR differs from growth factor RTKs in several respects. First, the latent IR is already dimerized by Cys-Cys bonds, and insulin binding induces a conformational change that leads to transphosphorylation of the cytoplasmic domains (Figure 1-17). A major recruited protein is the **insulin receptor substrate (IRS),** which is then phosphorylated on tyrosine residues by the IR. The pY residues on IRS recruit the Grb-2/SOS complex, thereby activating growth responses to insulin through the MAP kinase pathway. The pY residues on the IRS also recruit the lipid kinase, PI3 kinase, activating and concentrating the kinase near its substrate, PIP_2, in the cell membrane. As discussed earlier, this ultimately leads to activation of PKB, which is required for the metabolic responses to insulin. The IR also phosphorylates adaptor proteins that activate a small G protein-dependent pathway. The small G-protein–dependent pathway and

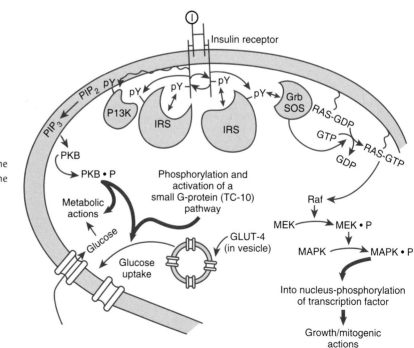

FIGURE 1-17 ■ Signaling from the insulin receptor (a receptor tyrosine kinase).

the PKB pathway are both required for the actions of insulin on glucose uptake (see Chapter 3).

RTKs are down-regulated by **ligand-induced endocytosis.** Additionally, the signaling pathways from RTKs, including the IR and IRSs, are inhibited by serine/threonine phosphorylation, tyrosine dephosphorylation, and by the suppressor of cytokine signaling proteins (see next section).

Receptors Associated with Cytoplasmic Tyrosine Kinases
Another class of membrane receptor falls into the **cytokine receptor family,** and includes receptors for growth hormone, prolactin, erythropoietin, and leptin. These receptors, which exist as dimers, do not have intrinsic protein kinase activity. Instead, the cytoplasmic domains are stably associated with members of the **JAK kinase** family (Figure 1-18). Hormone binding induces a conformational change, bringing the two JAKs associated with the dimerized receptor closer together and causing their transphosphorylation and activation. JAKs then phosphorylate tyrosine

residues on the cytoplasmic domains of the receptor. The pY residues recruit latent transcription factors called **STAT** (**signal transducers and activators of transcription**) proteins. STATs become phosphorylated by JAKs, which causes them to dissociate from the receptor, dimerize, and translocate into the nucleus, where they regulate gene expression.

A negative feedback loop has been identified for JAK/STAT signaling. STATs stimulate expression of one or more **suppressors of cytokine signaling (SOCS)** proteins. SOCS proteins compete with STATS for binding to the pY residues on cytokine receptors (Figure 1-19). This terminates the signaling pathway at the step of STAT activation. Recent studies show that a SOCS protein is induced by insulin signaling. SOCS 3 protein plays a role in terminating the signal from the IR, but also in reducing insulin sensitivity in hyperinsulinemic patients.

Receptor Serine/Threonine Kinases Receptors for the **transforming growth factor (TGF)-β family,** which includes the hormones anti-müllerian hormone and inhibin, are **receptor serine/threonine kinases.** Unbound receptors exist as dissociated heterodimers, called RI and RII (Figure 1-20). Hormone binding to RII induces dimerization of RII with RI, and RII activates RI by phosphorylation. RI then activates latent transcription factors called **Smads.** Activated Smads heterodimerize with a Co-Smad, enter the nucleus, and regulate specific gene expression.

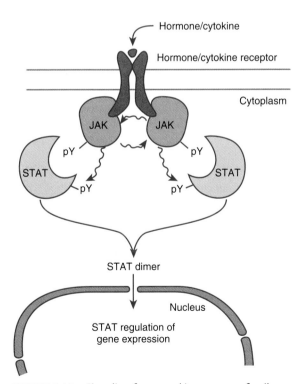

FIGURE 1-18 ■ Signaling from cytokine receptor family.

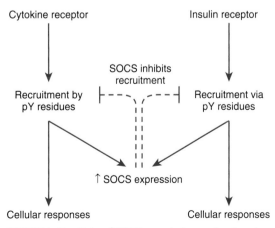

FIGURE 1-19 ■ Role of SOCS protein in terminating signals from cytokine family and insulin receptors.

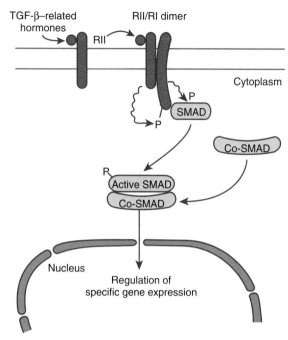

FIGURE 1-20 ■ Signaling from TGF-β–related receptors.

Receptors Regulating Ion Channels Hormone binding to these receptors opens ion channels, the most common of which are calcium channels (the calcium-calmodulin system). In the latter situation, hormone binding to the receptor opens the calcium channels and intracellular calcium levels rise (Figure 1-21).

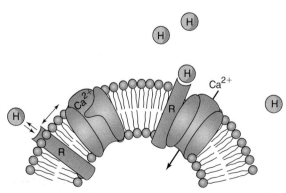

FIGURE 1-21 ■ Activation of calcium-calmodulin system. Hormone receptors (R) can bind hormone (H) and control opening of calcium channels in cell membrane.

The messenger role of intracellular Ca^{2+} was discussed earlier (see Figure 1-11).

Signaling from Intracellular Receptors

Steroid hormones, thyroid hormones, and 1,25-dihydroxyvitamin D act primarily through intracellular receptors. These receptors are structurally similar and are members of the **nuclear receptor superfamily** that includes receptors for steroid hormones, thyroid hormone, lipid-soluble vitamins, peroxisome proliferator–activated receptors (PPARs) and other "metabolic" receptors (liver X receptor, farnesyl X receptor).

Nuclear hormone receptors act as transcriptional regulators. This means that the signal of hormone-receptor binding is transduced ultimately into a change in the transcriptional rate of a subset of the genes that are expressed within a differentiated cell type. One receptor binds to a specific DNA sequence close to the promoter of one gene, and influences the rate of transcription of that gene in a hormone-dependent manner (see later). However, multiple hormone-receptor binding events are collectively transduced into the regulation of several genes. Moreover, regulation by one hormone usually includes activation and repression of the transcription of several genes in a given cell type.

Nuclear receptors have three major structural domains: the amino terminus domain, a middle DNA-binding domain, and a carboxyl terminus ligand-binding domain. The amino terminus domain contains a hormone-independent transcriptional activation domain. The DNA-binding domain contains two zinc finger motifs, which represent small loops organized by Zn^{2+} binding to four cysteine residues at the base of the each loop. The two zinc fingers and neighboring amino acids confer the ability to recognize and bind to specific DNA sequences, which are called **hormone-response elements (HREs)**. The carboxyl terminal ligand-binding domain contains several subdomains: (1) the site of hormone recognition and binding; (2) a hormone-dependent transcriptional activation domain; (3) a nuclear translocation signal; (4) a binding domain for heat-shock proteins; and (5) a dimerization subdomain.

There are numerous variations in the details of nuclear receptor mechanisms of action. Two generalized

Pathway 1 (Steroid hormones)

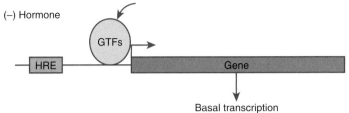

(−) Hormone

Basal transcription

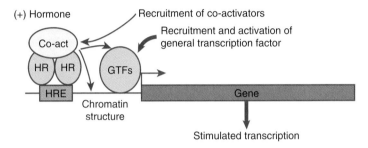

(+) Hormone

Recruitment of co-activators

Recruitment and activation of general transcription factor

Chromatin structure

Stimulated transcription

Pathway 2 (Thyroid hormones, vitamin D, PPARs)

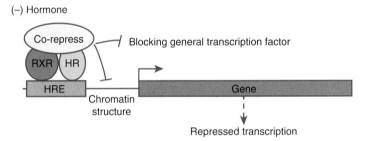

(−) Hormone

Blocking general transcription factor

Chromatin structure

Repressed transcription

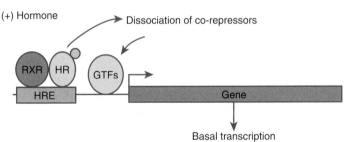

(+) Hormone

Dissociation of co-repressors

Basal transcription

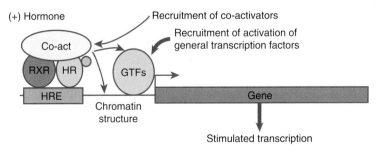

(+) Hormone

Recruitment of co-activators

Recruitment of activation of general transcription factors

Chromatin structure

Stimulated transcription

FIGURE 1-22 ■ Two general mechanisms by which nuclear receptor-hormone complexes increase gene transcription. HRE, hormone response element; co-repress, co-repressor proteins; GTFs, general transcription factors; HR, hormone receptor; RXR, retinoid X receptor; Co-act, co-activator proteins.

pathways by which nuclear hormone receptors increase gene transcription are the following (Figure 1-22):

Pathway 1: Unactivated receptor is cytoplasmic or nuclear, and binds DNA and recruits co-activator proteins upon hormone binding. This mode is observed for the ER, PR, GR, MR, and AR (i.e., steroid hormone receptors). In the absence of hormone, some of these receptors are held in the cytoplasm through an interaction with chaperone proteins (so called "heat-shock proteins" because their levels increase in response to elevated temperatures and other stresses). Chaperone proteins maintain the stability of the nuclear receptor in an inactive configuration. Hormone binding induces a conformational change in the receptor, causing its dissociation from heat-shock proteins. This exposes the nuclear localization signal and dimerization domains, so that receptors dimerize and enter the nucleus. Once in the nucleus, these receptors bind to their respective HREs. The HREs for the PR, GR, MR, and AR are inverted repeats with the recognition sequence, AGAACANNNTGTTCT. Specificity is conferred by neighboring base sequences and possibly by receptor interaction with other transcriptional factors in the context of a specific gene promoter. The ER usually binds to an inverted repeat with the recognition sequence, AGGTCANNNTGACCT. The specific HREs are also referred to as an **estrogen-response element (ERE), progesterone-response element (PRE), glucocorticoid-response element (GRE), mineralocorticoid-response element (MRE), and androgen-response element (ARE).** Once bound to their respective HREs, these receptors recruit other proteins, called **co-activators.** Co-activators act to recruit other components of the transcriptional machinery, and probably activate some of these components. Co-activators also possess intrinsic **histone acetlytransferase (HAT)** activity, which acetylates histones in the region of the promoter. Histone acetylation relaxes chromatin coiling, making that region more accessible to transcriptional machinery. Although the mechanistic details are beyond the scope of this chapter, the student should appreciate that steroid receptors can also repress gene transcription and that transcriptional activation and repression pathways are induced concomitantly in the same cell.

Pathway 2: Receptor is always in nucleus, and exchanges co-repressors with co-activators on hormone binding. This pathway is used by the thyroid hormone receptors (TR), vitamin D receptors, PPARs, and retinoic acid receptors. For example, the TR is bound, usually as a heterodimer with the retinoic acid X receptor (RXR). In the absence of thyroid hormone, the TR/RXR recruits **co-repressors.** Co-repressors, in turn, recruit proteins with **histone deacetylase (HDAC)** activity. In contrast to histone acetylation, histone deacetylation allows tighter coiling of chromatin, which makes promoters in that region less accessible to the transcriptional machinery. Thus, TR/RXR heterodimers are bound to **thyroid hormone response elements (TREs)** in the absence of hormone and maintain the expression of neighboring genes at a "repressed" level. Thyroid hormone (and other ligands of this class) readily move into the nucleus and bind to their receptors. Thyroid hormone binding induces dissociation of co-repressor proteins, thereby increasing gene expression to a "basal" level. The hormone-receptor complex subsequently recruits co-activator proteins, which further increase transcriptional activity to the "stimulated" level.

Termination of steroid hormone/receptor signaling is poorly understood, but appears to involve proteosomal degradation of receptors. The hormones are cleared as described earlier.

In summary, hormones signal to cells through membrane or intracellular receptors. Membrane receptors have rapid effects on cellular processes (e.g., enzyme activity, cytoskeletal arrangement) that are independent of new protein synthesis. Membrane receptors can also rapidly regulate gene expression through either mobile kinases (e.g., PKA, MAPKs) or mobile transcription factors (e.g., STATs, Smads). Steroid hormones have slower, longer term effects that involve chromatin remodeling and changes in gene expression. Increasing evidence points to rapid, nongenomic effects of steroid hormones as well, but these pathways are still being elucidated.

The presence of a functional receptor is an absolute requirement for hormone action, and loss of a receptor produces essentially the same symptoms as loss of hormone. In addition to the receptor, there are fairly complex pathways involving numerous intracellular messengers and effector proteins. Accordingly, endocrine diseases can arise from abnormal expression and/or activity of any of these signal transduction pathway components. Finally, hormonal signals can be terminated in several ways, including hormone/receptor internalization, phosphorylation/dephosphorylation, proteosomal destruction of receptor, and generation of feedback inhibitors (e.g., SOCS proteins).

HORMONAL RHYTHMS

Most endocrine secretion shows periodicity or rhythms. Frequently there are multiple, superimposed rhythms for a given hormone. The periods of these rhythms range from minutes to months (Figure 1-23).

These rhythms are important for normal endocrine function. Changes in endocrine rhythms are a major factor in the problems associated with jet lag.

These rhythms frequently are absent in disease states. The physician must be cognizant of normal endocrine rhythms. Many rhythms have a 24-hour cycle. These rhythms are called **circadian (diurnal) rhythms.** As can be seen in Figure 1-14, the normal serum cortisol, prolactin, or GH levels measured at 5 AM are different from the values obtained at 2 PM.

Pulsatile rhythms (usually a 1/2- to 2-hour period) frequently are superimposed on these circadian rhythms, and these pulsatile rhythms have functional significance. The role of pulsatile secretion is discussed in Chapters 8 and 9. These rhythms with a periodicity of less than 24 hours are referred to as **ultradian rhythms.** Figure 1-24 illustrates ultradian rhythms for LH, FSH, and testosterone.

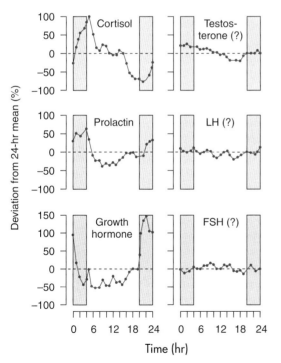

FIGURE 1-23 ■ Temporal patterns for plasma hormone levels. *Shaded areas* represent approximate sleep time. LH, luteinizing hormone; FSH, follicle-stimulating hormone. *(Redrawn from DeGroot LJ, et al: Endocrinology, vol 3, New York, 1979, Grune & Stratton.)*

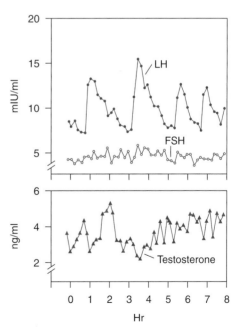

FIGURE 1-24 ■ Examples of ultradian rhythms. LH, luteinizing hormone; FSH, follicle-stimulating hormone. *(Redrawn from Naftolin F, et al: J Clin Endocrinol Metab 36:285, 1973.)*

SUMMARY

1. Knowledge of the chemical structure of a hormone can facilitate predicting how the hormone will be produced, carried, and act in a physiologic system.
2. Protein/peptide hormones are produced on ribosomes and stored in the endocrine cell in membrane-bound secretory granules. They typically do not readily cross cell membranes and act through membrane-associated receptors.
3. Catecholamines are synthesized in cytosol and secretory granules and do not readily cross cell membranes. They act through cell membrane-associated receptors.
4. Steroid hormones are not stored in tissues and generally cross cell membranes relatively readily. They act through intracellular receptors.
5. Thyroid hormones are synthesized in the follicular cells and are stored in the follicular colloid as thyroglobulin. They cross cell membranes and associate with nuclear receptors.
6. Some hormones act through membrane receptors, with their responses being mediated by G-protein–associated systems (adenylyl cyclase and phosphatidylinositol), calcium-calmodulin, tyrosine kinase-containing receptor, tyrosine kinase-associated systems, or serine/threonine kinase receptor.
7. Other hormones bind to nuclear receptors and act by directly regulating gene transcription.
8. Hormonal rhythms play a major role in physiologic response.

KEY WORDS AND CONCEPTS

- Exocrine gland
- Endocrine gland
- Hormone
- Receptor
- Target cell
- Target organ
- Ligand
- Agonist
- Antagonist
- Hormonal resistance
- Endocrine system
- Set-point
- Protein/peptide hormone
- Catecholamine
- Steroid hormone
- Iodothyronine
- Eicosanoids
- Signal peptide
- Signal recognition complex
- Docking protein
- Signal peptidase
- Prehormone
- Preprohormone
- Prohormone convertase
- Exocytosis
- Regulated secretory pathway
- Stimulus-secretion coupling
- Second messenger hypothesis
- Epinephrine
- Norepinephrine
- Adrenal cortex
- Ovary
- Testis
- Placenta
- Progestin
- Mineralocorticoid
- Glucocorticoid
- Androgen
- Estrogen
- Vitamin D
- Cycloperhydrophenanthrene ring
- Progesterone receptor
- Mineralocorticoid receptor
- Glucocorticoid receptor
- Androgen receptor
- Estrogen receptor
- Vitamin D receptor
- Steroidogenic cells
- Peripheral conversion
- Transport proteins
- Sex hormone-binding globulin
- Corticosteroid-binding globulin
- Glucuronide conjugation
- Sulfate conjugation
- Thyroid hormone-binding globulin

- Thyroid hormone receptor
- Prostaglandins
- Leukotrienes
- Thromboxanes
- Prostacyclin
- High-affinity receptor
- Signal transduction pathway
- Intracellular messengers
- Effector proteins
- Cellular response
- Covalent phosphorylation of proteins and lipids
- Tyrosine kinases and phosphatases
- Serine/threonine-specific kinases and phosphatases
- Mixed function kinases and phosphatases
- GTP-binding proteins (G proteins)
- G protein exchange factor (GEF)
- Intrinsic GTPase activity
- Regulators of G protein signaling (RGS proteins)
- Cyclic nucleotide monophosphates
- Cyclic AMP
- Cyclic GMP
- Adenylyl cyclase
- Guanylyl cyclase
- Protein kinase A (PKA)
- PKA regulatory subunit
- PKA catalytic subunit
- cAMP phosphodiesterase
- Nitric oxide (NO)
- Protein kinase G (PKG)
- CGMP phosphodiesterase
- Ca^{2+}
- Calmodulin
- Ca^{2+} channels
- Ca^{2+} ATPases
- Diacylglycerol (DAG)
- Inositol 1,4,5-triphosphate (IP_3)
- Phosphatidylinositol 3,4,5-triphosphate (PIP_3)
- Phosphatidylinositol-3-kinase (PI3K)
- Protein kinase B (PKB/Akt)
- G-protein–coupled receptor (GPCR)
- 7-Helix transmembrane receptors
- Heterotrimeric G proteins
- Ligand-activated GEF
- Ga
- $G\beta/\gamma$
- Gs-α
- Gi-α

- Gq-α
- Phospholipase C
- cAMP response element–binding protein (CREB)
- GPCR kinases (GRKs)
- β-Arrestins
- Hormonal desensitization
- Receptor tyrosine kinases (RTKs)
- Phosphotyrosine (pY)
- Grb2/SOS
- Ras
- Raf
- MEK
- Mitogen-activated protein kinase (MAPK)
- Insulin receptor (IR)
- Insulin receptor substrate (IRS)
- Ligand-induced endocytosis
- Cytokine receptor family
- JAK kinase family
- STAT
- Suppressors of cytokine signaling (SOCS) proteins
- Transforming growth factor (TGF)-β family
- Receptor serine/threonine kinases
- Smads
- Nuclear receptor superfamily
- Hormone response elements (HREs)
- Estrogen response element (ERE)
- Progesterone response element (PRE)
- Glucocorticoid response element (GRE)
- Mineralocorticoid response element (MRE)
- Androgen response element (ARE)
- Vitamin D response element (VRE)
- Co-activator proteins
- Histone acetlytransferase (HAT)
- Co-repressors
- Histone deacetylase (HDAC)
- Thyroid hormone–response element (TRE)
- Circadian (diurnal) rhythms
- Ultradian rhythms

SELF-STUDY PROBLEMS

1. What determines whether and how a cell responds to a specific hormone?
2. How do protein hormones differ from steroid hormones in terms of their storage within an endocrine cell?

3. How does binding to serum-transport proteins influence hormone metabolism and hormone action?

4. How would a large increase in the GTPase activity of Gs-α affect the cellular response to a hormone signaling through a cAMP/PKA pathway?

5. What role does the IRS protein play in transducing insulin receptor signaling into a growth response? a metabolic response?

6. In what fundamental way are cytokine and TGF-β–like hormones similar in their signaling pathways?

7. Compare the mechanisms by which the ER and the TR increase gene transcription.

BIBLIOGRAPHY

Baniahmad A: Nuclear hormone receptor co-repressors, *J Steroid Biochem Mol Biol* 93(2-5):89-97, 2005.

Grotzinger J: Molecular mechanisms of cytokine receptor activation, *Biochim Biophys Acta* 1592(3):215-223, 2002.

Habener JF: Genetic control of peptide hormone formation. In Larsen PR, Kronenberg HM, Melmed S, Polonsky KS, editors: *Williams' textbook of endocrinology*, ed 10, Philadelphia, 2003, WB Saunders.

Ilangumaran S, Rottapel R: Regulation of cytokine receptor signaling by SOCS1, *Immunol Rev* 192:196-211, 2003.

Javelaud D, Mauviel A: Mammalian transforming growth factor-betas: Smad signaling and physio-pathological roles, *Int J Biochem Cell Biol* 36(7):1161-1165, 2004.

Lazar MA: Mechanism of action of hormones that act on nuclear receptors. In Larsen PR, Kronenberg HM, Melmed S, Polonsky KS, editors: *Williams' textbook of endocrinology*, ed 10, Philadelphia, 2003, WB Saunders.

Leonard WJ, Lin JX: Cytokine receptor signaling pathways, *J Allergy Clin Immunol* 105(5):877-888, 2000.

Pattni K, Banting G: Ins(1,4,5)P3 metabolism and the family of IP3-3Kinases, *Cell Signal* 16(6):643-654, 2004.

Penela P, Ribas C, et al: Mechanisms of regulation of the expression and function of G protein-coupled receptor kinases, *Cell Signal* 15(11):973-981, 2003.

Spiegel AM, Weinstein LS: Inherited diseases involving g proteins and g protein-coupled receptors, *Annu Rev Med* 55:27-39, 2004.

Spiegel A, Carter-Su C, Taylor S: Mechanism of action of hormones that act at the cell surface. In Larsen PR, Kronenberg HM, Melmed S, Polonsky KS, editors: *Williams' textbook of endocrinology*, ed 10, Philadelphia, 2003, WB Saunders.

Taatjes DJ, Marr MT, et al: Regulatory diversity among metazoan co-activator complexes, *Nat Rev Mol Cell Biol* 5(5):403-410, 2004.

ten Dijke P, Hill CS: New insights into TGF-beta-Smad signaling, *Trends Biochem Sci* 29(5):265-273, 2004.

APPENDIX
DIFFERENT MODES OF CHEMICAL SIGNALING

Although this book is largely about endocrine signaling, the student will quickly come to appreciate that the distinctions between classical hormones and other chemical signals (neurotransmitters, neuropeptides, growth factors, morphogens, cytokines) become blurred. Similarly, essentially all cell types use chemical signaling at multiple levels. These can be classified into the following:

1. **Intracrine.** This involves production of an intracellular "chemical signal" that binds to an intracellular receptor without leaving the cell.

2. **Autocrine.** This involves secretion of a "chemical signal," which then regulates its cell of origin through a membrane receptor.

3. **Juxtacrine.** This involves signaling from one membrane-bound "ligand" to a membrane-bound receptor on an adjacent cell.

4. **Paracrine.** This involves release of a "chemical signal" into the extracellular fluid, and its regulation of surrounding cells by diffusion.

5. **Neurocrine.** This involves release of a "neurohormone" from axonal endings, and regulation of nearby cells by diffusion.

6. **Neuroendocrine.** This involves release of a "neurohormone" from axonal endings, its diffusion into capillaries, and regulation of distant cells.

7. **Endocrine.** This involves secretion of a hormone from an endocrine cell, its diffusion into capillaries, and regulation of distant cells.

2

THE ENDOCRINE FUNCTION OF THE GASTROINTESTINAL TRACT

OBJECTIVES

1. Understand the role of well-established GI hormones associated with the following four major aspects of GI physiology:

   - The regulation of gastric acid secretion and gastric motility in the regulation

   - The regulation of secretion from the exocrine pancreas and the gall bladder, and their associated ducts

   - The stimulation of GI tract growth (**an enterotropic action**)

   - The enhancement of nutrient-induced insulin secretion by the endocrine pancreas (**incretin action**)

Note: A fifth general function of GI hormones, the effect on appetite, will be discussed in the context of energy homeostasis in Chapter 3.

We begin our discussion of endocrine physiology with the hormonal function and regulation of the GI tract. The discovery of **secretin** in 1902 by Bayliss and Starling represented the first characterization of a **"hormone"** as a blood-borne chemical messenger—released at one site and acting at multiple other sites. Indeed, the epithelial layer of the mucosa of the GI tract harbors numerous **enteroendocrine cell** types, which collectively represent the *largest endocrine cell mass* in the body.

The diffuse enteroendocrine system is perhaps the most basic example of endocrine tissue in that it is composed of unicellular glands situated within a simple epithelium. Most enteroendocrine cells, called "open" cells, extend from the basal lamina of this epithelium to the apical surface (Figure 2-1), although there are also "closed" enteroendocrine cells, which do not extend to the luminal surface. The apical membranes of "open"

enteroendocrine cells express either receptors or transporters that allow the cell to "sample" the contents of the lumen. Luminal contents, called **secretogogues,** stimulate specific enteroendocrine cell types to secrete their hormones. This "sampling" or "nutrient tasting" is independent of osmotic and mechanical forces. The secretogogic mechanisms involved are poorly understood, but some appear to require the absorption of the nutrient. Additionally, different enteroendocrine cell types display distinct localizations along the GI tract (Table 2-1). We will see that these localizations are central to the function of each cell type.

In the simplest model of enteroendocrine cell function, a hormone is released from the basolateral membrane in response to the presence of a **secretogogue** at the luminal side of the cell. The secreted hormone diffuses into blood vessels in the underlying lamina propria, thereby gaining access to the general circulation.

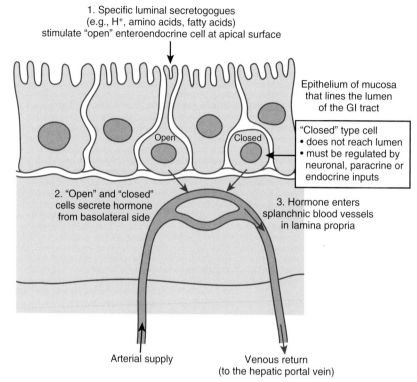

1. Specific luminal secretogogues
(e.g., H⁺, amino acids, fatty acids)
stimulate "open" enteroendocrine cell at apical surface

Epithelium of mucosa
that lines the lumen
of the GI tract

"Closed" type cell
• does not reach lumen
• must be regulated by
  neuronal, paracrine or
  endocrine inputs

Open   Closed

2. "Open" and "closed"
cells secrete hormone
from basolateral side

3. Hormone enters
splanchnic blood vessels
in lamina propria

Arterial supply

Venous return
(to the hepatic portal vein)

FIGURE 2-1 ■ Closed and open enteroendocrine cells. Enteroendocrine cells sit within the simple epithelium of the GI tract. "Open" cells extend from the basal lamina to the lumen. "Closed" cells do not reach the lumen. Both cells secrete hormones that enter capillaries in the lamina propria beneath the epithelium.

Circulating GI hormones regulate GI tract functions by binding to specific receptors at one or more sites within the GI tract and/or its extramural glands. In the classic model, the secretion of the hormone by an enteroendocrine cell is subsequently terminated when the luminal concentration of its secretogogue diminishes, thereby terminating the secretion of the hormone.

However, this simple model of the enteroendocrine system does not fully account for the integration with other systemic responses to a meal. In addition, both

TABLE 2-1				
Distribution of Enteroendocrine Cells along the GI Tract				
	STOMACH	DUODENUM	JEJUNUM	ILEUM	COLON
---	---	---	---	---	---
G cell (gastrin)	+	(+)			
S cell (secretin)		+	+		
I cell (CCK)		+	+	(+)	
K cell (GIP)		+	+		
L cell (GLP-1)				+	+
L cell (GLP-2)				+	+
M cell (motilin)		+	+		
Ghrelin-secreting cell	+	(+)	(+)	(+)	(+)

+, primary location of concentration; (+), less concentrated.

"open" and "closed" enteroendocrine cells are regulated by the **enteric nervous system (ENS)** and **paracrine** factors secreted by neighboring epithelial cells (**intrinsic regulators** of enteroendocrine cell function) (Figure 2-2). Additionally, there are **extrinsic regulators** of enteroendocrine cells, most notably the **autonomic nervous system** and **endocrine glands** that reside outside of the GI tract. Conversely, GI hormones can have local (i.e., paracrine) actions on the afferent nerves of autonomic or enteric reflexes, so that the response to a GI hormone can be mediated by a neurotransmitter. Thus, GI tract function is orchestrated through a complex interplay of neural and endocrine responses and actions. It is not surprising; therefore, that GI function is often perturbed in patients with mental disorders (e.g., depression) and endocrine disorders (e.g., hyperthyroidism).

The hormones secreted by the enteroendocrine system function to maintain the health of the GI tract and its extramural glands and provides an integrated response to the acquisition of nutrients. This integrated response to GI hormones is due, in part, to their ability to regulate multiple functions of the GI tract.

ENTEROENDOCRINE HORMONE FAMILIES AND THEIR RECEPTORS

All established GI hormones are peptides and bind to **G-protein–coupled receptors (GPCRs;** see Chapter 1) located on the plasma membrane of target cells.

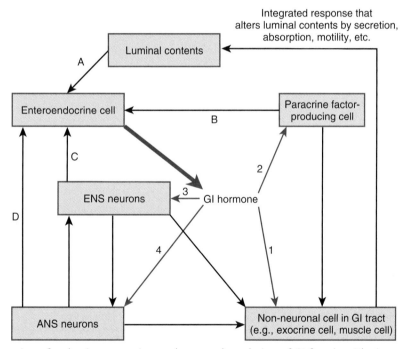

FIGURE 2-2 ■ Integration of endocrine, paracrine, and neuronal regulation of GI function. The integration of regulatory inputs (**A-D**) and outputs (1-4) of an enteroendocrine cell. The main input is the presence or absence of specific luminal contents (**A**). GI hormone secretion can also be influenced by the paracrine factors from neighboring cells (**B**), the enteric nervous system (ENS; **C**) or directly by the autonomic nervous system (ANS; **D**). The output is secretion of usually one hormonal peptide (but in some cases, the same cell secretes several peptides). The GI hormone can have a direct effect on non-neuronal cells of the GI tract and its extramural glands (**1**). This directly affects processes such as enzyme secretion or motility. GI hormones can also exert their effects through binding to receptors on neighboring paracrine cells (**2**), and on neurons of the ENS (**3**) and ANS (**4**).

GI hormones, as well as their cognate GPCRs, can be organized into gene families based on structural homologies. In this chapter, we will discuss members of three enteroendocrine hormone families: gastrin, secretin, and motilin (Table 2-2).

The gastrin family includes **gastrin** and **cholecystokinin (CCK),** which share a common stretch of 5 amino acids at the C-terminus. Gastrin binds with high affinity to the **CCK-2 receptor** (previously called the CCK-B/gastrin receptor). CCK binds with high affinity to the **CCK-1 receptor.**

The secretin family includes the hormones **secretin, glucagon,** and **glucagon-like peptides** (including **GLP-1** and **GLP-2**) and gastric inhibitory polypeptide (GIP; more recently referred to as **Glucose-dependent Insulinotropic Peptide**—see later). This family also includes the neurocrine factor, **vasoactive intestinal peptide (VIP).** The corresponding GPCRs for each member of the secretin family of peptides are also structurally related. These receptors are all primarily coupled to Gs signaling pathways that increase intracellular cAMP in target cells.

The motilin family includes the hormones **motilin** and **ghrelin.** Ghrelin was originally identified as a **growth hormone secretogogue (GHS),** but is most abundant in the fundus of the stomach. The receptors for motilin and ghrelin are GPCRs that are linked to phospholipase/IP$_3$ pathways, which, in turn, stimulate protein kinase C- and Ca^{2+}-dependent signaling pathways (see Chapter 1).

It is important to be aware of the fact that many GI peptides are also expressed by tissues outside of the GI tract. Pathophysiologically, GI peptides can be secreted in an uncontrolled manner from tumors. Other physiological sites of production include other endocrine glands (e.g., the pituitary gland) and reproductive structures (e.g., the acrosome of sperm). Several peptides are produced by the central (CNS) and peripheral (PNS) nervous systems where they are utilized as neurotransmitters or neuromodulatory factors.

TABLE 2-2
Enteroendocrine Hormone Families and Their Receptors

HORMONE FAMILY	MEMBERS OF FAMILY	RECEPTOR & PRIMARY SIGNALING PATHWAY	PRIMARY DISTRIBUTION OF RECEPTOR (RELATED TO GI FUNCTION)
Gastrin	Gastrin (G cell)	CCK2 Receptor Gq - ⇑ in Ca^{2+} and PKC	Gastric ECL cell & parietal cell
	CCK (I cell)	CCK1 Receptor Gq - ⇑ in Ca^{2+} and PKC	Gall bladder muscularis & sphincter of hepatopancreatic ampulla Pancreatic acinar cells Pancreatic ducts Vagal afferents and enteric neurons Stomach muscularis & pyloric sphincter Gastric D cells
Secretin	Secretin (S cell)	Secretin Receptor Gs - ⇑ in cAMP	Pancreatic ducts & biliary ducts Pancreatic acinar cells G cells & pancreatic cells
	GLP-1 (L cell)	GLP-1 Receptor Gs - ⇑ in cAMP	β cells of pancreatic islets
	GLP-2 (L cell)	GLP-2 Receptor Gs - ⇑ in cAMP	GI tract—especially small intestine
	GIP (K cell)	GIP Receptor Gs - ⇑ in cAMP	β cells of pancreatic islets Gastric mucosa & muscularis
Motilin	Motilin (M cell)	Motilin Receptor Gq - ⇑ in Ca^{2+} & PKC (also binds erythromycin)	Stomach & small intestines—especially in smooth muscle cells and enteric neurons
	Ghrelin (P/D1 cell)	GHS receptor type Ia (GHS-RIa) Gq - ⇑ in Ca^{2+} & PKC	Pituitary & hypothalamus

For example, CCK is expressed in the neocortical region of the CNS and the genitourinary-associated nerves of the PNS. As for its role in the CNS, CCK has been linked to anxiety and panic disorders. This also means that receptors for these peptides also reside within the CNS, the PNS, and probably other non-neural tissues. Thus, a pharmacologic agent (agonist or antagonist) related to a specific GI peptide can potentially have a wide range of effects, depending on its stability and whether it can cross the blood-brain barrier. The possibility also exists that extra-GI sites of synthesis can "spill over" into the general circulation and affect GI function.

THE REGULATION OF GASTRIC FUNCTION

The **stomach** acts as a food reservoir. People eat discontinuously, and typically eat more at one sitting than their GI tract can process immediately. Thus, the stomach holds the ingested food, and gradually releases partially digested food (chyme) into the first part of the small intestine, the duodenum. The layers of the stomach wall carry out two basic functions, secretion and contraction/relaxation.

Overview of Regulation of Gastric Secretion and Motility

The innermost layer of the stomach wall, the gastric mucosa, contains glandular and surface epithelia, and can be divided into proximal and distal segments. Two of the proximal portions of the stomach (**fundus** and **body**) contain the main gastric mucosal glands (Figure 2-3). Within these glands, the **parietal cells** secrete **HCl,** which is important for hydrolysis of macromolecules, activation of proenzymes, and the sterilization of ingested food. Parietal cells also secrete **intrinsic factor,** which is required for the efficient absorption of **vitamin B_{12}.** It should be noted that the parietal cells are also called **oxyntic cells,** and the region of the stomach in which they reside, is referred to as the oxyntic region.

The glands of the fundus and body also contain the **chief cells,** which secrete digestive enzymes (e.g., pepsinogen, gastric lipase). A third cell type, the mucous cell, is found in the neck of the gastric glands and on the surface throughout the stomach. Mucous cells secrete **mucigens,** which buffer and protect the lining of the stomach, particularly in the vicinity of the main gastric glands. Because gastric enzyme and mucus production is primarily under nervous control,

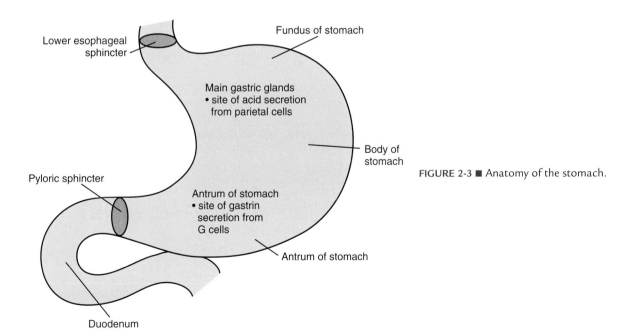

FIGURE 2-3 ■ Anatomy of the stomach.

with little endocrine input, we will focus here on gastric acid secretion and motility.

The distal part of the gastric mucosa, the **pyloric antrum,** has an important enteroendocrine function. This part of the stomach contains two types of "open" enteroendocrine cells. The G cells secrete **gastrin,** a hormone, and the D cells secrete **somatostatin,** a paracrine factor. These two peptides act antagonistically in a negative feedback loop to regulate gastric blood flow, cell growth, secretion, and motility (see later). D cells are also found within the oxyntic region, where they directly inhibit parietal cell secretion.

An outer layer of the stomach wall, the muscularis externa, is composed of smooth muscle. The relaxation of this muscle allows distention and storage, and its contractions ultimately move the partially digested food (chyme) into the duodenum. There are two gateways into and out of the stomach. These are the lower esophageal sphincter (LES) and the pyloric sphincter, respectively. The LES allows swallowed food particles to enter the stomach, and protects the esophagus from the reflux of acidic chyme. The pyloric sphincter operates in conjunction with the muscularis externa to allow only small particles of digested chyme to escape the stomach and enter the duodenum. The pyloric sphincter also prevents backflow of chyme into the stomach.

In general, regulation of gastric function involves the stimulation of secretion and motility as needed (i.e., in the presence of food), and the inhibition of gastric secretion and motility as acidic chyme reduces the pH of the stomach, or as chyme moves into the small intestine and colon. In this way, the stomach avoids excessive acid secretion in the absence of buffering foodstuffs. Further, the portion of the GI tract below the stomach protects itself from exposure to excessive amounts of acid, which is both damaging to the intestinal lining and inhibitory to the activity of intestinal enzymes. Additionally, the small intestine, in which the majority of digestion and absorption occurs, controls the flow rate of food into and through the small intestines in order to optimize digestion and absorption of nutrients, salts, and water. Inability to properly regulate acid secretion and its flow into the intestine usually gives rise to duodenal ulcers, although patients with a gastrin-producing tumor (**Zollinger-Ellison syndrome**) can present with ulceration of the esophagus, stomach, and duodenum.

The general model of gastric control in response to a meal can be organized into three phases. The **cephalic phase,** which accounts for about 20% of the response to a meal during the digestive period, is activated by the actual or imagined smell and sight of food, or by the presence of food in the mouth. The cephalic phase is associated with increased gastric secretion but decreased motility, in anticipation of the need to store and start digesting food. The **gastric phase,** which accounts for about 10% of the postprandial response, is activated by the presence of food in, and mechanical distention of, the stomach. During the gastric phase, secretion is strongly stimulated, and this is accompanied by an increase in peristaltic contractions and gastric emptying. The third phase is the **intestinal phase,** during which an acidic mixture of partially digested food (**chyme**) moves in a regulated manner through the pyloric sphincter into the small intestine and ultimately into the colon. The processes of enzymatic digestion and absorption that occur during the digestive phase account for 70% of the digestive period. The movement of food into the lower GI tract generally moderates both gastric secretion and emptying.

Gastrin and the Stimulation of Gastric Function

Gastric HCl secretion from parietal cells is stimulated by three pathways (1) paracrine stimulation by **histamine,** which is secreted by neighboring **enterochromaffin-like (ECL) cells;** (2) **enteric nervous system** and **vagal parasympathetic nervous system** stimulation via **gastrin-releasing peptide (GRP)** and **acetylcholine;** and (3) direct and indirect hormonal stimulation by the peptide hormone, **gastrin.**

Gastrin is produced by the **G cells** of the stomach antrum and proximal duodenum. In humans, the term "gastrin" refers to a 17-amino acid peptide which has modifications at both termini (**G-17**). In fact, the production of G-17 is an excellent example of how a peptide-encoding gene gives rise to multiple, larger precursors, which are also secreted into the blood. G-17 is the product of sequential posttranslational processing of **preprogastrin,** which can be generally characterized as three phases (Figure 2-4). In the first phase, sulfation and proteolysis generate a mixture of

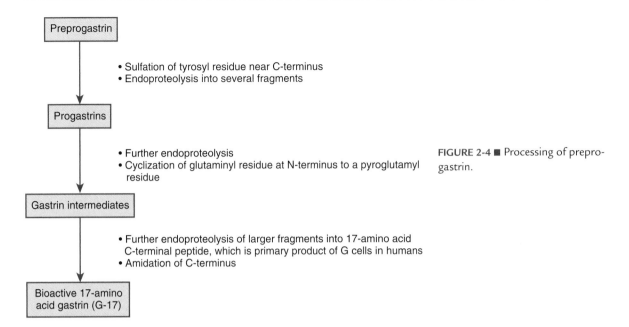

FIGURE 2-4 ■ Processing of prepro-gastrin.

gastrin precursors, called progastrins. The second phase involves proteolysis within secretory granules that generates C-termini peptides. Processing of these intermediates also includes the cyclization of the glutaminyl to a pyroglutamyl residue. The third stage involves the amidation of the C-terminus to produce **amidated gastrins**. The primary secreted bioactive product of human G cells is G-17 (i.e., 17 amino acids). The pyroGlu residue at the amino terminus and the amidation of the C-terminus protect G-17 from digestion by circulating aminopeptidases and carboxypeptidases. G-17 binds with high affinity to the CCK2 receptor, and is responsible for all of the gastrin effects on the stomach. The last four amino acids assign gastrin-like biological activity to G-17. A synthetic, clinically-used form of gastrin, **pentagastrin,** contains the last four amino acids, plus an alanine at the amino terminus that confers increased stability.

During the cephalic phase, gastric HCl secretion is stimulated by vagal (parasympathetic) inputs that directly stimulate the parietal cells, and stimulate the release of histamine from ECL cells, and gastrin from G cells (Figure 2-5). The former two effects are mediated by acetylcholine, which binds to the muscarinic receptor. Vagal stimulation of gastrin is mediated by the neurocrine factor, gastrin-releasing peptide (GRP).

During the gastric phase, gastrin secretion from G cells is primarily stimulated by the presence of peptides and amino acids in the lumen of the antrum (Figure 2-6). Gastrin secretion can also be stimulated by stomach distention during the gastric phase, through local neuronal pathways, and through a **vagovagal reflex.** Circulating gastrin levels increase by several-fold within 30 to 60 minutes after ingestion of a meal.

The primary action of gastrin is the stimulation of HCl secretion by the parietal cells of the gastric glands within the fundus and body of the stomach. To accomplish this, gastrin must enter and circulate through the general circulation and then exit capillaries and venules within the lamina propria of the gastric mucosa in the body and fundus (i.e., "upstream" of where gastrin is released within the stomach).

Gastrin evokes HCl secretion primarily through binding to the CCK2 receptor on enterochromaffin-like (ECL) cells. ECL cells, which reside in the lamina propria of the gastric mucosa, produce histamine in response to gastrin. Gastrin binding to the Gq-coupled CCK2 receptor on ECL cells increases intracellular Ca^{2+}, which leads to exocytosis of histamine-containing secretory vesicles. Gastrin also increases histamine synthesis and storage by increasing the expression of histidine decarboxylase, which generates histamine

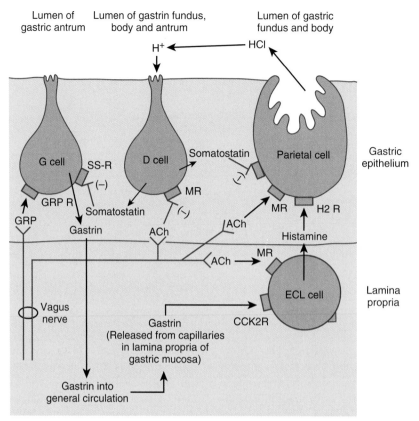

FIGURE 2-5 ■ Regulation of gastric HCl secretion during the cephalic phase. The thought, sight or smell of food, or the presence of food in the mouth, stimulates acid secretion through the vagus nerve. Intramural nerve fibers secreting acetylcholine (ACh) stimulate parietal cells directly, and through the release of histamine from enterochromaffin-like cells (ECL cells). Although luminal H+ potentially stimulates the inhibitory peptide, somatostatin from D cells, this is inhibited by neuronal ACh-mediated pathways. Gastrin is also stimulated by neuronal fibers that release gastrin-releasing peptide (GRP). As a hormone, gastrin levels increase in the general circulation. Gastrin stimulates gastric HCl secretion by binding to CCK2 receptors on ECL cells (and, to a lesser extent, on parietal cells—not shown) Thickness of arrows = relative importance. MR, stimulatory or inhibitory muscarinic receptor.

from histidine, and type 2 vesicular monoamine transporter (VMAT-2), which transports and concentrates histamine into the secretory vesicles. Thus, gastrin coordinates both the secretion and synthesis of histamine in ECL cells. Histamine, in turn, stimulates HCl secretion in a paracrine manner by binding to the H2 receptor on nearby parietal cells. Gastrin also has a direct, although less important, effect on parietal cells.

Inhibition of Gastric Function

Two negative feedback loops exist within the stomach to control gastrin release (Figure 2-7). A passive negative feedback loop involves the passage of stomach contents into the duodenum. This removes the stimulation of G cells by amino acids and peptides, and by distention-induced pathways. An active negative feedback loop involves the change in acidity of the stomach lumen. The removal of food reduces the buffering capacity of the gastric lumen. Thus, during the intestinal phase and the interdigestive period, the acidity of the stomach decreases. When the pH falls below 3, acid stimulates the D cells to secrete the paracrine peptide, **somatostatin.** Somatostatin acts through its receptors (SS-R) to inhibit gastrin secretion from neighboring G cells.

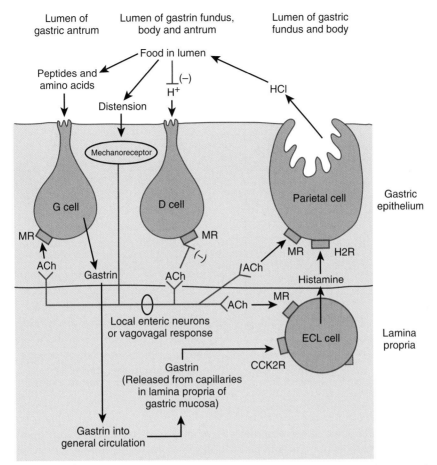

FIGURE 2-6 ■ Regulation of gastrin secretion during gastric phase. Luminal amino acids and peptides strongly stimulate G cells to secrete gastrin. Gastrin secretion and HCl secretion are also stimulated by stomach distention through local and autonomic (vagovagal) reflexes.

Gastrin release and gastric emptying is also inhibited during the intestinal phase by the release of hormones and neural signals from the small intestine and colon in response to acidity, hypertonicity, distention, and specific molecules (e.g., fatty acids). These hormones are collectively referred to as **enterogastrones.** The identity of the physiologic enterogastrones in humans which inhibit gastric acid secretion remains uncertain, but includes candidates such as secretin and GIP from the duodenum and jejunum, and peptide YY and GLP-1 from the distal ileum and colon. CCK is a well-established inhibitor of gastric motility and emptying. CCK is released from the duodenum and

jejunum in response to the presence of luminal fatty acids (Figure 2-8).

ENTEROENDOCRINE REGULATION OF THE EXOCRINE PANCREAS AND GALL BLADDER

The **exocrine pancreas** is an extramural gland that empties its secretory products through a main excretory duct into the GI tract at the duodenum (Figure 2-9). The exocrine pancreas produces enzymes necessary to digest macromolecules in the small intestine. Pancreatic enzymes have optimal activities at a neutral pH.

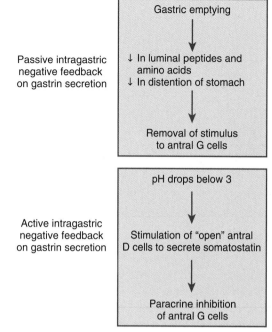

FIGURE 2-7 ■ Passive and active negative feedback loops on gastrin secretion.

Accordingly, the cells that line the pancreatic ducts secrete a bicarbonate-rich fluid, which serves to neutralize acidic chyme in the duodenum. The **gall bladder** is also an extramural organ. It receives bile that is secreted by the liver. Bile is both stored and concentrated in the gall bladder. Bile is released into small intestine through the common bile duct, which usually joins the main pancreatic duct to form the hepatopancreatic ampulla just before opening into the **duodenum** (see Figure 2-9). A major function of bile is the emulsification of triglycerides to increase their accessibility to pancreatic lipase. In order to perform this function, aggregates (called micelles) of bile acids and other lipids are required. Micelle formation requires neutral or slightly alkaline conditions. Accordingly, the epithelial cells of the common bile duct secrete a bicarbonate-rich fluid.

Pancreatic and gall bladder functions are primarily regulated by the autonomic nervous system during the interdigestive period (pancreatic secretion occurs in phase with the MMC in humans), and during the cephalic and gastric phases of the digestive period.

However, during the intestinal phase, when these glands are most active, they are predominantly under endocrine control by two GI hormones, **secretin** and **CCK.** Secretin primarily regulates ductal secretion of a bicarbonate-rich fluid from both pancreatic and bile ducts. CCK primarily stimulates enzyme secretion from pancreatic acinar cells and gall bladder contraction. This dual regulation allows for fine-tuning of the qualitative nature of the product (e.g., in terms of the percentage of bicarbonate and protein in pancreatic juice) that is finally secreted into the duodenum.

The classic model for secretin and CCK action on the pancreas is that the appearance of acid, long chain fatty acids, and glycine-containing dipeptides and tripeptides in the duodenum stimulates the "open" enteroendocrine cells to secrete the two hormones. Secretin and CCK then circulate in the blood and bind to their specific receptors on either ductal or acinar cells, respectively. However, there is evidence that secretin has permissive effects on CCK actions, and vice versa. Moreover, it is also clear that the autonomic and enteric nervous systems have a permissive effect on the secretin and CCK actions. The neurotransmitter, ACh, and a secretin-related enteric neurocrine peptide, VIP, stimulate pancreatic ductal and acinar cells, and synergize with secretin and CCK. Patients who have a VIPoma (i.e., a tumor producing high levels of VIP) suffer from pancreatic diarrhea because of a constant high level of pancreatic secretion into the gut.

Secretin

Secretin is produced by "open" **S cells** in the duodenum and jejunum. Similar to gastrin, secretin is produced by posttranslational processing of a larger preprosecretin molecule. Most secretin is a carboxyamidated 27-amino acid peptide.

The primary stimulus for secretin release is a decrease in duodenal pH. The threshold pH value for secretin release is 4.5. Circulating secretin levels increase rapidly (approximately 10 minutes) after acidified chyme passes through the pyloric sphincter into the duodenum. The exact mechanism by which H^+ induces secretin release from S cells is unclear. There is evidence for a direct action of H^+ on S cells, as well as evidence for indirect actions through enteric neurons and through a phospholipase A_2-like **secretin–releasing factor.**

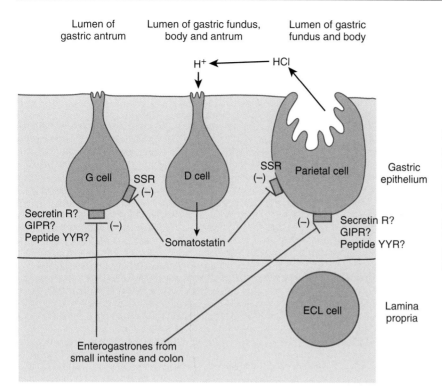

FIGURE 2-8 ■ Regulation of gastrin secretion during intestinal phase. The exact nature of physiologic enterogastrones in humans is not well established. Candidates include secretin and gastric-inhibitory peptide (GIP) from the small intestine, and peptide YY from the ileum and colon.

The primary short-term action of secretin is the stimulation of the secretion of a bicarbonate-rich fluid from the pancreatic and biliary ducts during the intestinal phase of the digestive period (Figure 2-10). Secretin acts through the secretin receptor, which is linked to cAMP-dependent pathways. In general, secretin increases the activity of transporters in the apical membrane of ductal cells, which increases the ability of these cells to transport Cl⁻ and water into the lumen, and then exchange Cl^- for HCO_3^-. This can occur through the activation of preexisting transporters in the apical membrane, and through the exocytotic insertion of transporter-containing vesicles into the membrane.

Secretin also binds to its receptor on the pancreatic acinar cells. Although secretin has a minimal effect on acinar cells by itself, secretin synergizes with the hormone CCK to further enhance pancreatic enzyme secretion over that achieved by CCK alone. Secretin may also function as an enterogastrone by inhibiting stomach acid secretion.

Cholecystokinin

CCK is a 33-amino acid peptide produced by the I cells of the duodenum and jejunum. CCK is structurally similar to gastrin, with the 5 amino acids at the carboxyl terminus identical to both hormones. CCK is also sulfated on a tyrosine that is the seventh amino acid from the carboxy terminus. CCK binds primarily to the CCK1 receptor (formerly called the CCKA receptor), whereas gastrin preferentially binds to the CCK2 receptor. Both hormones can weakly interact with the other's receptor, and desulfation of CCK increases its affinity for the CCK2 receptor. The CCK1 receptor is linked to protein kinase C-dependent and Ca^{2+}-dependent pathways.

The primary stimulus for CCK secretion is the presence of long chain fatty acids or monoglycerides in the small intestine. CCK secretion is also induced by glycine-containing dipeptides and tripeptides. The mechanism by which any of these act to stimulate CCK release is obscure, although there is some evidence for a postabsorptive effect of lipids after their

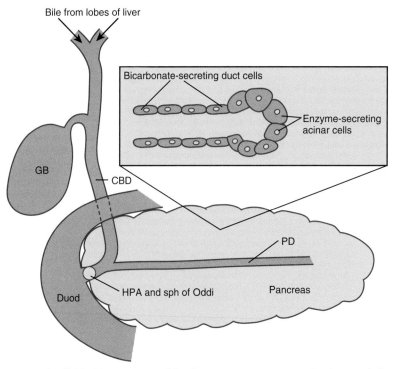

Bile from lobes of liver

Bicarbonate-secreting duct cells

Enzyme-secreting acinar cells

GB

CBD

PD

HPA and sph of Oddi

Duod

Pancreas

FIGURE 2-9 ■ Anatomy of gall bladder, common bile duct, pancreas, pancreatic duct and the duodenum. The gall bladder (GB) stores and concentrates bile from the liver. Contraction of the gall bladder and relaxation of the sphincter of Oddi (sph of Oddi) allows bile to flow down the common bile duct (CBD) into the duodenum (Duod). Pancreatic enzymes and bicarbonate reach the duodenum via larger and larger ducts that eventually form the main pancreatic duct (PD). This duct joins the common bile duct just before it reaches the duodenum, to form the hepatopancreatic ampulla (HPA). **Inset** shows a higher magnification of the exocrine pancreas. The termini of the secretory units are the pancreatic acini, which secrete enzymes. The ductal epithelium secretes a bicarbonate-rich fluid. Note that the ductal epithelium of the common bile duct also secretes a bicarbonate-rich fluid.

assembly into chylomicrons. Like secretin, CCK primarily regulates pancreatic and biliary function. In the pancreas, CCK stimulates enzyme secretion from the acinar cells (see Figure 2-10). The CCK1 receptor increases intracellular DAG and Ca^{2+}, which results in the exocytosis of enzyme-containing secretion granules. CCK also has a permissive effect on the ability of secretin to stimulate bicarbonate secretion. CCK is a strong stimulator of gall bladder contraction. CCK induces gall bladder contraction both directly and indirectly through activation of vagal afferent neurons. CCK also stimulates bile secretion into the duodenum through promoting relaxation of the sphincter of the hepatopancreatic ampulla (sphincter of Oddi). This latter action on hepatobiliary function

is likely due to the CCK-dependent release of inhibitory neurotransmitters, such as nitric oxide. As mentioned, CCK also inhibits gastric emptying, which reduces duodenal acidity and allows emulsification, digestion, and absorption of lipids.

Motilin and Stimulation of Gastric and Small Intestinal Contractions During the Interdigestive Period

Motilin is a 22-amino acid peptide produced from a 114-amino acid prepromotilin and secreted by the M cells of the small intestine. Motilin secretion is inhibited by the presence of food or acid in the small intestine, and is stimulated by alkalinization of the small intestine.

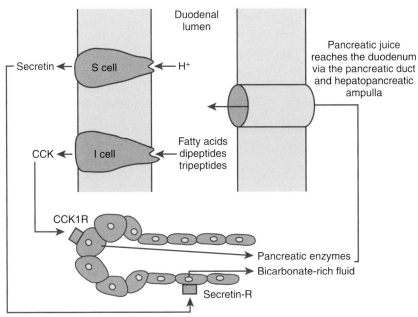

FIGURE 2-10 ■ Hormonal regulation of pancreatic secretion.

Circulating motilin levels peak every 1 to 2 hours in fasting individuals, in phase with the **migrating myoelectric complex (MMC).** The MMC is a set of organized contractions that move aborally from the stomach to the ileum, and clean the stomach and small intestines of indigestible particles. The MMC may also prevent the colonic bacteria from migrating into the small intestine. Motilin may function to either initiate or integrate the MMC.

The motilin receptor is a G-protein–coupled receptor that activates the phospholipase C signaling pathway. The motilin receptor also binds and is activated by the macrolide antibiotic, **erythromycin** (see Table 2-2). Erythromycin and other motilin receptor agonists are used in the treatment of delayed gastric emptying **(gastroparesis),** which is common in patients with diabetes mellitus and in some postsurgical patients.

THE INSULINOTROPIC ACTIONS OF GI PEPTIDES (INCRETIN ACTION)

Elevated circulating levels of nutrients, particularly blood glucose, are strong stimuli of insulin secretion from the pancreatic β cells (Chapter 3). The possibility that GI hormones also regulate the secretion of insulin was revealed by observations that oral administration of glucose caused a greater rise in insulin than did glucose administered by an intravenous route. This enteroinsular response gave rise to the concept of **incretins.** In this model, an enteroendocrine cell type(s) senses nutrients in the GI tract, and releases a hormone (an **incretin**), which, in turn, prepares the pancreatic β cells for the impending rise in blood nutrients (primarily blood glucose). There are two incretins in humans, gastric inhibitory peptide (GIP; also referred to as *g*lucose-dependent *i*nsulinotropic *p*eptide), and glucagon-like peptide-1 (GLP-1). These peptides (or analogs thereof) are currently being investigated for the treatment of type II diabetes mellitus (see Chapter 3). An important feature of incretins is that their ability to increase insulin secretion is strongly dependent on glucose levels. This means that incretin analogs pose a low risk of inducing severe hypoglycemia (low blood sugar) because once blood glucose falls, the effect of incretins is terminated.

In general, GIP and GLP-1 act through Gs-coupled receptors on β cells, which increase cAMP. This leads to an increase in intracellular Ca^{2+} that is required for glucose-dependent release of insulin. These hormones also enhance the synthesis of insulin and of proteins that sensitize the β cells to glucose levels, such as the glucose transporter, GLUT-2, and hexokinase.

Gastric Inhibitory Peptide/Glucose-Dependent Insulinotropic Peptide

GIP is a 42-amino acid peptide secreted by the K cells of the small intestine, and is a member of the secretin gene family. The primary stimulus for GIP release is the presence of long-chain fatty acids, triglycerides, glucose, and amino acids in the lumen of the small intestine.

GIP was first discovered as an enterogastrone in animal models, in which it inhibited gastric acid secretion and intestinal motility. However, physiologic levels of GIP have only a modest effect on stomach function in humans. In contrast, GIP has an important physiologic role as an incretin. GIP knockout mice display a reduced ability to maintain normal blood glucose levels after an oral glucose load (**impaired glucose tolerance**).

In rare cases, the GIP receptor is inappropriately expressed on cells of the zona fasciculata of the adrenal cortex (see Chapter 7). These patients display enlarged adrenals and **food-induced hypercortisolism.** In these patients, food in the small intestine stimulates the release of GIP, which then stimulates cortisol production by the adrenal cortex.

Glucagon-like Peptide-1

The glucagon gene is an example of a gene that encodes a large precursor protein (preproglucagon), which is proteolytically processed to form active and inactive peptides (Figure 2-11). Furthermore, the prohormone convertases that digest preproglucagon display cell-specific expression, so that different products are released from different cell types. In the α cells of the endocrine pancreas, the active product is glucagon (see Chapter 3). In contrast, intestinal L cells express preproglucagon, but secrete GLP-1 and GLP-2 as biologically-active peptides. GLP-1 is stimulated by the presence of free fatty acids and glucose in the lumen of the ileum and colon. GLP-1 secretion is also increased by neuronal pathways stimulated by free fatty acids and glucose in the upper small intestine. GLP-1 is co-secreted with the other glucagon-derived peptide, GLP-2 and **peptide YY** (which is not structurally related to glucagon). The tropic effect of GLP-2 will be discussed subsequently.

Like GIP, GLP-1 acts as an incretin. GLP-1 knockout mice have impaired glucose tolerance. GLP-1, along with peptide YY, also appears to be a component of the "ileal brake," in which free fatty acids and carbohydrates in the ileum inhibit gastric emptying through increased secretion of GLP-1 and peptide YY. This enterogastrone action of GLP-1 further enhances the ability of the organism to control excessive blood glucose excursions. A problem with the therapeutic use of native GLP-1 is the fact that it is rapidly degraded.

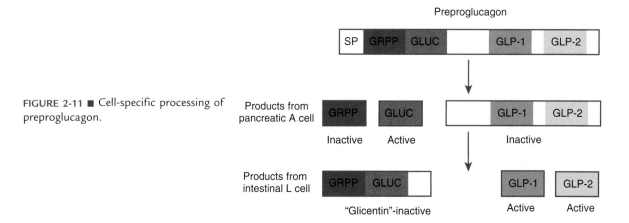

FIGURE 2-11 ■ Cell-specific processing of preproglucagon.

The use of more stable analogs, called **exendins,** and inhibitors of enzymatic degradation are currently under investigation for enhancing pancreatic β cell function in type 2 diabetics.

THE ENTEROTROPIC ACTIONS OF GI HORMONES

An important characteristic of most (if not all) hormones is their ability to promote the growth of their target tissues. This tropic effect helps to maintain the health and integrity of the target tissues, and optimizes the ability of target tissues to perform their differentiated functions. In addition to the actions of GI hormones on the maintenance of healthy GI structure and physiology, the tropic actions of GI hormones are of current clinical interest for several reasons, including (but not limited to):

1. The promotion of hypertrophy and hyperplasia of GI tissues, which sometimes progress to cancer, by the excessive secretion of a GI hormone (usually from a tumor);
2. The ability of the GI tract to adapt to a diseased portion of the tract, and/or corrective surgery that involves resection or bypass of a GI segment;
3. The ability to grow new pieces of GI tissue in vitro (i.e., tissue-engineered neointestine) from pluripotential or stem cells, which can be used for replacement of diseased or resected portions;
4. The ability to promote pancreatic islet growth and neogenesis in diabetic patients.

Gastrin

In addition to its well-established role in the regulation of gastric acid secretion, gastrin exerts several other effects on the stomach and GI tract. The second most important action of gastrin is its developmental and trophic effect on the gastric mucosa. Gastrin knockout mice display poorly differentiated gastric mucosa, with a reduced number of ECL and parietal cells. In contrast, patients suffering from **Zollinger-Ellison syndrome** (see earlier) exhibit hypertrophy and hyperplasia of the gastric mucosa, as well as submucosal rugal folds. Overgrowth is particularly true for the ECL cell population. Although ECL cell proliferation can progress to carcinoid tumor formation,

this is rare and usually requires other abnormalities. As discussed earlier, progastrin and glycine-extended gastrin (G-Gly) appear to promote the proliferation of colonic mucosa.

Gastric acid, through its effects on D cells and somatostatin release, inhibits the growth of G cells. Thus, long-term inhibition of gastric acid production (e.g., with pharmacologic proton pump inhibitors or H2 receptor blockers) can lead to an overgrowth of antral G cells.

Secretin and CCK

CCK has a direct effect on pancreatic acinar cells that promotes their maintenance and growth. Secretin inhibits pancreatic ductal cell growth through binding to the secretin receptor. In contrast, the secretin-related neurotransmitter, VIP, stimulates ductal growth through the VIP receptor (called $VPAC_1$ receptor). In some ductal pancreatic adenocarcinomas, the secretin receptor is defective, but the $VPAC_1$ receptor is intact. Thus, loss of secretin receptor function may shift the cell toward net proliferation.

GLP-1

One of the most exciting and promising aspects of enterotropic actions of GI hormones is the tropic effect that GLP-1 has on pancreatic islet development and growth, particularly with respect to the β cells. GLP-1 has been shown to induce differentiation of human islet stem cells into β cells in vitro. In mice and rats, GLP-1 and exendin-4 have protected against surgically- and chemically-induced diabetes, increased β-cell mass and neogenesis, and inhibited β-cell apoptosis. Further, GLP-1 receptor knockout mice do not display exendin-4–induced regeneration of islets after partial pancreatectomy. Thus, GLP-1 or analogs may become valuable reagents in the treatment of diabetics in whom their β-cell mass has been compromised.

GLP-2

GLP-2 is co-secreted with GLP-1 by the intestinal L cells. Unlike GLP-1, GLP-2 does not have an insulinotropic action. GLP-2 binds to its own receptor (the GLP-2 receptor), and has potent trophic effects on the intestines. In fact, evidence of this effect was first discovered in a patient who presented with a massive overgrowth of the small intestine. The patient was also found to have a tumor in the kidney that was producing large amounts of glucagon-related peptides. GLP-2 has been used to prevent mucosal atrophy in patients receiving total parenteral nutrition, and promotes intestinal growth and adaptation in patients undergoing resection of bowel. GLP-2 also has positive effects on hexose transport, and may enhance other absorptive functions of intestinal villi.

SUMMARY

1. Gastrointestinal (GI) hormones are produced by enteroendocrine cells. GI hormones are peptides or proteins and bind to G-protein–coupled receptors on their target cells. GI hormones are produced by specific cell types that reside in specific regions of the GI tract. The secretion of GI hormones is stimulated primarily by luminal secretogogues, and by neuronal and paracrine signals.

2. Gastrin plays a major role in the stimulation of gastric acid secretion. Gastrin is secreted by G cells in the stomach antrum in response to amino acids and peptides in the antral lumen and in response to neuronal stimulation. The primary secreted form of gastrin by the stomach is the 17-amino acid G-17 form. G-17 has a cyclized glutaminyl residue at its N-terminus and an amidated glycine at its C-terminus, which increase the biological half-life of secreted gastrin. Gastrin binds to the CCK2 receptor, and acts primarily by stimulating enterochromaffin-like cells (ECL cells) to secrete histamine. Histamine then stimulates the parietal cells of the stomach to secrete HCl.

3. The major enteroendocrine cells of the duodenum and jejunum are the S cells and the I cells, which secrete secretin and cholecystokinin (CCK), respectively. Secretin is released primarily during the "intestinal" phase of a meal in response to increased acidity in the duodenum. Secretin promotes the secretion of a bicarbonate-rich fluid from the bile duct and pancreatic ducts, which empty into the duodenum. CCK promotes the contraction of the gall bladder and relaxation of the sphincter of the hepatopancreatic ampulla, thus promoting the emptying of bile into the duodenum. CCK also stimulates enzyme secretion from pancreatic acinar cells.

4. Motilin is secreted by the M cells of the small intestine during the interdigestive phase (i.e., in between meals) in phase with the migrating myoelectric complex. Motilin promotes emptying of the stomach and small intestines. The motilin receptor is activated by erythromycin, which can be used to treat delayed gastric emptying (gastroparesis).

5. GI hormones called incretins are secreted in response to luminal nutrients (especially glucose) and increase the ability of blood glucose to stimulate insulin secretion from the pancreatic islets of Langerhans. Incretins include gastric inhibitory peptide (GIP), which has been named more recently for its incretin effect as glucose-dependent insulinotropic peptide. GIP is secreted from the K cells of the small intestine. Another important incretin is glucagon-like peptide-1 (GLP-1), which is secreted by the intestinal L cells. Due to their ability to sensitize insulin-producing β cells to glucose, incretins are being tested for the treatment of type 2 diabetes mellitus (T2DM; see Chapter 3).

6. GI hormones also have important trophic effects. Gastrin stimulates the growth of the gastric mucosa, especially the ECL cells and submucosa. Secretin and CCK promote the growth of exocrine pancreas tissue. GLP-1 promotes β-cell proliferation, which may prove an important function of GLP-1 in the treatment of T2DM. GLP-2, which is a related to, but a separate hormone from GLP-1, promotes GI mucosal growth and is used to treat patients at risk for GI mucosal atrophy.

7. Zollinger-Ellinger syndrome is caused by a gastrin-producing tumor. Patients have ulcerations of the esophagus, stomach, and duodenum and overgrowth of the stomach mucosa and rugal submucosal folds.

KEY WORDS AND CONCEPTS

- Secretin
- Hormone
- Enteroendocrine cell
- Secretogogues
- Enteric nervous system
- Paracrine
- Intrinsic regulators
- Extrinsic regulators
- Autonomic nervous system
- Endocrine glands
- Enterotropic action
- Incretion action
- G-protein–coupled receptors
- Gastrin
- Cholecystokinin (CCK)
- Glucose-dependent/insulinotropic peptide
- Vasoactive intestinal peptide
- Motilin
- Ghrelin
- Growth hormone secretogogue
- Stomach
- Fundus and body
- Parietal cells
- HCl
- Intrinsic factor
- Vitamin B_{12}
- Oxyntic cells
- Chief cells
- Mucigens
- Pyloric antrum
- Somatostatin
- Zollinger-Ellison syndrome
- Cephalic phase
- Gastric phase
- Intestinal phase
- Chyme
- Enterohistamine chromograffin-like
- (ECL) cells
- Enteric nervous system
- Vagal parasympathetic nervous system
- Gastrin-releasing peptide (GRP)
- Acetylcholine
- G-17
- Preprogastrin
- Amidated gastrins
- Pentagastrin
- Vagovagal reflex
- Enterogastrones
- Exocrine pancreas
- Gall bladder
- Duodenum
- CCK
- S cells
- Secretin-releasing factor
- I cells
- CCK1 receptor
- Migrating myoelectric complex (MMC)
- Erythromycin
- Gastroparesis
- Incretins
- Impaired glucose tolerance
- Food-induced hypercortisolism
- Peptide YY
- Exendins

SELF-STUDY PROBLEMS

1. What are the three phases of the digestive period? Which one has the greatest release of gastrin? Why?
2. When administered during the interdigestive period, what are the predicted effects on gastrin secretion of the following experimental agents?
   a. A somatostatin antagonist
   b. A mix of amino acids in the antral lumen
   c. Increased acidity in the antral lumen
   d. A muscarinic agonist
   e. Gastrin-releasing peptide
3. What is the relation between gastric emptying and secretion from duodenal S and I cells?
4. What are the effects of CCK on the following?
   a. Pancreatic bicarbonate secretion
   b. Pancreatic enzyme secretion
   c. Biliary bicarbonate secretion
   d. Contraction of the gall bladder muscularis
   e. Contraction of the sphincter of Oddi
5. What is the relation between GRP-1 and glucagon?
6. Define "incretin." Name two incretins.
7. What enterotropic effect is observed in patients with Zollinger-Ellison Syndrome?
8. Why does erythromycin promote gastric emptying?

BIBLIOGRAPHY

Buchan AM: Nutrient tasting and signaling mechanisms in the gut III. Endocrine cell recognition of luminal nutrients, *Am J Physiol* 277(6 Pt 1):G1103-1107, 1999.

Creutzfeldt W: The entero-insular axis in type 2 diabetes—incretins as therapeutic agents, *Exp Clin Endocrinol Diabetes* 109 Suppl 2:S288-303, 2001.

Dockray G J, A. Varro A, et al: The gastrins: their production and biological activities, *Annu Rev Physiol* 63:119-139, 2001.

Dowling RH: Glucagon-like peptide-2 and intestinal adaptation: an historical and clinical perspective, *J Nutr* 133(11):3703-3707, 2003.

Holst JJ: Gut hormones as pharmaceuticals. From enteroglucagon to GLP-1 and GLP-2, *Regul Pept* 93(1-3):45-51, 2000.

Johnson L: *Gastrointestinal Physiology*, ed 2, St. Louis, 2001, Mosby/Elsevier.

Konturek SJ, Zabielski R, et al: Neuroendocrinology of the pancreas: role of brain-gut axis in pancreatic secretion, *Eur J Pharmacol* 481(1):1-14, 2003.

Nielsen LL, Young AA, et al: Pharmacology of exenatide (synthetic exendin-4): a potential therapeutic for improved glycemic control of type 2 diabetes, *Regul Pept* 117(2):77-88, 2004.

Rehfeld JF: The new biology of gastrointestinal hormones, *Physiol Rev* 78(4):1087-1108, 1998.

Rozengurt E, Walsh JH: Gastrin, CCK, signaling, and cancer, *Annu Rev Physiol* 63:49-76, 2001.

Sachs G, Zeng N, et al: Physiology of isolated gastric endocrine cells, *Annu Rev Physiol* 59:243-256, 1997.

Solcia E, Rindi G, et al: Gastric endocrine cells: types, function and growth, *Regul Pept* 93(1-3):31-35, 2000.

3

ENERGY METABOLISM

■ ■ ■ ■ ■ ■ ■ ■ ■ ■ ■ ■

OBJECTIVES

1. Provide an overview of energy metabolism with emphasis on maintaining blood glucose within the normal range.
   - Relative to discontinuous caloric consumption
   - Relative to ever-changing expenditure of energy
2. Introduce the primary hormones involved in the regulation of energy metabolic homeostasis.

3. Cover the hormonal regulation of specific enzymatic pathways.
4. Discuss the emerging concepts concerning the role of adipose tissue as an endocrine organ.

We eat to live (although some of the less ascetic among us live to eat). Having discussed the role of hormones in the acquisition of food in Chapter 2, we now need to consider the role of hormones in the partitioning of food in order to maintain a constant supply of energy to all of the cells in the body during the digestive and interdigestive periods, and during fasting and exercising. Chapter 3 is organized into the following sections:

First, an overview of **energy metabolism** will be discussed with emphasis on the need to maintain blood glucose within a normal range, even in the face of discontinuous caloric consumption and an ever-changing expenditure of energy. This section will discuss how the **liver, skeletal muscle, adipose tissue,** and **brain** interact to maintain metabolic homeostasis.

Second, the primary hormones involved in the regulation of energy metabolic homeostasis will be introduced. These will include the **pancreatic islet hormones, insulin** and **glucagon,** the **adrenal hormone, epinephrine,** and the **sympathetic neurotransmitter, norepinephrine.**

Third, the regulation of specific enzymatic pathways by hormones will be covered.

Fourth, imbalances in metabolic homeostasis will be introduced. This section will examine **diet-induced obesity, insulin resistance,** and **type 1 diabetes mellitus (T1DM),** and **type 2 diabetes mellitus (T2DM),** and current concepts of the mechanisms by which glucotoxicity and lipotoxicity occur.

Emerging concepts concerning the role of adipose tissue as an endocrine organ will be discussed.

OVERVIEW OF ENERGY METABOLISM

Cells Must Make ATP to Function and Stay Viable

Cells continually perform work in order to maintain their integrity and internal environment, respond to stimuli, and perform their differentiated functions. Cells derive their energy to perform this work primarily from **adenosine triphosphate (ATP).** Thus, cells need a continual supply of ATP to the extent that humans synthesize well over one half of their own weight in ATP daily. This is done by oxidizing **glucose, nonesterified fatty acids (FFAs;** also called **"free fatty acids"**), **amino acids (AAs)**, and **ketone bodies.**

A critical feature of the utilization of different nutrients is cell specificity. Cells with no or very few mitochondria cannot utilize AAs and FFAs for energy, but must rely entirely on anaerobic glycolysis (see next page). Most importantly, because of the blood-brain barrier, the brain cannot access circulating FFAs for energy. The brain converts most of its amino acid pool into neurotransmitters instead of oxidizing them for energy. This means that the brain and some other tissues are obligate glucose users. In other words, the *function of the brain is critically dependent on circulating levels of blood glucose, much as it is on a continuous supply of oxygen.* An acute fall in blood glucose levels below 50 mg/100 ml (i.e., **hypoglycemia**) leads to impaired CNS functions, including the loss of vision, cognition, and muscle coordination, as well as lethargy and weakness (Figure 3-1). Severe hypoglycemia can ultimately lead to coma and death. Thus, a major role of the hormones involved in metabolic homeostasis is to maintain blood glucose levels above 60 mg/100 ml. Conversely, it is important that fasting blood glucose levels remain below 110 mg/100 ml. Indeed, the complications associated with poorly controlled DM has

taught us that not only is too little blood glucose incompatible with life, but that too much blood glucose imposes various stresses on cell functions, increasing morbidity and shortening life (see Figure 3-1).

A balance must be struck in which a discontinuous caloric intake is matched to the utilization or storage of energy substrates as required by an ever-present but fluctuating energy demand. This balance is achieved through the differential activation and inactivation of selective metabolic pathways during the fed state (i.e., during caloric surplus) versus during the interdigestive period, prolonged fasting, or exercise (i.e., during caloric deficit). *Importantly, all organs and tissues cannot simply transport glucose from the blood and oxidize it to the same extent at all times.* First, we will briefly review the primary metabolic pathways involved in the utilization and storage of glucose, FAs, and AAs. We will also discuss a nondietary fuel, the ketone bodies, which are made by the liver for use by other organs during a period of fasting.

Making ATP

Making ATP from Carbohydrates ATP is generated from the oxidation of carbohydrates, FFAs, and AAs. The primary carbohydrate utilized by cells is the

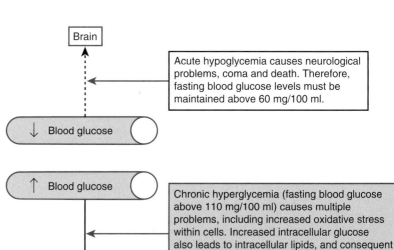

FIGURE 3-1 ■ The importance of maintaining blood glucose within the normal range.

Brain

Acute hypoglycemia causes neurological problems, coma and death. Therefore, fasting blood glucose levels must be maintained above 60 mg/100 ml.

↓ Blood glucose

↑ Blood glucose

Chronic hyperglycemia (fasting blood glucose above 110 mg/100 ml) causes multiple problems, including increased oxidative stress within cells. Increased intracellular glucose also leads to intracellular lipids, and consequent lipotoxicity. Ultimately, these stresses induce insulin-resistance and β-cell dysfunction, which further compromise glucose tolerance and lead to T2DM. High levels of blood glucose also create an osmotic burden on cells and the organism.

Vasculature, nerves, kidney, peripheral organs

6-carbon (hexose) monosaccharide, **glucose.** There are three main phases involved in the process of oxidizing glucose to the full extent: (1) transport and trapping of glucose inside the cell; (2) **glycolysis** (i.e., the splitting [lysis]) of the 6-carbon molecule, glucose (glycol), into the 3-carbon molecule, pyruvate (aerobic) or lactate (anaerobic); and (3) the **tricarboxylic acid (TCA) cycle,** which occurs in the inner mitochondrial matrix in proximity to the components of the electron transport chain (**ETC**) and **oxidative phosphorylation (OxPhos).**

In the first phase, glucose is transported across the cell membrane by bidirectional facilitative glucose transporters, called **GLUTs.** There are 14 different GLUT isoforms, but the ones that have been the most studied in metabolic homeostasis are listed in Table 3-1. Once inside the cell, glucose is prevented from exiting by phosphorylation to **glucose-6-phosphate (G-6-P).** This phosphorylation is catalyzed by **hexokinases.** The hexokinase found in the liver and pancreatic β cells has a low affinity for glucose (i.e., it transports glucose only when glucose is available at elevated concentrations) and is designated **glucokinase.**

The second phase involves **glycolysis** (Figure 3-2), which occurs in the cytoplasm. Glycolysis yields a net production of 2 moles of ATP/mole of glucose, while consuming the required cofactor, NAD^+, by reducing it to NADH. In the presence of robust oxidative phosphorylation (relative to the rate of glycolysis), NADH is converted back to NAD^+ in an O_2-dependent manner, and pyruvate is the primary product of glycolysis (oxidative glycolysis). If the cell has no or very few mitochondria (e.g., erythrocytes, lens of the eye), oxidative phosphorylation cannot be carried out and used to oxidize NADH back to NAD^+. In this case, the cell regenerates NAD^+ by reducing pyruvate to lactate by the process of anaerobic glycolysis.

During the third process (see Figure 3-2), pyruvate enters the mitochondria and is converted into acetyl coenzyme A (acetyl Co A). Acetyl Co A is then further metabolized in the **tricarboxylic acid (TCA) cycle** and the closely coupled process of **oxidative phosphorylation,** using the **electron transport chain.** This second stage of oxidation yields *almost 20 times more ATP than glycolysis.* Thus, the TCA cycle and oxidative phosphorylation are very efficient methods of generating ATP from glucose. However, this requires molecular oxygen (O_2). This is why humans need to breathe air and why oxidative phosphorylation can proceed only as fast as the respiratory and cardiovascular systems can deliver O_2 to tissues. Therefore, even tissues with mitochondria rely on anaerobic glycolysis for some needs. As discussed subsequently, the process of oxidative phosphorylation is also a major contributor to the generation of **reactive oxygen species (ROS),** which impose oxidative stress that is harmful to cells.

Making ATP from FFAs The other two energy substrates, FFAs and AAs, bypass glycolysis and ultimately enter the TCA cycle/oxidative phosphorylation as pyruvate, acetyl CoA, or as different components of the TCA cycle. FFAs are released from adipose tissue by lipolysis and circulate in the blood bound to serum albumin. Transport proteins then translocate FFAs into cells. FFAs are metabolized in the mitochondria by the repetitive, cyclic process of **β-oxidation** (see Figure 3-2). This requires the transport of FFAs into the inner mitochondrial matrix by the **carnitine palmitoyl–transferase** (**CPT-I** and **CPT-II**) system of transporters. Each cycle of β-oxidation removes 2-carbon moieties at a time from FFA chains. Each cycle of β-oxidation generates a molecule of acetyl-CoA, which is oxidized through the TCA cycle and oxidative phosphorylation. In addition to the generation of acetyl CoA, each cycle of β-oxidation generates 1 molecule each of $FADH_2$ and NADH, thereby

TABLE 3-1		
An Abridged List of Glucose Transporters		
TRANSPORTERS	DISTRIBUTION	CHARACTERISTICS
GLUT-1	Ubiquitous	High affinity—transports basal levels of glucose
GLUT-2	Pancreatic β cell, liver	Low affinity—important during fasting-to-fed transition
GLUT-3	Ubiquitous	High affinity—primary Glut in neuronal tissue
GLUT-4	Skeletal muscle and adipose tissue	Dependent on insulin signalling for translocation to cell membrane from intracytoplasmic site
GLUT-5	Small intestine and spermatozoa	Fructose transporter

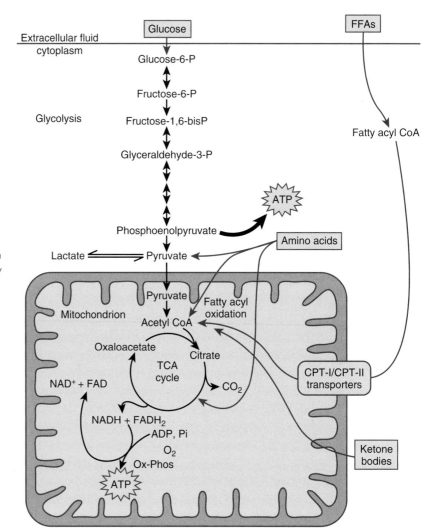

FIGURE 3-2 ■ ATP is made from glucose, amino acids, free fatty acids (FFAs), and ketone bodies.

producing up to 17 ATPs. Thus, FFAs are a more efficient source of energy storage than CHOs because the cell can obtain more ATPs/carbon from FFAs than from glucose.

Making ATP from Amino Acids AAs can be also be oxidized after transamination (transfer of their amino group to another molecule). The carbon skeletons of AAs converge on the TCA cycle by conversion to intermediates, including pyruvate, acetyl CoA, α-ketoglutarate, succinyl CoA, fumarate, and oxaloacetate (see Figure 3-2).

Making ATP from Ketone Bodies Ketone bodies are 4-carbon molecules that include **acetoacetate** and **β-hydroxybutyrate.** Ketone bodies do not exist in significant levels in the diet, as do carbohydrates, fats, and amino acids. Rather, ketone bodies represent a fourth class of fuels that are synthesized from acetyl CoA in the liver and exported into the bloodstream for other organs to use. Extrahepatic tissues convert ketone bodies back to acetyl CoA using succinyl CoA as a CoA donor and the enzyme **thiophorase** (Figure 3-3). The liver itself lacks thiophorase, and thus cannot utilize ketone bodies for its own energy needs.

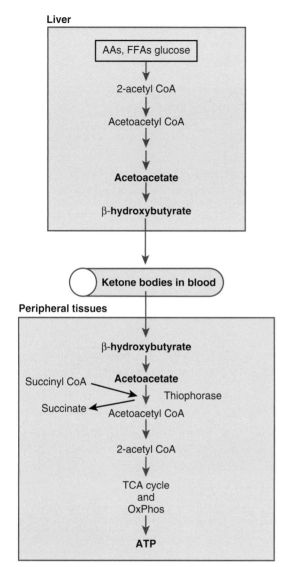

Liver

AAs, FFAs glucose

↓

2-acetyl CoA

↓

Acetoacetyl CoA

↓

Acetoacetate

↓

β-**hydroxybutyrate**

↓

(Ketone bodies in blood)

Peripheral tissues

↓

β-**hydroxybutyrate**

↓

Succinyl CoA   **Acetoacetate**

Thiophorase

Succinate ←   Acetoacetyl CoA

↓

2-acetyl CoA

↓

TCA cycle
and
OxPhos

↓

ATP

FIGURE 3-3 ■ Production of ketone bodies in liver and their utilization by peripheral tissues.

Storage Forms of Energy

Glycogen In general, nutrients are stored during the fed state. Glucose can be stored as **glycogen,** which is a large polymer of glucose molecules. Once glucose is trapped as glucose-6-phosphate, it can be converted to glucose-1-phosphate by the enzyme, phosphoglucomutase. Glucose-1-phosphate is then added to glycogen chains by two repetitive reactions. The primary,

regulated enzyme in glycogenesis is **glycogen synthase** (Figure 3-4).

During the interdigestive period, individual glucose moieties can be cleaved from glycogen and metabolized back to glucose-6-phosphate (see Figure 3-4). The primary enzyme in glycogenolysis is called **glycogen phosphorylase.** In the liver, glucose-6-phosphate can be further converted to glucose by **glucose-6-phosphatase,** and the glucose which is generated can be transported out of the cell by the bidirectional GLUT-2 transporter. Thus, liver glycogen can directly contribute to blood glucose levels. Muscle does not express glucose-6-phosphatase, so that glycogenolysis is linked to intramyocellular glycolysis. Lactate produced by muscle glycolysis can be converted to glucose in the liver by gluconeogenesis (see later). In this manner, muscle glycogen can contribute indirectly to blood glucose levels.

Triglyceride The **triglycerides (TGs)** can be stored in most tissues, but only **adipose tissue** has evolved as an efficient storage depot for TG. Significant TG accumulation in other organs (cardiac muscle, liver) can compromise their physiologic functions and cause cell death. Thus, the body has developed mechanisms for transport of dietary TGs and endogenously synthesized TGs to adipose tissue.

Dietary TG Most of the TG stored in adipose tissue originates from the diet. Dietary TGs are digested by lipases in the intestinal lumen, and are absorbed by intestinal cells as FFAs and 2-monoglycerides. These components are reassembled into TGs within the enterocytes. However, TGs are extremely hydrophobic and would partition into nearby cell membranes if they were secreted into the blood as free TGs. Instead, intestinal cells package TGs into a **lipoprotein particle,** called a **chylomicron,** which enters villar lymphatics (Figure 3-5). The intestinal lymphatics bypass the hepatic portal circulation and the liver and empty into the general circulation. Once in the blood, chylomicrons travel to adipose (and other) tissue.

A chylomicron contains a core of TG and a small amount of cholesterol esters (both hydrophobic), and an outer shell of amphipathic phospholipids and free cholesterol. Chylomicrons are called lipoprotein particles because, in addition to the lipids, they contain surface proteins, called **apoproteins (Apos).** A primary

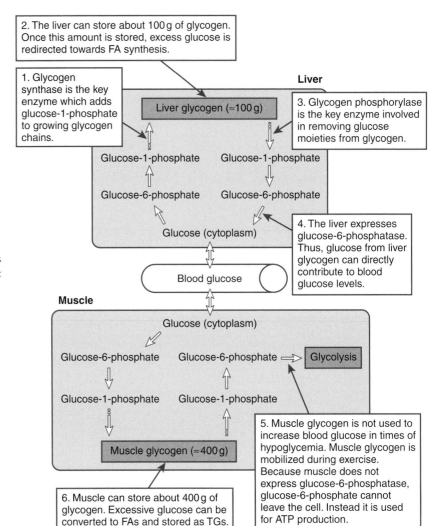

FIGURE 3-4 ■ Glycogen synthesis and breakdown serve different needs in liver and muscle.

apoprotein on chylomicrons is **ApoB48.** Secreted chylomicrons acquire additional apoproteins from **high-density lipoproteins (HDLs).** For example, **ApoCII** is an apoprotein that is exchanged between HDL and chylomicrons. Apo CII acts an activator/cofactor of the enzyme, **lipoprotein lipase (LPL),** which digests circulating chylomicrons. LPL is synthesized by adipose (and other) cells. LPL is secreted and ultimately translocated to the apical surface of the endothelium lining of neighboring capillaries, to which LPL remains noncovalently attached by heparin-sulfate proteoglycans. Dozens of LPL molecules attach to and digest lipoprotein particles, releasing FFAs and glycerol (see Figure 3-5). Several proteins are involved in the transport of FFAs from the apical surface of the endothelia to the cytoplasm of the adipocyte. Once FFAs enter any cell, they are immediately converted to acyl CoAs. The glycerol is recycled to the liver, which can convert glycerol into glycerol-3-phosphate. Note that the adipocyte does not express glycerol kinase; consequently it cannot make glycerol-3-phosphate from glycerol. Instead, adipocytes generate the glycerol-3-phosphate that is required for re-esterification of FFAs and TG synthesis from glycolysis. It should be

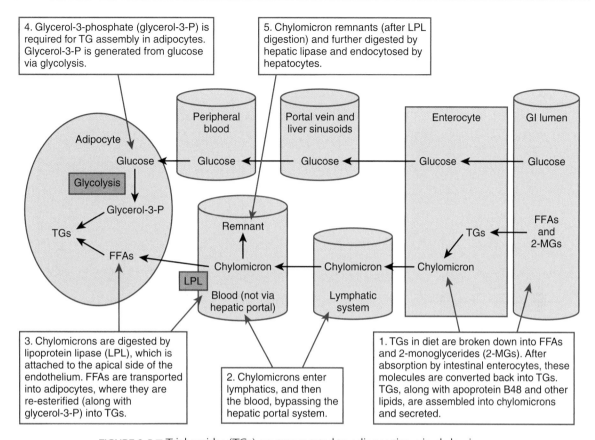

4. Glycerol-3-phosphate (glycerol-3-P) is required for TG assembly in adipocytes. Glycerol-3-P is generated from glucose via glycolysis.

5. Chylomicron remnants (after LPL digestion) and further digested by hepatic lipase and endocytosed by hepatocytes.

3. Chylomicrons are digested by lipoprotein lipase (LPL), which is attached to the apical side of the endothelium. FFAs are transported into adipocytes, where they are re-esterified (along with glycerol-3-P) into TGs.

2. Chylomicrons enter lymphatics, and then the blood, bypassing the hepatic portal system.

1. TGs in diet are broken down into FFAs and 2-monoglycerides (2-MGs). After absorption by intestinal enterocytes, these molecules are converted back into TGs. TGs, along with apoprotein B48 and other lipids, are assembled into chylomicrons and secreted.

FIGURE 3-5 ■ Triglycerides (TGs) are transported to adipose tissue in chylomicrons.

noted that numerous other tissues (e.g., muscle) express LPL, and can take up FFAs from chylomicrons and oxidize them for energy. Partially digested, TG-depleted chylomicrons are called **chylomicron remnants.** These are cleared by the liver through the process of receptor-mediated endocytosis that requires another apoprotein, **apoE.**

Endogenously-Synthesized TG TGs can also be synthesized from glucose and other precursors of acetyl CoA (Figure 3-6). This occurs most during high-caloric intake when liver and muscle glycogen stores are saturated and the supply of glucose exceeds the need for ATP synthesis. The primary site of endogenous fatty acid synthesis in humans is the liver, usually in response to high levels of glucose. Glucose is metabolized to acetyl CoA, and then to citrate in the first reaction of the TCA cycle. However, the presence

of high ATP and NADH levels in the well-fed state inhibit progression of the TCA cycle, causing intramitochondrial levels of citrate to accumulate. Citrate is then translocated to the cytoplasm, where it is converted back to cytosolic acetyl CoA and oxaloacetate. Once in the cytoplasm, acetyl CoA can enter fatty acyl CoA and TG synthesis (see Figure 3-6). Fatty acyl CoAs are esterified to glycerol-3-phosphate to form monoglycerides, diglycerides, and finally TGs. TGs are not normally stored in the liver to a large extent, but in adipose tissue. Thus, TGs must be packaged by the liver into lipoprotein particles called **very-low-density lipoproteins (VLDLs)** before being secreted into the blood. Like chylomicrons, VLDLs contain a core of TG and cholesterol esters (very hydrophobic), and a covering of phospholipids and free cholesterol (amphipathic). The VLDL particle also contains **apoprotein B100.**

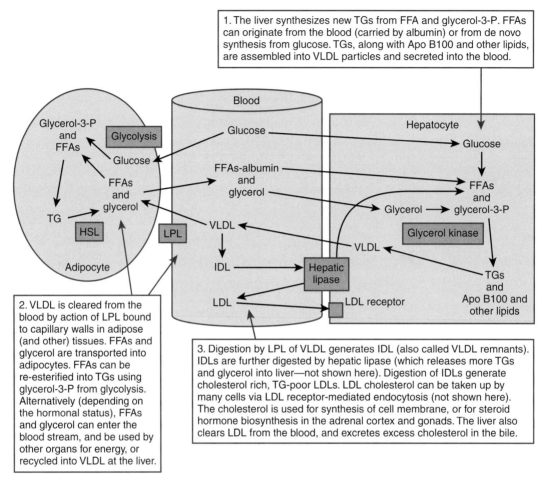

1. The liver synthesizes new TGs from FFA and glycerol-3-P. FFAs can originate from the blood (carried by albumin) or from de novo synthesis from glucose. TGs, along with Apo B100 and other lipids, are assembled into VLDL particles and secreted into the blood.

2. VLDL is cleared from the blood by action of LPL bound to capillary walls in adipose (and other) tissues. FFAs and glycerol are transported into adipocytes. FFAs can be re-esterified into TGs using glycerol-3-P from glycolysis. Alternatively (depending on the hormonal status), FFAs and glycerol can enter the blood stream, and be used by other organs for energy, or recycled into VLDL at the liver.

3. Digestion by LPL of VLDL generates IDL (also called VLDL remnants). IDLs are further digested by hepatic lipase (which releases more TGs and glycerol into liver—not shown here). Digestion of IDLs generate cholesterol rich, TG-poor LDLs. LDL cholesterol can be taken up by many cells via LDL receptor-mediated endocytosis (not shown here). The cholesterol is used for synthesis of cell membrane, or for steroid hormone biosynthesis in the adrenal cortex and gonads. The liver also clears LDL from the blood, and excretes excess cholesterol in the bile.

FIGURE 3-6 ■ Endogenous synthesis of triglycerides (TGs) in the liver is coupled to the synthesis of very low-density lipoprotein (VLDL) particles and transport of TGs to adipose tissue for storage.

After secretion, VLDLs acquire other proteins from circulating high-density lipoprotein (HDL) particles, including apo CII, and are digested by LPL within capillary beds (see Figure 3-6).

Partial Digestion of VLDL Generates Cholesterol-Rich Low-Density Lipoprotein

Partially LPL-digested VLDL particles are called **VLDL remnants,** or **intermediate-density lipoprotein particles (IDLs)** (see Figure 3-6). These particles are further processed by the ectoenzyme, **hepatic lipase,** into **low-density lipoprotein particles (LDLs).** LDLs have lost much of their TG, and are rich in cholesterol

(primarily cholesterol esters). LDL particles can receive cholesterol esters from HDL particles by the action of **cholesterol ester transfer protein (CETP),** which is associated with HDLs. LDLs and HDLs are the primary carriers of cholesterol in the blood. LDLs and HDLs provide cholesterol to cells that are making membrane (i.e., growing and proliferating cells), to cells that are making steroid hormones, and to the liver, where cholesterol is used to make bile acids or is excreted into the intestine. LDL particles are susceptible to oxidation. **Oxidized LDL** particles are endocytosed by **scavenger receptors** on macrophages, a process that contributes to **atherogenic** changes in the wall of blood vessels.

Release of Triglycerides in Adipose Cells

TGs are catabolized back to FFAs and glycerol. This is initiated by the action of a **hormone-sensitive lipase,** followed by additional lipases that remove the second and third fatty acyl groups (see Figure 3-6). The net amount of TG versus FFAs in adipose is thus determined by the balance of TG synthesis and lipolysis, which is extremely sensitive to hormonal signals (see later). Hydrophobic FFAs are carried in the blood noncovalently associated with albumin. FFAs are actively transported into cells, which divert FFAs into β-oxidative pathways for energy, or, in the case of the liver, into ketone bodies (see Figure 3-3). This latter fate of FFAs is important during a prolonged fast, because unlike FFAs, ketone bodies in sufficient levels can cross the blood-brain barrier.

Protein

Unlike TG stored in depot fat, proteins perform many dynamic functions other than storage of energy. Nevertheless, proteins are hydrolyzed when needed to produce amino acids. Amino acids can then be oxidized for energy, or used to make glucose (see Gluconeogenesis later), FFAs, or ketone bodies. This involves **transamination** of an amino acid, whereby its amino group is transferred to α-ketoglutarate to form glutamate. Glutamate can accept an NH_3 group from other amino acids to form glutamine. After transport to the liver, glutamine is converted back to glutamate. Glutamate then undergoes oxidative deamination, yielding ammonia (NH_3). Ammonia is detoxified, primarily in the liver, by conversion to urea by the **urea cycle.** In skeletal muscle, glutamate can donate its amino group to pyruvate, regenerating α-ketoglutarate, and producing alanine. Alanine is a major amino acid transferred to the liver for glucose production (see next section).

Gluconeogenesis—Making Glucose from Glycerol, Lactate, and Amino Acids

The breakdown of glycogen is a transient way by which the liver can contribute directly to blood glucose levels. The liver, and to a lesser extent the kidney, can also produce glucose for a much longer period of time by converting glycerol, lactate, and amino acids into glucose.

Certain amino acids (especially alanine) and lactate can be converted to pyruvate, and the liver and kidney have the ability to convert pyruvate to glucose. This is accomplished by the carboxylation of pyruvate to oxaloacetate by **pyruvate carboxylase** (Figure 3-7). Oxaloacetate escapes the mitochondria as malate, which is then reoxidized to oxaloacetate. Oxaloacetate is then converted to phosphoenolpyruvate (PEP) by the enzyme, **PEP carboxykinase (PEPCK).** PEP is then converted to fructose 1,6-bisphosphate via the reversible reactions of glycolysis. In the presence of a high ATP/AMP ratio, the enzyme **fructose-1,6-bisphosphatase** is active, thereby generating fructose-6-phosphate. Fructose-6-phosphate is reversibly converted to glucose-6-phosphate, which is dephosphorylated by **glucose-6-phosphatase** and released into the blood through the bidirectional GLUT-2 transporter. Glycerol can also be used to make glucose. The liver expresses glycerol kinase, which converts glycerol to glycerol-3-phosphate, which can enter glycolytic and gluconeogenic pathways.

Importantly, acetyl CoA cannot be used to make net glucose. This means that FFAs, ketone bodies, and certain amino acids cannot directly contribute to blood glucose levels. However, the utilization of FFAs by tissues spares blood glucose (i.e., it has a **glucose-sparing** effect) for use by the brain and cells without mitochondria. Additionally, ketone bodies eventually reach levels sufficient to be used by the brain, thereby reducing glucose utilization by the brain.

Summary of Key Metabolic Pathways

ATP is the primary source of energy in all cells. The body can make ATP from carbohydrates (primarily after converting them to glucose), FFAs, amino acids, and ketone bodies. However, the brain is exclusively dependent on glucose, except after days of fasting when it can metabolize ketone bodies. Humans can store excess calories as glycogen, TGs, and protein during a meal, and release stored energy substrates as needed during a fast or for physical activity. Additionally, in times of a fast, the liver can convert energy substrates to ketone bodies for use by other organs (especially the brain). The enzymatic pathways that coordinate the partitioning of energy stores during a meal, and their utilization between meals,

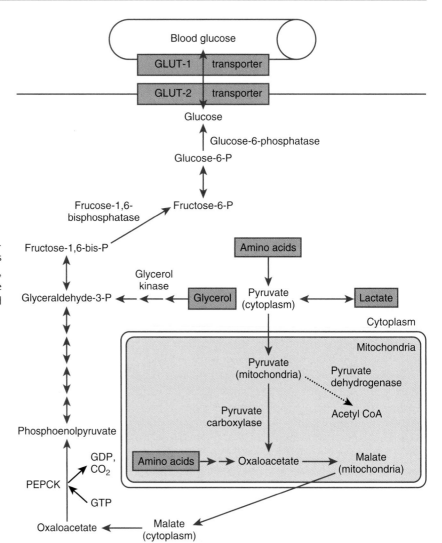

FIGURE 3-7 ■ Gluconeogenesis. The liver expresses key enzymes that can utilize amino acids, glycerol, and lactate to synthesize glucose to maintain blood glucose levels.

are regulated by both nutrient status and by key hormones. Before discussing how hormones regulate these pathways, we first need to learn about the hormones themselves.

KEY HORMONES INVOLVED IN METABOLIC HOMEOSTASIS

The Endocrine Pancreas

The islets of Langerhans constitute the endocrine portion of the pancreas (Figure 3-8). Approximately 1 million islets, making up about 1% to 2% of total

pancreatic mass, are spread throughout the pancreas. The islets are composed of several cell types, each producing a different hormone. In islets situated in the body, tail, and anterior portion of the head of the pancreas (all of which have a common embryologic origin), the most abundant cell type is the β cell (also called B cell). β cells make up about three fourths of these cells of the islets, and produce the hormone, insulin. The α (A) cells make up about 10% of these islets, and secrete glucagon. The third major cell type of the islets within these regions are the δ (D) cells, which make up about 5% of the cells and produce the

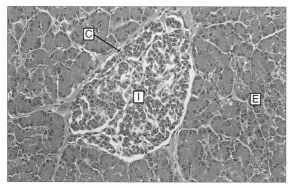

FIGURE 3-8 ■ Islet of Langerhans (I) surrounded by exocrine pancreatic tissue (E), but separated by a connective tissue capsule (C).

peptide, somatostatin. A fourth cell type, the F cell, represents about 80% of the cells in the islets situated within the posterior portion of the head of the pancreas (including the uncinate process) and secretes the peptide, **pancreatic polypeptide.** Because the physiologic function of pancreatic polypeptide in humans remains obscure, it will not be further discussed.

Blood flow through the islets passes from β cells, which predominate in the center of the islet, to α and δ cells, which predominate in the periphery. Consequently, the first cells affected by circulating insulin are the α cells, in which insulin inhibits glucagon secretion.

Insulin

Insulin (Box 3-1) is the primary anabolic hormone that is responsible for maintaining the upper limit of blood glucose and FFA levels. Insulin achieves this by promoting glucose uptake and utilization by muscle and adipose tissue, increasing glycogen storage in liver and muscle, and reducing glucose output by the liver. Insulin promotes protein synthesis from amino acids

---

BOX 3-1
OVERVIEW OF INSULIN'S ACTIONS

Insulin is an anabolic hormone secreted in times of excess nutrient availability. It allows the body to use carbohydrates as energy sources and store nutrients.

---

and inhibits protein degradation in peripheral tissues. Insulin also promotes TG synthesis in the liver and adipose tissue and represses lipolysis of adipose TG stores. Finally, insulin regulates metabolic homeostasis through effects on satiety.

Insulin Structure, Synthesis, and Secretion Insulin is a protein hormone that belongs to a gene family that also includes insulin-like growth factors I and II (IGF-I, IGF-II), relaxin, and several insulin-like peptides. Organized, functional islets appear in the human pancreas at the beginning of the third trimester of gestation. Insulin gene expression and islet cell biogenesis are dependent on several transcription factors that are specific to the pancreas and liver. Heterozygous mutations of one of these factors result in progressively inadequate production of insulin. This leads to a condition called mature onset diabetes of the young (MODY), which typically manifests before age 25.

The insulin gene encodes preproinsulin. Insulin is synthesized on the polyribosome as preproinsulin, and microsomal enzymes cleave the N-signal peptide to produce proinsulin as the peptide enters the endoplasmic reticulum. **Proinsulin** is packaged in the Golgi apparatus into membrane-bound secretory granules. Proinsulin contains the amino acid sequence of insulin plus the 31-amino acid **C** (**connecting**) **peptide** and four linking amino acids. The proteases that cleave proinsulin (proprotein convertases 2 and 3) are packaged with proinsulin within the secretory granule. The mature hormone consists of two chains, an α chain and a β chain, connected by two disulfide bridges (Figure 3-9). A third disulfide bridge is contained within the α chain. Insulin is stored in secretory granules in zinc-bound crystals. On stimulation, the granule's contents are released to the outside of the cell by exocytosis. Release requires a functional microtubular system and is Ca^{2+}-dependent. Because the entire contents of the granule are released, equimolar amounts of insulin and C peptide are secreted, as are small amounts of proinsulin. When insulin secretion is rapid, the percentage of proinsulin secreted tends to rise. C peptide has no known biological activity, and proinsulin has about 7% to 8% of the biological activity of insulin. Measurements of C peptide in the blood are used to quantify endogenous insulin production in

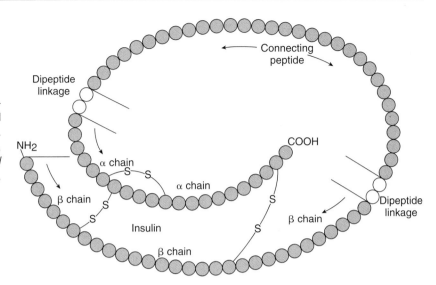

FIGURE 3-9 ■ Structure of proinsulin. Two dipeptides are cleaved to produce C peptide and insulin. *(Modified from Greenspan FS, Strewler GJ, editors: Basic and clinical endocrinology, ed 5, Norwalk, Conn, 1997, Appleton & Lange.)*

patients receiving exogenous insulin, which has been purified from C peptide.

Unlike most protein hormones, insulin shows minimal species variability; consequently, bovine and porcine insulin can be used to treat humans. Insulin has a 5- to 8-minute half-life ($t_{1/2}$) and is cleared rapidly from the circulation. It is degraded by insulinase in the liver, kidney, and other tissues. Because insulin is secreted into the portal vein, it is exposed to liver insulinase before it enters the peripheral circulation. Consequently, almost one half of the insulin is degraded before leaving the liver. Thus, the peripheral tissues are exposed to only one half the serum insulin concentration as the liver. Recombinant human insulin and insulin analogs are now available, with different characteristics of onset and duration of action and peak activity.

Serum insulin levels normally begin to rise within 10 minutes after food ingestion and reach a peak in 30 to 45 minutes. The higher serum insulin level rapidly lowers blood glucose to baseline values. When insulin secretion is stimulated, insulin is released rapidly (within minutes). If the stimulus is maintained, insulin secretion falls within 10 minutes and then slowly rises over a period of about 1 hour (Figure 3-10). The latter phase is referred to as the **late phase of insulin release**. The **early phase of insulin release** probably involves release of preformed insulin, whereas the late phase represents the release of newly formed insulin.

Glucose is the primary stimulus of insulin secretion. Glucose entry into β cells is facilitated by the GLUT-2 transporter. Once glucose enters the β cell, it is phosphorylated to glucose-6-phosphate (glucose-6-P) by the low affinity hexokinase, **glucokinase.** Glucokinase is referred to as the "**glucosesensor**" of the β cell, because the rate of glucose entry is correlated to the rate of glucose phosphorylation which, in turn, is directly related to insulin secretion. Heterozygous mutations in glucokinase are another defect that leads to inadequate insulin release in patients with MODY (see earlier). Glucose-6-P is metabolized by β cells, increasing the intracellular ATP/ADP ratio and closing an **ATP-sensitive K+ channel** (Figure 3-11). This results in depolarization of the β cell membrane, which opens **voltage-gated**

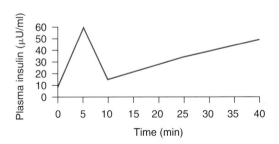

FIGURE 3-10 ■ Insulin release after perfusion of pancreas with 300 mg/dl glucose.

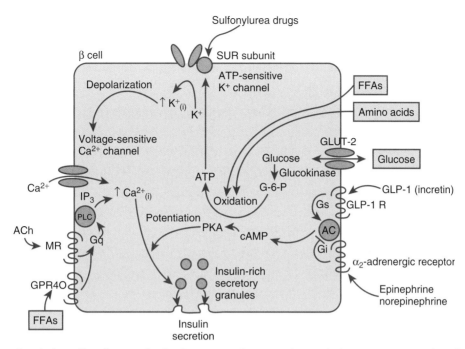

FIGURE 3-11 ■ Regulation of insulin secretion by the energy substrates, glucose (primary secretogogue), amino acids, and free fatty acids (FFAs), and by neurotransmitters and hormones, acetylcholine (ACh), norepinephrine, epinephrine, and glucagon-like peptide-1 (GLP-1).

Ca²⁺ channels. Increased intracellular Ca²⁺ levels activate microtubule-mediated exocytosis of insulin/proinsulin-containing secretory granules. The ATP-sensitive K⁺ channel is a protein complex, which contains an ATP-binding subunit called **SUR**. This subunit is also activated by **sulfonylurea drugs**, which are widely used as oral agents to treat hyperglycemia in patients with partially-impaired β-cell function. It should also be noted that nutrients (glucose, amino acids) can stimulate insulin secretion independent of the SUR protein pathway.

Glucose is a major regulator of insulin secretion (Table 3-2). When serum glucose levels rise, insulin secretion is stimulated; when the levels fall, insulin secretion is inhibited. Certain amino acids and vagal (parasympathetic) cholinergic innervation (i.e., in response to a meal) also stimulate insulin through increasing intracellular Ca²⁺ levels (see Figure 3-11). Long-chain FFAs also increase insulin secretion, although to a lesser extent than glucose and amino acids. FFAs may act through a G-protein–coupled receptor

TABLE 3-2	
Regulators of Insulin Secretion	
STIMULATORS OF INSULIN SECRETION	**INHIBITORS OF INSULIN SECRETION**
↑ Serum glucose	↓ Glucose
↑ Serum amino acids	↓ Amino acids
↑ Serum free fatty acids	↓ Free fatty acids
↑ Serum ketone bodies	
Hormones	Hormones
Gastroinhibitory peptide (GIP)	Somatostatin
Glucagon-like peptide-1 (GLP-1)	Epinephrine (α-receptor)
Gastrin	Leptin
Cholecystokinin (CCK)	
Secretin	
Vasoactive intestinal peptide (VIP)	
Epinephrine (β-receptor)	
Autonomic Nervous System	
Parasympathetic nervous system	Autonomic Nervous System

(GPR40) on the β-cell membrane, or as a nutrient that increases ATP through β-oxidation (see Figure 3-11).

As discussed in Chapter 2, nutrient-dependent stimulation of insulin release is enhanced by the incretin hormones, GLP-1 and GIP, and possibly other GI hormones (CCK, secretin, gastrin). These act primarily by raising intracellular cAMP, which amplifies the intracellular Ca^{2+} effects of glucose (see Figure 3-11). However, these agents do not increase insulin secretion in the absence of glucose. Targeted disruption of the insulin receptor (IR) in β cells caused reduced insulin release and fewer β cells in transgenic mice. Thus, insulin may play an autocrine role in its own production. This may partially explain the finding that impaired insulin signaling in insulin resistance and T2DM is often associated with impaired β-cell function.

Insulin secretion is inhibited by α_2-adrenergic receptors, which are activated by epinephrine (from the adrenal medulla) and norepinephrine (from postganglionic sympathetic fibers). Alpha-2 receptors act by decreasing cAMP, and possibly by closing Ca^{2+} channels

(see Figure 3-11). Adrenergic inhibition of insulin serves to protect against hypoglycemia, especially during exercise. Although somatostatin from D cells inhibits both insulin and glucagon, its physiologic role in pancreatic islet function is unclear.

The Insulin Receptor The **insulin receptor (IR)** is a member of the **receptor tyrosine kinase (RTK)** family, which includes receptors for several other growth factors (e.g., IGFs, platelet-derived growth factor (PDGF), and epidermal growth factor (EGF). The IR is expressed on the cell membrane as a homodimer composed of α/β monomers (Figure 3-12). The α/β monomer is synthesized as one protein, which is then proteolytically cleaved—with the two fragments connected by a disulfide bond. The two α/β monomers are also held together by a disulfide bond between the α subunits. The α subunits are external to the cell membrane and contain the hormone-binding sites. The β subunits span the membrane and contain tyrosine kinase on the cytosolic surface. Insulin binding to the receptor induces the β subunits to cross-phosphorylate each

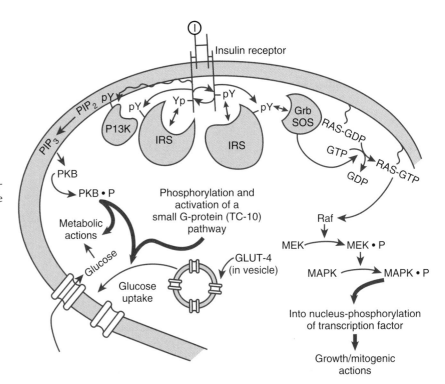

FIGURE 3-12 ■ Intracellular signaling pathways coupled to the insulin receptor.

other on three tyrosine residues. These phosphotyrosine residues recruit three classes of adaptor proteins: the **insulin-receptor substrates (IRSs), SHC protein,** and **APS protein.** The IRS proteins are phosphorylated, which in turn, recruit PI3 kinase to the membrane, where it phosphorylates its substrates and activates a pleiotropic **protein kinase B (PKB)-dependent pathway** that is largely involved in the metabolic effects of insulin. One important effect of insulin is to induce the insertion of GLUT-4 glucose transporters into the cell membranes of muscle and adipose tissue (see later). This action requires both the IRS/PI3K-dependent signaling and an additional APS adaptor protein–dependent pathway that activates a small GTPase pathway. The SHC protein is linked to the mitogen-activated protein kinase (MAPK) pathway, which mediates the growth and mitogenic actions of insulin.

The termination of insulin/IR signaling is a topic of high interest, because these mechanisms potentially play a role in insulin resistance. Insulin induces the down-regulation of its own receptor by receptor-mediated endocytosis and degradative pathways. Additionally, there are several serine/threonine protein kinases that are activated by insulin and that subsequently inactivate IRS proteins. A third mechanism appears to involve the activation of the **"suppressor of cytokine signaling" (SOCS)** family of proteins, which reduces activity and/or levels of the IR and IRS proteins.

Glucagon

Glucagon (Box 3-2) is the primary "counter-regulatory" hormone that increases blood glucose levels through its effects on liver glucose output. Glucagon promotes the production of glucose through elevated glycogenolysis and gluconeogenesis, and through decreased glycolysis and glycogenolysis. Glucagon also inhibits hepatic FFA synthesis from glucose.

Glucagon Structure, Synthesis, and Secretion As discussed in Chapter 2, glucagon is a member of the secretin gene family. Preproglucagon is proteolytically cleaved in the α cell in a cell-specific manner to produce the 29 amino acid glucagon (refer to Figure 2-11). Glucagon is highly conserved among mammals.

Like insulin, glucagon circulates in an unbound form, and has a short $t_{1/2}$ (about 6 minutes). The predominant site of glucagon degradation is the liver, which degrades as much as 80% of the circulating glucagon in one pass. Because glucagon (either from the pancreas or the gut) enters the hepatic portal vein and is carried to the liver before reaching the systemic circulation, a large portion of the hormone never reaches the systemic circulation. The liver is the primary target organ of glucagon, with only small effects on peripheral tissues.

As discussed later, glucagon opposes the actions of insulin. Thus, several factors that stimulate insulin inhibit glucagon (Table 3-3). Indeed, it is the insulin/glucagon ratio that determines the net flow of hepatic metabolic pathways. A major stimulus for glucagon secretion is a drop in blood glucose, which is primarily an indirect effect of the removal of inhibition by insulin. Circulating catecholamines, which inhibit insulin secretion via α2-adrenergic receptors, stimulate glucagon secretion via β2-adrenergic receptors. Serum amino acids also stimulate glucagon secretion. This means that a protein meal will increase postprandial levels of both insulin and glucagon,

---

BOX 3-2
OVERVIEW OF GLUCAGON'S ACTIONS

Glucagon is a catabolic hormone. Levels rise during periods of food deprivation, and stored nutrient reserves are mobilized. It mobilizes glycogen, fat, and even protein to serve as energy sources.

TABLE 3-3	
Effects on Glucagon Secretion	
STIMULI FOR GLUCAGON SECRETION	**INHIBITORS OF GLUCAGON SECRETION**
↓ Blood glucose	Somatostatin
↑ Serum amino acids (arginine, alanine)	Insulin
Sympathetic nervous system stimulation	↑ Blood glucose
Stress	
Exercise	

which protects against hypoglycemia, whereas a carbohydrate meal only stimulates insulin.

The Glucagon Receptor The glucagon receptor is a 7-transmembrane receptor primarily linked to Gs. Consequently, glucagon increases intracellular cAMP levels in the liver. The increase in cAMP initiates the cascade of metabolic changes associated with enzyme phosphorylation. Note that several of insulin's effects in the liver involve the activation of an opposing phosphatase.

Epinephrine and Norepinephrine

The other major counter-regulatory factors are the catecholamines, **epinephrine,** and **norepinephrine.** Epinephrine and norepinephrine are secreted by the adrenal medulla (see Chapter 7), whereas only norepinephrine is released from postganglionic sympathetic nerve endings. The direct metabolic actions of catecholamines are mediated primarily by β-adrenergic receptors located on muscle, adipose, and liver. Like the glucagon receptor, β-adrenergic receptors (β2 and β3) are linked to a Gs signaling pathway that increases intracellular cAMP. Catecholamines are released from sympathetic nerve endings and the adrenal medulla in response to decreased glucose concentrations, stress, and exercise. Decreased glucose levels (i.e., hypoglycemia) are primarily sensed by hypothalamic neurons, which initiate a sympathetic response to release catecholamines.

METABOLIC HOMEOSTASIS—THE INTEGRATED OUTCOME OF HORMONAL AND SUBSTRATE/PRODUCT REGULATION OF METABOLIC PATHWAYS

The levels of blood glucose, which must be maintained within a specific range, are determined by the absorption of food and the flow of recently absorbed or stored energy substrates through different metabolic pathways, which must also meet the energy demands of all cells. The relative flow of carbon through different pathways is determined at key enzymatic reactions. The enzymes involved are regulated by substrate and product concentrations, and by endocrine and

autonomic regulation of enzyme gene expression and/or activity. The hormonal regulation of these key enzymatic steps will by emphasized in this section.

The Fasting-to-Fed State Transition Involves Anabolic Pathways that Store Energy

Insulin Promotes the Storage of Glucose as Glycogen and TGs in the Liver Ingestion of a mixed meal stimulates β cells to release insulin (see earlier) and insulin rapidly inhibits glucagon release from the adjacent α-cells. This results in an increased insulin/glucagon ratio in the hepatic portal vein as it enters the liver. The liver responds to this signal by increasing hepatic glucose utilization (Box 3-3)—first through enhanced glycogen synthesis. Once hepatic glycogen stores (80 to 100 g) are replenished, excess glucose is used for TG synthesis (the liver meets its own energy needs primarily from oxidation of unbranched amino acids in the fed state). Glucose is directed into glycolysis, which in the liver can be thought of as an accessory pathway to TG synthesis. Glycolysis promotes accumulation of citrate, which transports the acetyl group of acetyl CoA into the cytoplasm, where fatty acyl CoA synthesis originates. Glucose is also directed into the nonoxidative pathway, the hexose monophosphate shunt, which is a major supplier of the NADPH required for fatty acyl CoA synthesis. In addition to these glucose-utilizing anabolic pathways of glycogenesis and lipogenesis, the high insulin/glucagon ratio inhibits the hepatic glucose-producing pathways of glycogenolysis and gluconeogenesis and inhibits hepatic fatty acyl CoA oxidation. This is achieved by the stimulation of key enzymes and the concomitant inhibition of

---

BOX 3-3
ACTIONS OF INSULIN ON LIVER

↑ Glucose uptake (if blood glucose level is high)
↑ Glucose use
↑ Glycogenesis, ↓ glycogenolysis
↑ Glycolysis, ↓ gluconeogenesis
↑ Fatty acid synthesis and very-low-density lipoprotein formation, ↓ ketogenesis
↓ Urea cycle activity

opposing enzymes. This coordinated activation and repression minimizes the generation of futile cycles.

Some of the key metabolic steps that are regulated by insulin in the liver are as follows:

1. *Trapping intracellular glucose* (Step 1) (Figure 3-13). Although glucose enters the hepatocytes through the insulin-independent GLUT-2 transporter, insulin increases hepatic retention and utilization of glucose by increasing the expression of **glucokinase.** Insulin increases glucokinase expression through increased expression and activation of the transcription factor, **sterol-responsive element binding protein-1C (SREBP-1C),** which acts as a "master

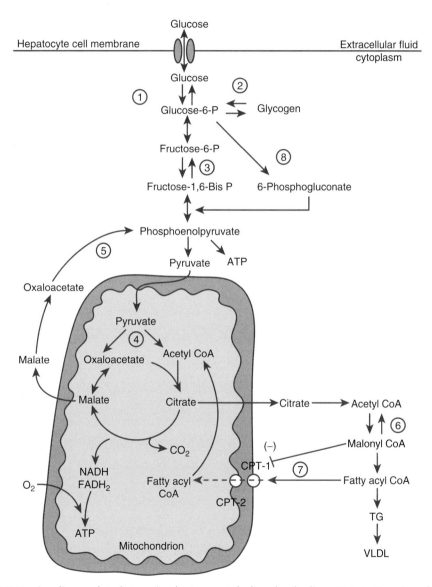

FIGURE 3-13 ■ Key insulin-regulated steps in glucose metabolism by the liver. *Step 1*: Trapping glucose as glucose-6-phosphate (glucose-6-P). Forward reaction: Catalyzed by glucokinase (GK). Insulin increases the transcription of the GK gene through the transcription factor, SREBP-1C. Note that GK is allosterically activated by glucose.

Continued

FIGURE 3-13—*Continued*

Reverse reaction: Catalyzed by glucose-6-phosphatase. Insulin represses expression of the glucose-6-phosphatase gene. *Step 2*: Converting glucose-6-P into glycogen. Forward reaction: Catalyzed by glycogen synthase. Insulin activates glycogen synthase by promoting its dephosphorylation, primarily through activation of protein phosphatase 1. Reverse Reaction: Catalyzed by glycogen phosphorylase. Insulin inhibits glycogen phosphorylase by promoting its dephosphorylation. *Step 3*: Commitment to glycolysis. Forward reaction: Catalyzed by phosphofructokinase-1 (PFK-1). Insulin increases PFK-1 gene expression through the transcription factor, SREBP-1C. Insulin also promotes the dephosphorylation by protein phosphatase-1 of the bifunctional enzyme, phosphofructokinase-2/fructose-2,6-bisphosphatase. This increases the kinase activity of this enzyme, which generates fructose-2,6-bisphosphate (fructose-2,6-bisP). Fructose-2,6-bisP is a strong allosteric activator of PFK-1. Reverse reaction: Catalyzed by fructose-1,6-bisphosphatase. Insulin represses fructose-1,6-bisphosphatase gene expression. Also, fructose-2,6-bisP (which is increased by insulin) is an allosteric inhibitor of fructose-1,6-bisphosphatase. *Step 4:* Partitioning of carbons (as pyruvate) into lipogenic versus gluconeogenic pathways. Lipogenic reaction: Pyruvate is converted to acetyl CoA by the enzyme, pyruvate dehydrogenase (PDH). Insulin activates PDH by promoting its dephosphorylation. Acetyl CoA negatively feeds back as an allosteric inhibitor of PDH. However, lipogenic pathways (see Step 7) inhibit oxidation of FFAs, thereby keeping acetyl CoA levels relatively low. The further metabolism of citrate during the digestive period is inhibited by relatively high ATP and NADH levels, so that citrate accumulates, and ultimately leaves the mitochondria. The insulin-inducible enzyme ATP-citrate lyase converts cytoplasmic citrate into cytoplasmic acetyl CoA—a key substrate for lipogenesis. Gluconeogenic reaction: Pyruvate is converted to oxaloacetate by pyruvate carboxylase. Oxaloacetate can be reversibly converted to malate, which can leave the mitochondria and be converted back to cytoplasmic oxaloacetate—a key substrate for gluconeogenesis. *Step 5:* Flow of carbons into pyruvate versus phosphoenolpyruvate (PEP). Forward reaction: Catalyzed by pyruvate kinase (PK). Insulin stimulates PK activity by promoting its dephosphorylation (by protein phosphatase-1). Reverse reaction: As shown *above*, the reverse reaction is not simply converting pyruvate to PEP. Instead, carbons that ultimately flow into cytoplasmic oxaloacetate are converted to PEP by the gluconeogenic enzyme, PEP carboxykinase (PEPCK). PEPCK gene expression is repressed by insulin. *Step 6*: Commitment to fatty acyl-CoA synthesis: generation of malonyl CoA. Forward reaction: Catalyzed by acetyl CoA carboxylase (ACC). Insulin increases ACC gene expression through the SREBP-1C transcription factor, and increases ACC activity by promoting its dephosphorylation (by protein phosphatase-1). Reverse reaction: Catalyzed by malonyl CoA decarboxylase (MCD). MCD expression is repressed by insulin. *Step 7:* Commitment to fatty acyl-CoA synthesis. Forward reaction: Catalyzed by fatty acid synthase (FAS). Insulin increases FAS gene expression through SREBP-1C. Catabolism (oxidation) of newly synthesized long chain fatty acyl CoAs. Rate-limiting transport of long chain fatty acyl-CoAs into mitochondria (where oxidation occurs) requires carnitine: palmitoyl transferase I (CPT I). Insulin inhibits oxidation of fatty acyl CoAs indirectly by promoting the generation of malonyl CoA. Malonyl CoA is a strong allosteric inhibitor of CPT I. *Step 8:* Commitment to the hexose monophosphate shunt: generation of NADPH for lipogenesis. Forward (irreversible) reaction: Catalyzed by glucose-6-phosphate dehydrogenase. Insulin increases glucose 6-phosphate dehydrogenase gene expression through SREBP-1C.

switch" in the fed state to coordinately increase the levels of several enzymes involved in glucose utilization and TG synthesis. Insulin prevents the futile cycle of glucose phosphorylation ⇔ dephosphorylation by repressing gene expression of enzyme, **glucose-6-phosphatase.**

2. *Increasing glycogen synthesis* (Step 2)(see Figure 3-13). Insulin increases the activity of glycogen synthase in several ways. Insulin indirectly increases

glycogen synthase through increased expression of glucokinase because high levels of G-6-P allosterically increase glycogen synthase activity. Insulin also increases the activity of **protein phosphatase-1,** which dephosphorylates and thereby activates **glycogen synthase.** Insulin also inactivates **glycogen synthase kinase-3,** which promotes the accumulation of dephosphorylated (active) glycogen synthase. Insulin also prevents the futile cycle of glycogen synthesis ⇔ glycogenolysis through inhibition of **glycogen phosphorylase.** Protein phosphatase-1 also dephosphorylates **phosphorylase kinase** and **glycogen phosphorylase.** In contrast to glycogen synthase, dephosphorylation reduces the enzymatic activity of these two catabolic enzymes.

3. Increasing glycolysis.
   - *Increasing phosphofructokinase-1* (Step 3) (see Figure 3-13). Insulin increases the activity of the rate-limiting and irreversible reaction of phosphorylating fructose-6-phosphate to fructose-1,6-bisphosphate that is catalyzed by the enzyme, **phosphofructokinase-1** (**PFK-1**). Insulin promotes the dephosphorylation of the bifunctional enzyme **phosphofructokinase-2/fructose bisphosphatase-2,** thereby activating the kinase function and lessening the phosphatase function. This results in increased levels of **fructose-2, 6-bisphosphat**e, which is an allosteric activator of phosphofructokinase-1. Fructose-2,6-bisphosphatase also competitively inhibits the gluconeogenic enzyme, **fructose-1,6-bisphosphatase,** thereby blocking the futile cycle of fructose-6-phosphate fructose-1,6-bisphosphate.
   - *Increasing pyruvate kinase and pyruvate dehydrogenase* (Steps 4 and 5) (see Figure 3-13). Fructose-1,6-bisphosphate activates the downstream irreversible reaction of converting phosphoenolpyruvate to pyruvate that is catalyzed by **pyruvate kinase.** Thus, insulin activates pyruvate kinase indirectly through a feed-forward mechanism that is initiated by dephosphorylation of phosphofructokinase-2/fructose bisphosphatase. Insulin also promotes the dephosphorylation of pyruvate kinase, which increases activity of the enzyme. Insulin increases pyruvate dehydrogenase activity, which converts pyruvate into acetyl CoA, an important building block for fatty acid synthesis. Insulin represses gene expression of the gluconeogenic enzyme, **phosphoenolpyruvate carboxykinase (PEPCK),** which converts pyruvate, by way of the oxaloacetate-malate-oxaloacetate transfer out of the mitochondria, to phosphoenolpyruvate. By repressing PEPCK, insulin blocks the futile cycle of pyruvate ⇔ phosphoenolpyruvate.

- *Increasing triglyceride synthesis* (Steps 6 through 9) (see Figure 3-13). In the presence of excess amounts of glucose and amino acids, excess acetyl CoA is not used for ATP synthesis by the liver. Instead, acetyl CoA is transferred from the mitochondria to the cytosol in the form of citrate, which is then converted back to acetyl CoA and oxaloacetate by the cytosolic enzyme, **ATP-citrate lyase.** Insulin increases ATP-citrate lyase gene expression through the transcription factor, SREBP-1C.

Once in the cytoplasm, acetyl CoA can enter fatty acid synthesis. The first step involves the conversion of acetyl CoA to malonyl CoA by the enzyme, **acetyl CoA carboxylase.** Insulin stimulates acetyl CoA carboxylase gene expression through the transcription factor, SREBP-1C. Insulin also promotes the dephosphorylation of acetyl CoA carboxylase, which activates the enzyme. Finally, by promoting pathways (especially glycolysis) that generate high levels of citrate, insulin increases acetyl CoA carboxylase activity indirectly through allosteric activation by citrate.

Malonyl CoA is converted to the 16-carbon fatty acid, palmitate, by repetitive additions of acetyl groups (contributed by malonyl CoAs) by the **fatty acid synthase complex (FAS).** Fatty acid synthase gene expression is enhanced by insulin through the transcription factor, SREBP-1C. Palmitate synthesis also requires NADPH. A major source of NADPH is the **pentose phosphate shunt.** The first reaction of this pathway converts glucose-6-phosphate to 6-phosphogluconolactone by the enzyme **glucose-6-phosphate dehydrogenase,** and generates NADPH. Insulin increases glucose-6-phosphate dehydrogenase gene expression through the transcription factor, SREBP-1C. Insulin also stimulates **palmitoyl CoA desaturase,** which produces unsaturated fatty acids.

By activating steps that lead to the generation of malonyl CoA, insulin indirectly inhibits oxidation of FFAs. Malonyl CoA inhibits carnitine palmitoyltransferase I activity. Thus, FFAs that are synthesized cannot be transported into the mitochondria, where they undergo β-oxidation. Increased malonyl CoA prevents the futile cycle of FFA synthesis more than FFA oxidation.

FFA are converted to TGs by the liver, and are either stored in the liver or transported to adipose and muscle in the form of VLDL. TG synthesis requires the presence of glycerol-3-phosphate. In the liver, glycerol-3-phosphate is derived from insulin-enhanced glycolysis, or from the phosphorylation of glycerol by the enzyme, **glycerol kinase.** Insulin acutely promotes the degradation of the VLDL apoprotein, apoB100. This keeps the liver from secreting VLDL during a meal, when the blood is rich with chylomicrons. Thus, the lipid made in response to insulin during a meal is released as VLDL during the interdigestive period, and provides an important source of energy to skeletal and cardiac muscle.

Insulin Promotes Utilization of Glucose by Skeletal Muscle and Adipose (Boxes 3-4 and 3-5) The glucose that is not captured by the liver contributes to the postprandial rise in glucose levels in the peripheral circulation. **Glucose tolerance** refers to the ability of an individual to minimize the excursions of blood glucose concentrations. A primary way in which insulin promotes glucose tolerance is the activation of glucose transporters in skeletal muscle (Figure 3-14). Insulin stimulates the translocation of preexisting GLUT-4 transporters to the cell membrane. Insulin also promotes the storage of intramyocellular glucose by stimulating glycogen synthesis in muscle. However, the relative amount of glucose used for replenishing glycogen stores versus the amount used for energy is dependent on the amount of the physical activity that an individual is engaged in during or soon after a meal. In the presence of excessive carbohydrate intake, insulin increases TG synthesis from glucose in skeletal

---

BOX 3-4
ACTION OF INSULIN ON MUSCLE

↑ Glucose uptake by increasing GLUT-4 availability
↑ Glucose use
↑ Glycogenesis, ↓ glycogenolysis
↑ Glycolysis
↑ Amino acid uptake (particularly branched-chain amino acids)
↑ Protein synthesis, ↓ proteolysis

BOX 3-5
ACTION OF INSULIN ON ADIPOSE TISSUE

↑ Glucose uptake by increasing GLUT-4 availability
↑ Glucose use
↑ Glycolysis
↑ Production of α-glycerol phosphate
↑ Esterification of fats
↓ Lipolysis

---

muscle, which may lead to lipotoxicity and insulin resistance (see later).

Insulin also stimulates GLUT-4–dependent uptake of glucose and subsequent glycolysis in adipose tissue (see Figure 3-14). Adipose tissue utilizes glycolysis for energy needs, but also for the generation of glycerol-3-phosphate, which is required for the re-esterification of FFAs into TGs. As in the liver and skeletal muscle, excessive carbohydrate intake can also lead to insulin-stimulated lipogenesis in adipose tissue.

Insulin Promotes Storage of Ingested Lipids in Adipose Tissue Insulin stimulates the expression of lipoprotein lipase within adipose parenchyma and its migration to the apical side of endothelia of adipose capillary beds (see Figure 3-14). This action of insulin thereby promotes the release of FFAs from chylomicrons within adipose tissue. Insulin also stimulates translocation of fatty acid transport proteins into the cell membrane. Fatty acid transport proteins facilitate the movement of FFAs into the adipocyte and the activation of FFAs by their conversion to fatty acyl CoAs. Insulin stimulates glycolysis in adipocytes, which generates the glycerol-3-phosphate required for re-esterification of FFAs into TGs. Insulin also inhibits hormone-sensitive lipase through stimulating protein phosphatases, which, in turn, dephosphorylate hormone-sensitive lipase and perilipins.

Insulin Promotes Protein Synthesis in Many Tissues Insulin promotes protein synthesis at several levels in muscle and adipose tissue. Insulin stimulates amino acid uptake and mRNA translation in muscle and adipose tissue. Insulin blocks a futile cycle by also inhibiting proteolysis. Although the liver utilizes amino acids for

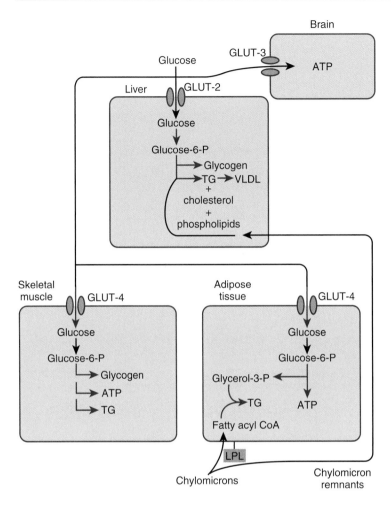

FIGURE 3-14 ■ Partitioning of glucose and triglyceride (TG) during the digestive period (high insulin/glucagon ratio). Highlighted pathways are stimulated by insulin.

ATP synthesis, insulin also promotes the synthesis of hepatic proteins during the digestive period. Consistent with its effects on protein synthesis and proteolysis, insulin attenuates the activity of urea cycle enzymes in the liver.

Release of Energy During the Interdigestive Period or an Extended Fast

Insulin Levels Fall as Circulating Nutrient Levels Decline, Whereas Those of Glucagon and Epinephrine Rise Several hours after a meal, nutrient levels fall, leading to lower levels of insulin secretion. Consequently, the stimulatory and inhibitory effects of insulin on hepatic, muscle, and adipose tissue are attenuated. The decrease in insulin also relieves inhibition

of glucagon secretion. Thus, the liver is exposed to an increasingly larger glucagon/insulin ratio during the interdigestive period and fasting, which has the following effects on hepatic metabolism:

1. Glycogen phosphorylase is activated through a cAMP-dependent kinase cascade, involving protein kinase A (PKA) and phosphorylase kinase (Step 2) (see Figure 3-13). Conversely, glycogen synthase is inhibited through phosphorylation. Thus, glycogenolysis exceeds glycogen synthesis and supports hepatic glucose output for about 12 hours at the beginning of a fast.

2. Gluconeogenic enzymes are increased over glycolytic enzymes (Steps 1, 3, 4 and 5) (see Figure 3-13). Glucagon increases PEPCK at a transcriptional level,

while inhibiting pyruvate kinase by phosphorylation. The increased glucagon/insulin ratio also increases fructose-1,6-bisphosphatase and glucose-6-phosphatase, while inhibiting the opposing enzymes, phosphofructokinase-1, and glucokinase, respectively. Gluconeogenesis takes over after glycogenolysis as the primary pathway of hepatic glucose production and continues to support blood glucose levels for days during an extended fast.

3. Lipogenesis is inhibited, in part by the phosphorylation-dependent inhibition of acetyl CoA carboxylase and the activation of the opposing enzyme, malonyl CoA decarboxylase (Step 6, see Figure 3-13). The reduction of malonyl CoA also relieves inhibition on the carnitine palmitoyltransferase I (CPT I)

transporter (Step 7) (see Figure 3-13). This allows for more efficient transport of fatty acyl CoAs into the mitochondria. The liver can then use circulating FFAs for energy and also synthesize ketone bodies (Figure 3-15). Ketogenesis supplements blood glucose in that the brain can utilize ketone bodies after several days of a fast.

Hepatic Metabolism is Supported by and Integrated with Changes in Skeletal Muscle and Adipose During a Fast As liver glycogen is depleted, the liver shifts to gluconeogenesis to maintain blood glucose levels. However, the ability of the liver to generate glucose is dependent on the ability of the liver to obtain sufficient levels of substrates (lactate, amino acids, and glycerol)

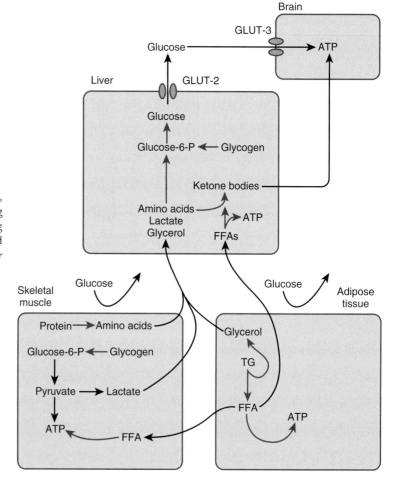

FIGURE 3-15 ■ Utilization of glucose, triglyceride (TG) and protein during the interdigestive period or fasting (low insulin/glucagon ratio). Highlighted steps are promoted by glucagon and or epinephrine/norepinephrine.

for gluconeogenesis. These substrates originate primarily from skeletal muscle and adipose tissue (see Figure 3-15). Most of the glucagon is inactivated by the liver, and has only minor effects on extrahepatic tissues. Thus, the release of gluconeogenic substrates is promoted by the lack of insulin combined with elevated levels of the catecholamines, epinephrine, and norepinephrine. Epinephrine and norepinephrine are released in response to vigorous exercise and in response to relatively severe hypoglycemia through an autonomic mechanism that originates in the hypothalamus. Catecholamines amplify the effects of glucagon at the liver and act as the primary counter-regulatory hormones (or neurotransmitter in the case of norepinephrine) at skeletal muscle and adipose tissue.

In the skeletal muscle, a high catecholamine/insulin ratio promotes increased proteolysis and decreased protein synthesis (see Figure 3-15). This results in the release of gluconeogenic and ketogenic amino acids. Because skeletal muscle shifts to the use of FFAs for energy during a fast, pyruvate dehydrogenase is inhibited by the relatively abundant acetyl CoA generated by β-oxidation. Thus, more pyruvate is converted to lactate, which is released to be used by the liver for gluconeogenesis.

In adipose tissue, a high catecholamine/insulin ratio stimulates phosphorylation of **hormone-sensitive lipase (HSL)** and **perilipin proteins** that surround fat droplets (see Figure 3-15). Phosphorylated perilipins dissociate from the triglyceride-cytoplasm interface and allow access to hormone-sensitive lipase, which is activated by phosphorylation. Complete de-esterification of TGs results in FFAs and glycerol. FFAs circulate in the blood as FFA-albumin complexes, and are used by several tissues (including skeletal muscle, liver, and adipose) for energy. This use of FFAs, especially by skeletal muscle, plays an essential "**glucose-sparing**" role. This means that FFAs compete for the enzymes involved in oxidation of glucose, so that less glucose is consumed by muscle and other tissues. The high catecholamine/insulin ratio also minimizes the ability of skeletal muscle to take up glucose through GLUT-4 transporters. Consequently, the glucose-sparing action of FFAs indirectly increases blood glucose availability to cell types that are obligate glucose users.

As stated, the liver does not use all of the FFAs it internalizes for its own energy. Rather, the liver generates ketone bodies from FFAs (and from some amino acids). After several days of fasting, circulating ketone bodies can be utilized by the brain. This places less demand on the liver to maintain normal levels of glucose.

In summary, both skeletal muscle and adipose tissue contribute to circulating blood glucose through the release of gluconeogenic substrates (lactate, amino acids, glycerol), and indirectly through the release of FFAs, which allow skeletal muscle and other tissues to consume less glucose. Finally, release of FFAs and ketogenic amino acids supports ketogenesis by the liver.

DIABETES MELLITUS

Diabetes mellitus (DM) is a disease in which insulin levels and/or responsiveness of tissues to insulin is insufficient to maintain normal levels of plasma glucose. Although the diagnosis of DM is based primarily on plasma glucose, DM also causes **dyslipidemia.** Normal fasting (i.e., no caloric intake for at least 8 hours) plasma glucose levels should be below 110 mg/dl A patient is considered to have impaired glucose control if the fasting plasma glucose is between 110-126 mg/dl, and the diagnosis of diabetes mellitus is made if the fasting plasma glucose exceeds 126 mg/dl on 2 successive days. Another approach to the diagnosis of diabetes is the oral glucose tolerance test. After overnight fasting, the patient is given a bolus amount of glucose (usually 75 g) orally, and blood glucose levels are measured at 2 hours. The glucose is administered orally rather than intravenously (IV) because the insulin response to an oral glucose load is faster and greater than the response to an IV load (i.e., the incretin effect, Chapter 2). A 2-hour plasma glucose greater than 200 mg/dl on 2 consecutive days is sufficient to make the diagnosis of diabetes. The diagnosis of diabetes is also indicated if the patient presents with symptoms associated with diabetes (see later) and has a nonfasting plasma glucose of greater than 200 mg/dl.

Diabetes mellitus is currently classified as **type 1 (T1DM)** or **type 2 diabetes mellitus (T2DM).** T2DM is by far the more common form, accounting for 90% of diagnosed cases. However, T2DM is usually a progressive disease that remains undiagnosed in a significant percentage of patients for several years. T2DM is often associated with visceral obesity and lack of exercise—indeed, obesity-related T2DM is reaching epidemic proportions worldwide. Usually, there are multiple causes for the development of T2DM in a given individual that are associated with defects in the ability of target organs to respond to insulin (i.e., **insulin resistance**), along with some degree of β cell deficiency. Insulin sensitivity can be compromised at the level of the insulin receptor (IR), or more commonly, at the level of postreceptor signaling. T2DM appears to be the consequence of insulin resistance, followed by reactive hyperinsulinemia, but ultimately by **relative hypoinsulinemia** (i.e., inadequate release of insulin to compensate for the end-organ resistance). Although "insulin resistance" specifically refers to an inability of insulin to maintain blood glucose levels below normal upper limits, the underlying causes of insulin resistance may differ among patients. Three major underlying causes of obesity-induced insulin resistance are due to the following:

1. A decreased ability of insulin to increase GLUT-4-mediated uptake of glucose, especially by

skeletal muscle. This function, which is specifically a part of the **glucometabolic** regulation by insulin, may be due to the excessive accumulation of TG in the muscle in obese individuals. Excessive caloric intake induces hyperinsulinemia. Initially, this leads to excessive glucose uptake into skeletal muscle. Just as in the liver (see Figure 3-13), excessive calories in the form of glucose promote lipogenesis and, through the generation of malonyl CoA, repression of fatty acyl CoA oxidation. Byproducts of fatty acid and TG synthesis, such as diacylglycerol and ceramide, may accumulate and stimulate signaling pathways (e.g., protein kinase C–dependent pathways) that antagonize signaling from the insulin receptor and/or IRS proteins (Figure 3-16). Thus, insulin resistance in the skeletal muscle of obese individuals may be due to **lipotoxicity.**

2. A decreased ability of insulin to repress hepatic glucose production. The liver makes glucose by glycogenolysis in the short term, and by gluconeogenesis in the long term. The ability of insulin to repress key hepatic enzymes in both of these pathways (see Figure 3-13) is attenuated in insulin-resistant individuals. Insulin resistance in the liver

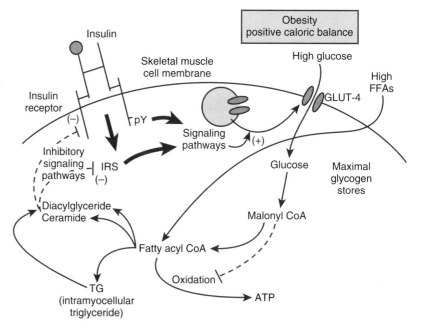

FIGURE 3-16 ■ Role of lipotoxicity in the development and progression of insulin resistance. In states of caloric excess, fatty acids accumulate in muscle from the uptake of FFAs and from de novo lipogenesis from excessive glucose. An intermediate of lipogenesis, malonyl CoA, inhibits the transport of fatty acyl CoA into the mitochondria, thereby inhibiting fatty acyl CoA oxidation. Excessive accumulation of cytoplasmic fatty acyl CoA and TG gives rise to byproducts (diacylglycerol, ceramide), which stimulate signaling pathways that inhibit the insulin receptor and downstream components of the insulin signaling pathway.

may also be due to lipotoxicity in obese individuals (e.g., **fatty liver** or **hepatic steatosis**). The degree of insulin-resistance is correlated to degree of visceral (e.g., abdominal) obesity (as opposed to subcutaneous or peripheral obesity—see p 73). Note that secreted products of visceral adipose tissue enter the hepatic portal system, conveying these products directly to hepatocytes. Visceral adipose tissue is likely to affect insulin signaling at the liver in several ways, in addition to the effects of lipotoxicity. For example, visceral adipose tissue releases the cytokine, **tumor necrosis factor-α** (**TNF-α;** see p 75), which has been shown to antagonize insulin signaling pathways. Also, TG in visceral adipose tissue has a high rate of turnover (possibly owing to a rich sympathetic innervation), so that the liver is exposed to high levels of FFAs, which further exacerbates hepatic lipotoxicity.

3. An inability of insulin to repress hormone-sensitive lipase and/or increase LPL in adipose tissue. High HSL and low LPL are major factors in the dyslipidemia associated with insulin-resistance and diabetes. The dyslipidemia is characterized as hypertriglyceridemia and large TG-rich VLDL particles produced by the liver. Because of their high TG content, large VLDLs give rise to small dense LDL particles, which are very atherogenic, and low levels of HDL particles, which normally play a protective role against vascular disease. Insulin resistance in adipose tissue is likely due to the production of anti-insulin local factors, such as TNF-α.

There are numerous other factors that promote insulin resistance and may act at skeletal muscle, liver, and adipose tissue. Hyperinsulinemia per se causes down-regulation of the IR and components of the IR signaling pathway, and activates intracellular negative feedback pathways such as the "suppressor of cytokine signaling" (SOCS) pathway. Glucocorticoids, which are released in response to stress and acute hypoglycemia, are diabetogenic. Sex steroids also antagonize insulin signaling. Growth hormone, prolactin, and its homolog, human placental lactogen (which is also high during pregnancy) also induce insulin resistance.

Exercise and weight loss are effective treatments for obesity-related insulin-resistance and T2DM. The beneficial effects from exercise are due, in part, to the activation of **AMP kinase.** which acts as an intracellular energy sensor. In the presence of elevated AMP levels, AMP kinase activates oxidative pathways while inhibiting lipogenic and gluconeogenic (i.e., ATP-consuming) pathways. The oral hypoglycemic agent, **metformin,** appears to act, in part, through activation of AMP kinase. Although T2DM is also referred to as **non–insulin-dependent diabetes mellitus,** it should be stressed that T2DM is usually associated with some degree of compromised β-cell function; patients with T2DM may require insulin therapy at some point in their life. Patients with T2DM can also benefit from agents that optimize β-cell function, such as sulfonylurea drugs or GLP-1 (see Figure 3-11).

Type 1 diabetes mellitus (T1DM) is characterized by the destruction, almost always by an autoimmune mechanism, of the β cells. T1DM is also termed "insulin-dependent diabetes mellitus." The characteristics of this disorder are as follows:

1. People with T1DM need exogenous insulin to maintain life and prevent ketosis; there is virtually no pancreatic insulin production.
2. There is histologic damage to the pancreatic beta cells; insulinitis with pancreatic mononuclear cell infiltration is a characteristic feature at the onset of the disorder. Cytokines may be involved in the early destruction of the pancreas.
3. People with T1DM are prone to ketosis.
4. Ninety percent of the cases begin in childhood, mostly between 10 and 14 years of age. This common observation led to application of the term *juvenile diabetes* to the disorder. This term is no longer used because T1DM can present at any time of life, although juvenile onset is the typical pattern.
5. Islet cell autoantibodies are frequently present around the time of onset. People demonstrating autoantibodies only transiently may have virally induced diabetes. Occasionally, antibodies will persist long term, particularly if they are associated with other autoimmune disorders. The persistence of autoantibodies suggests an autoimmune disorder.

BOX 3-6
SYMPTOMS OF DIABETES MELLITUS

Hyperglycemia
Polyuria
Polydipsia
Polyphagia
Ketoacidosis (IDDM)
Hyperlipidemia
Muscle wasting
Electrolyte depletion

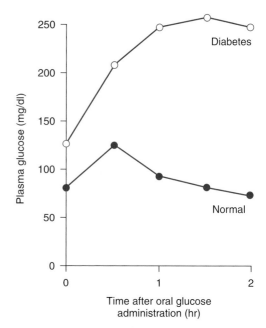

FIGURE 3-17 ▪ Oral glucose tolerance test. Fasting glucose should be less than 115 mg/dl; when measured at 2 hours, level should be less than 140 mg/dl and not greater than 200 mg/dl. If 2-hour measurement plus level at one other measurement exceeds 200 mg/dl, preliminary diagnosis of diabetes is made. *(Redrawn from Ganong WF: Review of medical physiology, ed 18, Norwalk, Conn, 1997, Appleton & Lange.)*

6. About 50% of T1DM is related to problems with the major histocompatibility complex on chromosome 6. It is correlated with increased frequencies of certain human leukocyte antigen (HLA) alleles. The HLA types DR3 and DR4 are most commonly associated with diabetes mellitus.

Symptoms of Diabetes Mellitus

Box 3-6 lists the symptoms of diabetes mellitus.

Hyperglycemia Hyperglycemia, or high blood glucose concentration, occurs due to decreased glucose uptake and utilization, and increased liver glucose production. This results in an elevated fasting plasma glucose, or an abnormally high 2-hour plasma glucose (Figure 3-17). Diabetes mellitus is characterized by hyperglycemia and the "three polys"—**polyuria, polydipsia,** and **polyphagia.**

Polyuria Polyuria refers to excessive urine production. As serum glucose levels rise, glucose is presented to the renal tubules (filtered load) at a rate that exceeds the glucose tubular maximum (Tm). As the renal threshold is exceeded, glucose begins to appear in the urine (glucosuria) and acts as an osmotic diuretic. **Glucosuria** generally becomes evident at blood sugar levels between 150 and 200 mg/dl. As dehydration progresses, polyuria eventually leads to hemoconcentration and circulatory failure because of decreased circulating blood volume. **Oliguria,** or scant urination, results from reduced glomerular filtration because of decreased glomerular hydrostatic pressure.

Polydipsia Polydipsia, or increased thirst, is a result of the dehydration that results from the osmotic diuresis.

Polyphagia Polyphagia, or excessive eating, occurs because the areas of the hypothalamus that regulate appetite (ventrolateral and ventromedial nuclei) have insulin-sensitive transport systems. Consequently, intracellular glucose levels remain low although serum glucose levels are high; intracellular glucose availability is a regulator of appetite and satiety.

Ketoacidosis Many diabetic symptoms resemble those associated with starvation; these symptoms result from the inability of many cells to take up and use glucose appropriately. Ketoacidosis is acidosis caused by excessive ketone body production. It is a symptom of T1DM that results from both low serum insulin levels and high (relative to blood glucose) glucagon levels. These endocrine changes *increase HSL activity,* which mobilizes lipids, and produce an *elevated level of serum FFA.* Liver FFA uptake and beta oxidation increase. The low I/G ratio inhibits glycolysis and hence the production of malonyl CoA, which is the first committed intermediate in fatty acid synthesis. Malonyl CoA is a competitive inhibitor of carnitine palmitoyltransferase I. When malonyl CoA levels drop, carnitine palmitoyltransferase I activity increases. This enzyme transesterifies fatty acyl CoA to fatty acyl carnitine. In this form, it can traverse the inner mitochondrial membrane, thereby becoming accessible to the enzymes for beta oxidation and ketogenesis. The elevated acetyl CoA production accompanied by a decreased TCA cycle activity (the result of NAD depletion) increases ketone body production. Because production exceeds the peripheral use, ketosis, or abnormally high ketone body levels, results. Ketosis is not thought to be a problem in patients with T2DM because these patients have some insulin. The insulin present is adequate to prevent ketosis but not to maintain normal carbohydrate metabolism.

The high serum ketone body level reduces serum pH (acidosis) because ketone bodies are acidic. In addition, as hypovolemia (low blood volume) leads to circulatory collapse, tissue perfusion decreases. This results in hypoxia (low tissue oxygenation) and subsequent increased lactic acid production. The majority of the metabolic acidosis and the increased anion gap result from high ketone body levels.

Hyperlipemia Hyperlipemia (abnormally high serum lipid levels) is typical of T1DM. VLDL levels rise because of decreased clearance resulting from lower lipoprotein lipase activity. High serum FFA levels reflect the increase in HSL activity and resultant fat mobilization. Insulin deficiency decreases LDL receptor availability, which decreases serum cholesterol clearance. This decreased clearance produces hypercholesterolemia, or high blood cholesterol.

Protein Wasting Net protein loss occurs because insulin is needed for normal amino acid uptake into cells and protein synthesis. Furthermore, because cellular glucose uptake is impaired, proteins are mobilized as an energy source. Serum branched-chain amino acids (leucine, isoleucine, valine) increase because their use in muscle protein synthesis decreases.

Electrolyte Depletion When insulin is deficient, there is a net shift of potassium from the intracellular compartment to the extracellular compartment. This potassium is lost in the urine, so serum potassium levels may appear normal but total body potassium is low. The glucosuria and ketonuria produce diuresis, which results in obligatory loss of many electrolytes. Additional sodium is lost as a result of renal acid secretion and cellular dehydration. Additional phosphate is lost in association with acid excretion and because acidosis lowers the phosphate tubular maximum. Bicarbonate is lost because of acidosis. A physician must be careful when beginning to treat a patient with poorly controlled diabetes. Insulin administered too rapidly and not supplemented with potassium can produce hypokalemia as potassium shifts intracellularly.

Acute Complications of Diabetes Mellitus

Diabetic Ketoacidosis Diabetic ketoacidosis is a serious consequence (Figure 3-18) of poorly controlled T1DM. It is characterized by elevated blood glucose level, ketonemia, increased serum osmolarity (because of the high serum glucose concentration), and elevated stress hormone levels (the counter-regulatory hormones to insulin—cortisol, GH, glucagon, epinephrine). These elevated hormones aggravate the metabolic disorder. The patients have acidosis and decreased vascular volume. The neurologic symptoms can include an altered cognitive state, but the patients may not lose consciousness.

Nonketotic Hyperosmolar Coma A nonketotic hyperosmolar coma can occur with either T1DM or T2DM. People with nonketotic hyperosmolar coma have extremely high serum hyperosmolarity and glucose. When they become dehydrated to the point of oliguria, the last significant route for disposing of excess glucose is lost, so serum glucose levels rise more rapidly. The hyperosmolarity causes cellular dehydration. By definition, ketoacidosis is not present. This type of coma is characterized by extreme dehydration. When ketoacidosis occurs, the patient frequently becomes

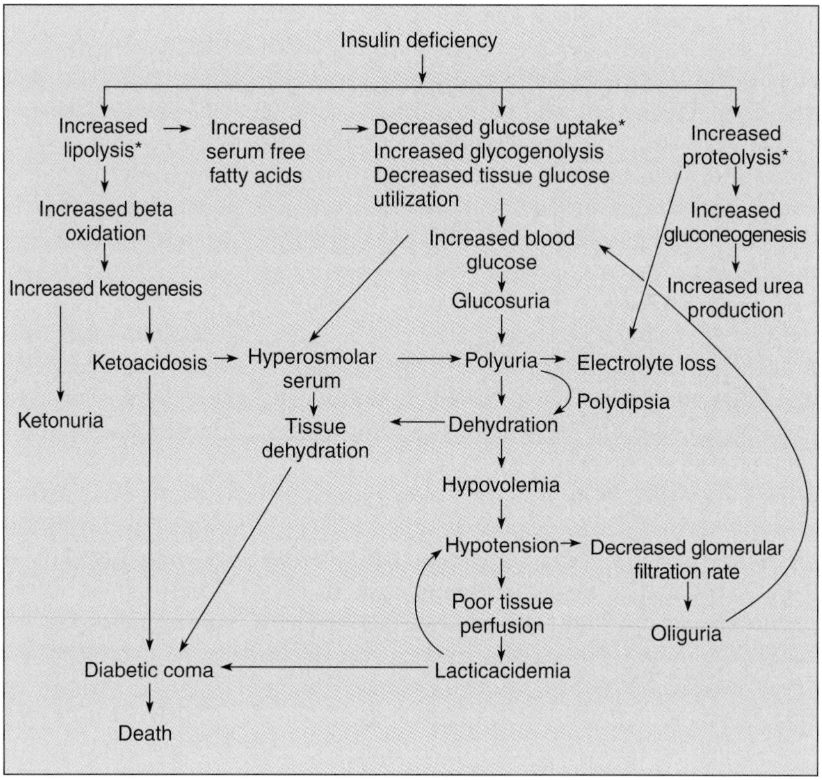

FIGURE 3-18 ■ Summary of biological effects of insulin deficiency. *Asterisk*, Point at which elevated stress hormone levels will aggravate problem.

nauseated, vomits, and exhibits obvious signs of acidosis, such as increased ventilation. Consequently, patients with ketosis frequently receive medical attention sooner than patients without. However, people in nonketotic hyperosmolar coma are likely to have more severe cellular dehydration by the time they receive medical care.

Insulin Shock Administering excessive amounts of insulin can lead to hypoglycemia, which can cause confusion, convulsions, loss of consciousness, and even death.

Long-Term Sequelae of Diabetes Mellitus

Hyperglycemia leads to elevated intracellular glucose in specific cell types, especially endothelial cells in the retina, kidney, and capillaries associated with peripheral nerves. This **glucotoxicity** alters cell function in several ways that may contribute to pathological changes.

These include increased synthesis of **polyols, hexosamines** and **diacylglycerol** (which activates protein kinase C). Although the exact mechanisms by which intracellular accumulation of these molecules causes abnormal cell function remain unclear, current thinking indicates that these changes lead to increased oxidative stress within the cell. Additionally, intracellular **nonenzymatic glycation** of proteins gives rise to advanced glycation end products (AGEs). Intracellular AGEs have altered function, whereas secreted AGEs in the extracellular matrix interact abnormally with other matrix components and matrix receptors on cells. Finally, some secreted AGEs interact with receptors on macrophages and endothelial cells. Endothelial receptors for AGEs (RAGE) leads to proinflammatory gene expression.

An important circulating product of glycation is **hemoglobin A_{1c} (HbA$_{1c}$),** which is a useful marker for long-term glucose regulation. A red blood cell has a

120-day life span; once glycation occurs, the hemoglobin remains glycated for the remainder of the red blood cell's life span. The proportion of HbA$_{1c}$ present in a nondiabetic person is low. However, a diabetic patient who has had prolonged periods of hyperglycemia over the last 8 to 12 weeks will have elevated levels. HbA$_{1c}$ measurements are clinically useful for checking treatment compliance.

Retinopathies **Retinopathies** are various forms of retinal abnormalities that develop in diabetic patients. Retinopathies are the major cause of new-onset blindness in preretirement adults in the United States. Hyperglycemia results in high intracellular glucose concentrations in retinal endothelial cells and pericytes (capillary supportive cells). This is due to the inability of these cells specifically to adapt to hyperglycemia by decreasing GLUT expression. As discussed earlier, elevated intracellular glucose probably initiates multiple mechanisms that ultimately lead to **endothelial cell dysfunction,** leading to increased resistance, hypertensive-induced changes, and cell death (Figure 3-19). These microvascular changes lead to microaneurysms, increased capillary permeability, small retinal hemorrhages, and excessive microvascular proliferation. Proliferative retinopathy is caused by impaired blood flow to the retina and subsequent tissue hypoxia. Subsequent vascular degeneration can produce vitreal hemorrhage, retinal detachment, and neovascular glaucoma, all of which can lead to severe visual loss.

Neuropathies Peripheral nerve damage (**neuropathy**) can occur as a result of metabolic, oxidative or immune-related damage to neurons or Schwann cells. Additionally, the microvasculature of peripheral nerves undergoes changes similar to those seen in retinopathies, and may represent an event that is concurrent with, or causal to, peripheral neuropathy. Schwann cells (supportive cells involved in myelination) are among those shown to accumulate sorbitol as a result of hyperglycemia. Diabetic patients can exhibit sensory loss, paresthesias, and even pain as a result of the neurologic damage. Neuropathies of the autonomic nerves also develop in diabetics, which can lead to numerous symptoms in multiple organ systems, including erectile dysfunction, postural hypotension, and heat intolerance. The sensory loss is more apparent in the extremities, particularly the lower portions of the legs and feet. This poses particular problems because, as diabetic patients lose cutaneous sensation in the feet, they become unaware of poorly fitting shoes and are more prone to injuries. Poor peripheral circulation aggravates this problem. Because diabetic patients have impaired wound healing, foot ulcerations can become a serious threat.

Nephropathies Diabetes is a common cause of impairment of renal function (**nephropathy**), and is the greatest cause of end-stage renal disease in North America. Clinical or overt diabetic nephropathy is characterized by the loss of greater than 300 mg of albumin in the urine over a 24-hour period (**albuminuria**) and progressive decline of renal function. Nephropathies develop from microvascular changes that occur in the glomerular capillaries. The glomerular capillary basement membrane thickens, resulting in thicker walls and narrower lumina (**glomerulosclerosis**), and expansion of the supportive mesangial cells. Poor renal filtration also leads to activation of the renin-angiotensin system (see Chapter 7), inducing hypertension.

Macroangiopathies Atherosclerosis develops in diabetic patients at an accelerated rate (macroangiopathies). Diabetic patients are more likely to have coronary artery disease and myocardial infarction than are nondiabetic individuals. Many diabetics with coronary artery disease have the additional risk factors of hypertension, abdominal obesity, insulin resistance, and dyslipidemia. This cluster of factors has been identified as the **metabolic syndrome** (also called **syndrome X, insulin resistance syndrome, and cardiovascular dysmetabolic syndrome**). Some of the consequences of visceral obesity, insulin resistance, and dyslipidemia are discussed earlier.

Nonretinal Visual Problems As blood glucose and therefore blood osmolarity rise, the volume of the lens changes, distorting vision. Diabetic patients commonly have cataracts, and sorbitol and glycosylated protein accumulation have been proposed as mechanisms for inducing cataract formation.

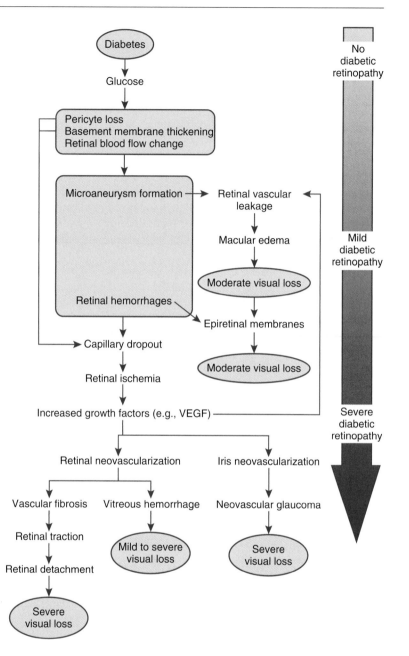

FIGURE 3-19 ■ Diabetic retinopathy flow chart. The schematic flow chart represents the major preclinical and clinical findings associated with the full spectrum of diabetic retinopathy and macular edema. VEGF, vascular endothelial growth factor. *(From Brownlee M, Aiello LP, Friedman E, et al: Complications of diabetes mellitus. In Larsen PR, Kronenberg HM, Melmed S, Polonsky KS, editors: Williams' textbook of endocrinology, ed 10, Philadelphia, 2003, WB Saunders, p 1524.)*

Problems Associated with Diabetes Management

Sometimes a diabetic patient will awaken in the morning with hyperglycemia, even before eating. One cause of this preprandial hyperglycemia is the **Somogyi effect,** which results from nocturnal hypoglycemia that stimulates secretion of the stress or counter-regulatory hormones (glucagon, cortisol, GH, and epinephrine) that act to elevate blood glucose. People with this problem generally need a lower nighttime insulin dose. The **dawn phenomenon** is thought to be a result of sleep-induced GH secretion that antagonizes insulin's effect, thereby producing hyperglycemia. This problem can sometimes be prevented by administering the evening insulin dose at bedtime rather than at dinnertime.

EMERGING CONCEPTS IN ENERGY HOMEOSTASIS: ADIPOSE TISSUE AS AN ENDOCRINE ORGAN

Adipose tissue is not contiguous, but spread throughout the body. There are two forms of adipose tissue, **brown adipose tissue (BAT)** and **white adipose tissue (WAT)**. BAT plays an important role in thermogenesis in the newborn, but BAT is much reduced in adult humans. WAT plays three general roles. First, WAT is used for cushioning (e.g., in the orbits surrounding the eyeballs). Second, the vast majority of WAT is used as a metabolic storage depot, which can be called on to release FFAs and glycerol in times of fasting. Third, the WAT involved in nutrient storage also functions as a classic endocrine organ (Box 3-7).

WAT is composed of several cell types. The TG-storing cell is called the **adipocyte.** These cells

develop during gestation in humans from preadipocytes. This process of adipocyte differentiation, which may continue throughout life, is promoted by several transcription factors. One of these factors is **sterol regulatory binding element protein–1C (SREBP-1C).** As discussed earlier, SREBP-1C is an example of a transcription factor that coordinately regulates several genes involved in a common metabolic outcome. In the case of SREBP-1C, these genes are involved in FFA and TG synthesis. SREBP-1C is activated by lipids, as well as insulin and several growth factors and cytokines. Another important transcription factor in WAT is **peroxisome proliferator–activated receptor-gamma (PPAR-γ).** PPAR-γ is a member of the nuclear receptor superfamily, which includes steroid hormone receptors (see Chapter 1). PPAR-γ heterodimerizes with the retinoid X receptor (RXR). The natural ligands for PPAR-γ are FFAs and their derivatives. Activated PPAR-γ promotes expression of genes involved in TG storage. Thus, an increase in food consumption leads to SREBP-1C and PPAR-γ activation, which increase preadipocyte differentiation into small adipocytes, and an upregulation of enzymes within these cells to allow storage of the excess fat. The **thiazolidinediones (TZDs)** are pharmacologic activators of PPAR-γ, and are being used to treat insulin resistance and T2DM.

In addition to adipocytes, about 50% of WAT is composed of nonadipocyte cells, including resident connective tissue cells (e.g., fibroblasts, macrophages) and a connective tissue matrix, cells associated with blood vessels, and cells associated with inflammatory and immune responses. WAT also receives a rich autonomic innervation. Several cell types contribute to the integrated endocrine function of WAT.

WAT tissue is divided into subcutaneous and intra-abdominal (visceral) depots. Intra-abdominal WAT refers primarily to omental and mesenteric fat, and is the smaller of the two depots. These depots receive different blood supplies that are drained in a fundamentally different way, in that the venous return from the intra-abdominal fat leads into the hepatic portal system. Thus, intra-abdominally–derived FFAs are mostly cleared by the liver, whereas subcutaneous fat is the primary site for providing FFAs to muscle during exercise or fasting. The regulation of intra-abdominal and subcutaneous adipose tissue also differs. These depots

---

BOX 3-7
ADIPOSE TISSUE HORMONES

Leptin
- Increases with adiposity
- Signals to hypothalamus to regulate appetite and to link energy-requiring
- Processes (e.g., reproduction) to adequate energy supplies
- Increases FFA oxidation in peripheral tissue
- Increases insulin sensitivity

Adiponectin
- Decreases with adiposity
- Increases FFA oxidation in peripheral tissue
- Increases insulin sensitivity
- Has direct antiatherogenic changes in vasculature

TNFα
- Increases with adiposity
- Promotes release of FFA from adipose tissue (represses genes involved in adipogenesis and lipogenesis)
- Decreases insulin sensitivity

are innervated by distinct sets of neurons within autonomic nuclei in the spinal cord and brain stem, and are influenced differently by sex steroids. Men tend to gain fat in the intra-abdominal depot (**android [apple-shaped] adiposity**), whereas women tend to gain fat in the subcutaneous depot, particularly in the thighs and buttocks (**gynecoid [pear-shaped] adiposity**). Finally, these two depots display differences in hormone production and enzyme activities.

Three protein factors produced by WAT will be discussed: **leptin, adiponectin,** and **TNF-α.** In humans, leptin and adiponectin have true endocrine functions. TNF-α may also act as a true hormone, especially at the liver, but evidence in humans presently suggest that TNF-α is also an important paracrine factor (much like somatostatin in the stomach), which indirectly influences other tissues through effects on adipose release of FFAs, leptin and adiponectin. The student should be aware that other factors are produced by WAT, including resistin, interleukin-6 (IL-6), angiotensinogen, and acylation stimulating protein (ASP). The role of these factors in humans are still being established, and thus they will not be considered in this edition.

Leptin

Leptin was discovered in 1994 as an adipocyte-derived protein that signals to the hypothalamus information about the degree of adiposity and nutrition, which in turn controls eating behavior and energy expenditure. Leptin-deficient mice and humans become morbidly obese. These findings originally raised hopes that leptin therapy could be used to combat morbid obesity. However, leptin administration to individuals who suffer from diet-induced obesity does not have a significant anorectic or energy-consuming effect. In fact, obese individuals already have elevated endogenous circulating levels of leptin and appear to have developed **leptin resistance.** *Thus, it is more likely that the importance of leptin in eating behavior is in the signal that diminished leptin levels send to the hypothalamus concerning the loss of energy stores, which promotes eating behavior and decreases energy expenditure.*

More recent studies have demonstrated an important peripheral role of leptin. Leptin has an important role in **liporegulation** in peripheral tissues.

Leptin protects peripheral tissues (i.e., the liver, skeletal muscle, cardiac muscle, β cells) from the accumulation of too much lipid and directs storage of excess caloric intake into adipose tissue. This action of leptin, while opposing the lipogenic actions of insulin, contributes significantly to the maintenance of insulin sensitivity (as defined by insulin-dependent glucose uptake) in peripheral tissues. Leptin also acts as a signal that the body has sufficient energy stores to allow for reproduction and to enhance erythropoiesis, lymphopoiesis, and myelopoiesis. For example, in women suffering from anorexia nervosa, leptin levels are extremely low, resulting in low ovarian steroids, amenorrhea (lack of menstrual bleeding), anemia due to low red blood cell production, and immune dysfunctions.

Leptin Structure, Synthesis, and Secretion Leptin is a 16-kDa protein secreted by mature adipocytes. It is encoded by the Lep^{ob} gene and is structurally related to cytokines. Thus, it is sometimes referred to as an **adipocytokine.** The circulating levels of leptin show a direct relationship with adiposity and nutritional status. Subcutaneous WAT secretes more leptin than intra-abdominal WAT. Leptin output is increased by insulin, which prepares the body for the correct partitioning of incoming nutrients. Leptin is inhibited by fasting and weight loss, and by lipolytic signals (e.g., increased cAMP and β3 agonists).

The Leptin Receptor Several membrane-bound (long and short forms) and circulating forms of the leptin receptor exist owing to splicing variations and proteolytic cleavage. The fully active form of the leptin receptor (LR) is the long form, also called **LRb.** The short forms may play a role in transport of leptin across the blood-brain barrier, whereas the circulating form may regulate the levels of free leptin. The LR is a member of the cytokine receptor family (see Chapter 1).

Diet-induced obesity, advanced age and T2DM are associated with leptin resistance. Thus, mechanisms that turn off leptin signaling are potential therapeutic targets. One negative regulator of LRb signaling is SOCS (see **the insulin receptor** earlier). There is also evidence for termination of JAK activity through a phosphotyrosine phosphatase that removes the activating phosphotyrosine from JAK.

Adiponectin

Adiponectin (also called Acrp30, adipoQ, and apM1) was discovered in 1995 and 1996 by several independent laboratories. Adiponectin regulates metabolism in a manner similar to leptin, in that it improves insulin sensitivity in terms of glucose uptake, but opposes insulin in terms of FFA utilization/storage. *Adiponectin stimulates FFA oxidation and reduces intramyocellular TG content, which in turn is associated with enhanced insulin-dependent glucose uptake (i.e., increases insulin sensitivity). Adiponectin also increases FFA oxidation in the liver and decreases hepatic glucose output. Adiponectin also has direct positive effects on blood vessels, which collectively decrease the risk of cardiovascular disease.*

Adiponectin Structure, Synthesis, and Secretion
Adiponectin is a 30-kDa protein expressed by adipocytes. It has homology to a complement component and collagens. Adiponectin contains a globular domain at its C-terminus, which is proteolytically cleaved from the parent protein. The globular domain fragment also circulates at significant levels and has biological activity.

Unlike leptin, adiponectin levels decrease with obesity. As adipocytes enlarge with stored TG, they secrete less adiponectin. Adiponectin levels increase after weight loss, including in morbidly obese patients who lose weight after gastric bypass surgery. Patients who have inactivating mutations in PPAR-γ have very low levels of adiponectin and severe insulin resistance, and agonists of PPAR-γ (e.g., thiazolidinediones) increase adiponectin release from adipose tissue. These findings suggest that adiponectin is dependent on differentiation of preadipocytes into small adipocytes, whereas excessive growth of mature adipocytes inhibits adiponectin production.

The Adiponectin Receptor
Two adiponectin receptors have been characterized in humans, **AdipoR1** and **AdipoR2.** Both receptors bind full-length and globular adiponectin. AdipoR1 and AdipoR2 are 7-transmembrane domain receptors (Chapter 1). However, they are not linked to Gs and do not increase cAMP. Both receptors have been shown to increase the activity of signaling molecules, including **PPAR-α** and AMP-dependent kinase, both of which promote FFA oxidation.

PPAR-α is structurally related to PPAR-γ, in that it is a member of the nuclear hormone receptor family. PPAR-α is expressed in nonadipose tissue (cardiac and skeletal muscle, liver) and increases fatty acyl CoA oxidation, thereby lowering lipids and increasing insulin sensitivity. Drugs of the **fibrate** family (e.g., clofibrate) act as ligands for PPAR-α.

Tumor Necrosis Factor-α (TNF-α)

TNF-α, which was originally identified as an endotoxin-induced peptide that caused tumor necrosis (hence the name, TNF), is an important component of the acute inflammation response, and a regulator of the innate immune system. TNF-α became linked to metabolism by its identification as the macrophage-derived "**cachexin.**" **Cachexia** is a wasting syndrome that represents a profound metabolic imbalance within certain patients (often with widespread cancer), in which increased metabolic demands are mismatched with loss of appetite, a progressive loss of fat and lean body mass, weakness, and anemia. *More recently, TNF-α and its two receptors have been shown to be expressed in adipose tissue. TNF-α strongly opposes the lipogenic and antilipolytic actions of insulin on adipose tissue, and suppresses production of leptin and adiponectin. By decreasing leptin and adiponectin, and increasing circulating levels of FFAs, TNF-α also indirectly reduces the insulin sensitivity of liver and muscle. In animals (and possibly humans), TNF-α also has direct anti-insulin effects at the liver and muscle.*

TNF-α Structure, Synthesis, and Secretion
TNF-α belongs to the TNF-ligand family. TNF-α precursor is synthesized as a 26-kDa transmembrane protein. A 17-kDa extracellular fragment is released by proteolytic cleavage by the membrane metalloprotease.

TNF-α production by adipose tissue increases with obesity, and TNF-α acts in an autocrine/paracrine manner to repress the expression of genes encoding proteins involved in the uptake of FFAs and glucose, and in lipogenesis. TNF-α reduces insulin sensitivity through increased serine phosphorylation of the IRS-1 and decreased expression of GLUT-4 and IRS-1. TNF-α also represses expression of PPAR-γ, thereby further inhibiting adipocyte differentiation and lipogenesis. Conversely, agonists of PPAR-γ

(thiazolidinediones) inhibit TNF-α, thereby increasing insulin sensitivity.

The TNF-α Receptor TNF-α binds to two receptors that are members of the **TNF/nerve growth factor family.** Among the several downstream signals is the activation of a kinase (IKK) which phosphorylates the inhibitor (I-κB) of the family of transcription factors referred to as NF-κB. Phosphorylation of I-κB targets it for degradation, allowing NF-κB to translocate to the nucleus. NF-κB-mediated transcription is involved in several of the TNF-α-induced changes in adipose tissue, including repression of PPAR-γ expression.

SUMMARY

1. Cells make ATP to meet their energy needs. ATP is made by glycolysis, and by the TCA cycle coupled to oxidative phosphorylation.

2. Cells can oxidize carbohydrate (primarily in the form of glucose), amino acids, and FFAs to make ATP. Additionally, the liver makes ketone bodies for other tissues to oxidize for energy in times of fasting.

3. Some cell types are limited in what energy substrates they can oxidize for energy. The brain is normally exclusively dependent on glucose for energy. Thus, blood glucose must be maintained above 60 mg/dl for normal autonomic and CNS function. Conversely, inappropriately high levels of glucose (i.e., fasting glucose above 110 mg/dl) promote glucotoxicity in specific cell types, leading to the long-term complications of diabetes.

4. The endocrine pancreas produces the hormones insulin, glucagon, somatostatin, gastrin, and pancreatic polypeptide.

5. Insulin is an anabolic hormone that is secreted in times of excess nutrient availability. It allows the body to use carbohydrates as energy sources and store nutrients.

6. Major stimuli for insulin secretion include increased serum glucose and certain amino acids. Cholinergic (muscarinic) receptor activation also increases insulin secretion, whereas α2-adrenergic receptors inhibit insulin secretion. The GI tract releases incretin hormones that stimulate pancreatic insulin secretion. GLP-1 and GIP are particularly potent in augmenting glucose-dependent stimulation of insulin secretion.

7. Insulin binds to the insulin receptor, which is linked to multiple pathways that mediate metabolic and growth effects of insulin.

8. During the digestive period, insulin acts on the liver to promote trapping of glucose to glucose-6-phosphate. Insulin also increases glycogenesis, glycolysis, and fatty acid synthesis in the liver. Insulin regulates hepatic metabolism by both regulating gene expression and by posttranslational dephosphorylation events.

9. Insulin increases GLUT-4-mediated glucose uptake in muscle and adipose tissue. Insulin increases glycogenesis, glycolysis, and—in the presence of caloric excess—lipogenesis in muscle and adipose tissue. Insulin increases muscle amino acid uptake and protein synthesis. Insulin also increases fatty acid esterification, lipoprotein lipase activity, and decreases hormone-sensitive lipase (HSL) activity in the adipocyte.

10. Glucagon is a catabolic hormone. Its secretion increases during periods of food deprivation, and it acts to mobilize nutrient reserves. It also mobilizes glycogen, fat, and even protein.

11. Glucagon is released in response to decreased serum glucose (and therefore insulin) and increased serum amino acid levels and β-adrenergic signaling.

12. Glucagon binds to the glucagon receptor, which is linked to Gs/PKA-dependent pathways.

13. The primary target organ for glucagon is the liver. Glucagon increases liver glucose output by increasing glycogenolysis and gluconeogenesis. It increases beta oxidation of fatty acids and ketogenesis.

14. Glucagon regulates hepatic metabolism by both regulating gene expression, and through posttranslational PKA-dependent phosphorylation events.

15. The major counter-regulatory factors in muscle and adipose is the adrenal hormone, epinephrine, and the sympathetic neurotransmitter, norepinephrine. These two factors act through β2- and β3-adrenergic receptors to increase cAMP levels. Epinephrine and norepinephrine increase glycogenolysis and fatty acyl oxidation in muscle and increase hormone-sensitive lipase in adipose tissue.

16. Diabetes mellitus (DM) is classified as Type 1 DM (T1DM) and Type 2 DM (T2DM). T1DM is characterized by the destruction of pancreatic β cells and requires exogenous insulin for treatment. T2DM can be due to numerous factors, but usually is characterized as insulin resistance coupled to some degree of β-cell deficiency. Patients with T2DM may require exogenous insulin at some point to maintain blood glucose levels.

17. Obesity-associated T2DM is currently at epidemic proportions worldwide. Obesity-associated T2DM is characterized by insulin resistance due to lipotoxicity, hyperinsulinemia, and inflammatory cytokines produced by adipose tissue. T2DM is often associated with obesity, insulin resistance, hypertension, and coronary artery disease. This constellation of risk factors is referred to as **metabolic syndrome.**

18. Major symptoms of diabetes mellitus include hyperglycemia, polyuria, polydipsia, polyphagia, muscle wasting, electrolyte depletion, and ketoacidosis (in T1DM).

19. Long-term complications of poorly controlled diabetes is due to excess intracellular glucose (glucotoxicity) in specific cells, especially in the retina, kidney, and peripheral nerves. This leads to retinopathies, nephropathies, and neuropathies.

20. It is increasingly well-established that adipose tissue has an endocrine function, especially in terms of energy homeostasis. Hormones produced by adipose tissue include leptin, adiponectin, and TNF-α.

KEY WORDS AND CONCEPTS

- Energy metabolism
- Liver
- Skeletal muscle
- Adipose tissue
- Brain
- Pancreatic islet
- Insulin
- Glucagon
- Adrenal hormone epinephrine
- Sympathetic neurotransmitter norepinephrine
- Diet-induced obesity
- Insulin resistance
- Type 1 diabetes mellitus (T1DM)
- Type 2 diabetes mellitus (T2DM)
- Adenosine triphosphate (ATP)
- Glucose
- Nonesterified fatty acids
- Free fatty acids (FFAs)
- Amino acids (AAs)
- Ketone bodies
- Hypoglycemia
- Glycolysis
- Tricarboxylic acid (TCA) cycle
- Oxidative phosphorylation
- Electron transport chain
- Reactive oxygen species (ROS)
- β-oxidation
- Carnitine palmitoyl-transferase (CPT-I and CPT II)
- Acetoacetate
- β-hydroxybutyrate
- Thiophorase
- Glycogen
- Glycogen synthase
- Glycogen phosphorylase
- Triglycerides (TGs)
- Lipoprotein particle
- Chylomicron
- Apoproteins (Apos)
- Apo B48
- High-density lipoproteins (HDLs)
- Apo CII
- Lipoprotein lipase (LPL)
- Chylomicron remnants
- Apo E
- Very low-density lipoproteins (VLDLs)
- Apoprotein B100
- VLDL remnants
- Intermediate-density lipoprotein particles (IDLs)
- Hepatic lipase

- Low-density lipoprotein particles (LDLs)
- Cholesterol ester transfer protein (ETP)
- Oxidized LDL
- Scavenger receptors
- Atherogenic
- Hormone-sensitive lipase
- Transamination
- Urea cycle
- Pyruvate carboxylase
- PEP carboxykinase (PEPCK)
- Fructose-6-phosphatase
- Glucose-6-phosphatase
- Pancreatic polypeptide
- Proinsulin (connecting) peptide
- Late-phase of insulin release
- Early-phase of insulin release
- Glucokinase
- Glucose sensor
- ATP-sensitive K^+ channel
- Voltage-gated Ca^{2+} channels
- SUR
- Sulfonylurea drugs
- Insulin-receptor substrates (IRSs)
- Shc protein
- APS protein
- Protein Kinase B (PKB)-dependent pathway
- Suppressor of cytokine signaling (SOCS)
- Epinephrine
- Norepinephrine
- Glucokinase
- Sterol-responsive element binding protein-1C (SREBP-1C)
- Protein phosphatase 1
- Glycogen synthase
- Glycogen synthase kinase 3
- Glycogen phosphorylase
- Phosphorylase kinase
- Phosphofructokinase-1 (PFK-1)
- Phosphofructokinase-2 (PFK-2)
- Fructose-bisphosphate-2
- Fructose-2,6-bisphosphate
- Fructose-1,6-bisphosphate
- Pyruvate kinase
- Phosphoenolpyruvate carboxylase (PEPCK)
- ATP-citrate lyase
- Acetyl CoA carboxylase

- Fatty acid synthase complex (FAS)
- Pentose phosphate shunt
- Glucose-6-phosphate dehydrogenase
- Palmitoyl CoA desaturase
- Glycerol kinase
- Glucose tolerance
- Glucometabolic
- Lipotoxicity
- Fatty liver
- Hepatic steatosis
- Tumor necrosis factor-α (TNF-α)
- AMP kinase
- Metformin
- Non–insulin-dependent diabetes mellitus
- Polyuria
- Polydipsia
- Polyphagia
- Glucotoxicity
- Polyols
- Hexosamines
- Diacylglycerol
- Nonenzymatic glycation
- Hemoglobin A_{1c} (HbA_{1c})
- Endothelial cell dysfunction
- Neuropathy
- Nephropathy
- Albuminuria
- Somogyi effect
- Dawn phenomenon
- Brown adipose tissue (BAT)
- White adipose tissue (WAT)
- Adipocyte
- Peroxisome proliferation–activated receptor-gamma (PPAR-γ)
- Thiazolidinediones (TZDs)
- Android (apple-shaped) adiposity
- Gynecoid (pear-shaped) adiposity
- Leptin
- Adiponectin
- AdipoR1
- AdipoR2
- Fibrate
- Cachexin
- Cachexia
- Leptin resistance
- Liporegulation

- Adipocytokine
- Leptin receptor (LR); long form (LRb)
- Pyruvate dehydrogenase (PDH)

SELF-STUDY PROBLEMS

1. During the fed state, how does the role of glycolysis in the liver differ from the role of glycolysis in adipose tissue?

2. How does the function of glycogen differ in the liver versus the skeletal muscle?

3. Normally, the brain is dependent on glucose. What other energy substrate is used by the brain during a prolonged fast? What is the origin of this substrate?

4. What is the relation between mitochondrial citrate levels and lipogenesis?

5. What two enzymes are dysregulated in DM that contribute to high levels of circulating TGs?

6. What is the relation of lipoprotein lipase to the following: chylomicrons, VLDL, LDL?

7. Why does loss of the LDL receptor give rise to high blood cholesterol?

8. What futile cycle does high levels of malonyl CoA prevent?

9. What is the difference between insulin released in the early phase of secretion and that released in the late phase?

10. How would a mutant glucokinase with decreased activity affect insulin secretion?

11. How does insulin regulate the following hepatic enzymes: glucokinase, frutose-1, 6-bisphosphatase, pyruvate kinase, pyruvate dehydrogenase, acetyl CoA carboxylase, PEPCK?

12. What is meant by the term *hypoglycemic hormone?*

13. What is the basis for ketoacidosis in patients with poorly managed diabetes mellitus?

14. How is obesity related to insulin resistance?

15. How do AGEs alter cell function? What is meant by endothelial dysfunction?

16. Visceral adiposity is associated with increased levels of TNF-α. How does this alter hepatic function?

BIBLIOGRAPHY

Barthel A, Schmoll D: Novel concepts in insulin regulation of hepatic gluconeogenesis, *Am J Physiol Endocrinol Metab* 285(4):E685-692, 2003.

Collier JJ, Scott DK: Sweet changes: glucose homeostasis can be altered by manipulating genes controlling hepatic glucose metabolism, *Mol Endocrinol* 18(5):1051-1063, 2004.

De Meyts P: Insulin and its receptor: structure, function and evolution, *Bioessays* 26(12):1351-1362, 2004.

Ferre P: The biology of peroxisome proliferator-activated receptors: relationship with lipid metabolism and insulin sensitivity, *Diabetes* 53 Suppl 1:S43-50, 2004.

Foufelle F, Ferre P: New perspectives in the regulation of hepatic glycolytic and lipogenic genes by insulin and glucose: a role for the transcription factor sterol regulatory element binding protein-1c, *Biochem J* 366(Pt 2):377-391, 2002.

Holm C: Molecular mechanisms regulating hormone-sensitive lipase and lipolysis, *Biochem Soc Trans* 31(Pt 6):1120-1124, 2003.

Kershaw EE, Flier JS: Adipose tissue as an endocrine organ, *J Clin Endocrinol Metab* 89(6):2548-2556, 2004.

Meier JJ, Nauck MA: Glucagon-like peptide 1(GLP-1) in biology and pathology, *Diabetes Metab Res Rev* 21(2):91-117, 2005.

Moller DE, Kaufman KD: Metabolic syndrome: a clinical and molecular perspective, *Annu Rev Med* 56:45-62, 2005.

Muller-Wieland. Kotzka DJ: SREBP-1: gene regulatory key to syndrome X? *Ann N Y Acad Sci* 967:19-27, 2002.

Pirola LA, Johnston M, Van Obberghen: Modulation of insulin action, *Diabetologia* 47(2):170-184, 2004.

Ruan H, Lodish HF: Insulin resistance in adipose tissue: direct and indirect effects of tumor necrosis factor-alpha, *Cytokine Growth Factor Rev* 14(5):447-455, 2003.

Ruderman N, M. Prentki M: AMP kinase and malonyl-CoA: targets for therapy of the metabolic syndrome, *Nat Rev Drug Discov* 3(4):340-351, 2004.

Shulman GI: Cellular mechanisms of insulin resistance, *J Clin Invest* 106(2):171-176, 2000.

Taskinen MR: Diabetic dyslipidaemia: from basic research to clinical practice, *Diabetologia* 46(6):733-749, 2003.

Unger RH: Minireview: weapons of lean body mass destruction: the role of ectopic lipids in the metabolic syndrome. *Endocrinology* 144(12):5159-5165, 2003.

Yan SF, Ramasamy R, Naka, Schmidt AM: Glycation, inflammation, and RAGE: a scaffold for the macrovascular complications of diabetes and beyond, *Circ Res* 93(12):1159-1169, 2003.

RECOMMENDED READING

For a more in-depth and more clinical discussion of energy metabolism and diabetes mellitus, the student is encouraged to read selected parts of Chapters 29 through 34 in Larsen PR, Kronenberg HM, Melmed S, Poloinsky KS, editors: *Williams' Textbook of Endocrinology*, ed 10, Philadelphia, 2003, WB Saunders.

4 CALCIUM AND PHOSPHATE HOMEOSTASIS

OBJECTIVES

1. Describe the structure and synthesis of PTH, the regulation of PTH secretion and the nature of the PTH receptor.

2. Describe the structure and synthesis of 1,25-dihydroxyvitamin D, the regulation of 1,25-dihydroxyvitamin D production, and the receptor for 1,25-dihydroxyvitamin D.

3. Discuss the role of the GI tract, bone, and kidneys in Ca^{2+}/Pi homeostasis.

4. Discuss the actions of calcitonin, PTHrP, FGF 23, and gonadal and steroid hormones on Ca^{2+}/Pi metabolism.

5. Discuss the pathophysiology associated with imbalances in PTH and 1,25-dihydroxyvitamin D.

Calcium (Ca^{2+}) and phosphate (Pi) are essential to human life, playing important structural roles in hard tissues (i.e., bones and teeth), and important regulatory roles in metabolic and signaling pathways. The two primary sources of circulating Ca^{2+} and Pi are the diet and the skeleton (Figure 4-1). Two hormones, **1,25-dihydroxyvitamin D** (also called **calcitriol**) and **parathyroid hormone** (**PTH**) regulate intestinal absorption of Ca^{2+} and Pi, and the release of Ca^{2+} and Pi into the circulation following bone resorption. The primary processes for removal of Ca^{2+} and Pi from the blood are renal excretion and bone formation (see Figure 4-1), and 1,25-dihydroxyvitamin D and PTH regulate these processes as well. Other hormones and paracrine growth factors also have clinical relevance to Ca^{2+} and Pi homeostasis.

CALCIUM AND PHOSPHORUS ARE IMPORTANT DIETARY ELEMENTS THAT PLAY MANY CRUCIAL ROLES IN CELLULAR PHYSIOLOGY

Calcium is an essential dietary element. In addition to getting calcium from the diet, humans contain a vast store (i.e., >1 kg) of calcium in their bones, which can be called on to maintain normal circulating levels of calcium in times of dietary restriction and during the increased demands of pregnancy and nursing. Circulating calcium exists in three forms (Table 4-1): free ionized calcium (Ca^{2+}), protein-bound calcium, and calcium complexed with anions (e.g., phosphates, bicarbonate, and citrate). The ionized form represents about 50% of circulating calcium, and because this form is so critical to many cellular functions, Ca^{2+}

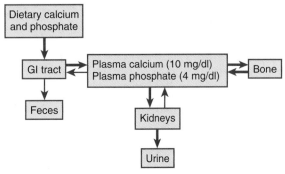

FIGURE 4-1 ■ Daily Ca^{2+} and Pi fluxes.

levels in both extracellular and intracellular compartments are tightly controlled (see Chapter 1 for discussion Ca^{2+}-dependent signaling pathways). Circulating Ca^{2+} is under direct hormonal control and is normally maintained in a relatively narrow range. Either too little Ca^{2+} (**hypocalcemia;** total serum Ca^{2+} below 8.5 mg/dl [2.1 mM]) or too much Ca^{2+} (**hypercalcemia;** total serum Ca^{2+} above 10.5 mg/dl [2.6 mM]) in the blood can lead a broad range of pathophysiologic changes, including neuromuscular dysfunction, CNS dysfunction, renal insufficiency, calcification of soft tissue, and skeletal pathologies.

Phosphorus is also an essential dietary element and is stored in large quantities in bone complexed with calcium. In the blood, most phosphorus exists in the ionized form of phosphoric acid, which is called **inorganic phosphate (Pi)**. Most circulating Pi is in the free ionized form, but some Pi (<20%) circulates as a protein-bound form or complexed with cations (see Table 4-1). Phosphorus also exists as pyrophosphate (two Pi groups in a covalent linkage). Unlike Ca^{2+},

phosphate is incorporated covalently as single or multiple phosphate groups into many molecules and, consequently, soft tissues contain about 10-fold more phosphate than Ca^{2+}. This means that significant tissue damage (e.g., crush injury with massive muscle cell death) can result in **hyperphosphatemia,** which can then complex with Ca^{2+} to cause acute hypocalcemia. Phosphate represents a key intracellular component. Indeed, it is the high energy phosphate bonds of ATP that maintain life. Phosphorylation/dephosphorylation of proteins, lipids, second messengers and cofactors represent key regulatory steps in numerous metabolic and signaling pathways, and phosphate also serves as the backbone for nucleic acids.

PHYSIOLOGICAL REGULATION OF CALCIUM AND PHOSPHATE: PARATHYROID HORMONE (PTH) AND 1,25-DIHYDROXYVITAMIN D

PTH and **1,25-dihydroxyvitamin D** represent the two physiologically important hormones that are dedicated to the maintenance of normal blood Ca^{2+} and Pi levels in humans. As such, they are referred to as calciotropic hormones. The structure, synthesis, and secretion of these two hormones, and their receptors will be discussed. In the following section, the detailed actions of PTH and 1,25-dihydroxyvitamin D on the three key sites of Ca^{2+}/Pi homeostasis (i.e., gut, bone, and kidney) will be discussed.

Parathyroid Hormone

PTH is a key hormone that protects against a hypocalcemic challenge. The primary targets of PTH are bone and kidneys. PTH also functions in a positive feedforward loop by stimulating 1,25-dihydroxyvitamin D production.

The Parathyroid Glands

The **parathyroid glands** develop from the endodermal lining of the third and fourth branchial pouches. They usually develop into four, loosely organized glands: two superior and two inferior parathyroid glands. The embryonic anlage of the parathyroids become associated with the caudal migration of the thyroglossal duct, so that the parathyroid glands usually become situated

		TABLE 4-1		
		Forms of Ca^{2+} and Pi in Plasma		
ION	**mg/dl**	**IONIZED (%)**	**PROTEIN BOUND (%)**	**COMPLEXED (%)**
Ca^{++}	10 mg/dl	50	45	5
Pi	4 mg/dl	84	10	6

Ca^{++} is bound (i.e., complexed) to various anions in the plasma, including HCO_3^-, citrate, Pi, and SO_4^-. Pi is complexed to various cations, including Na^+ and K^+.
From Koeppen BM, Stanton BA: *Renal physiology,* ed 4, Philadelphia, 2007, Mosby.

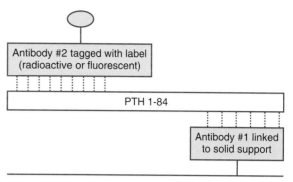

FIGURE 4-3 ■ Double-antibody PTH assay. Antibodies #1 and #2 are generated against peptides corresponding to the C-terminus and N-terminus, respectively, of full-length PTH. Lack of either terminus will give a negative reading.

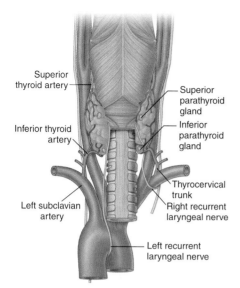

FIGURE 4-2 ■ Anatomic position of the parathyroid glands. *(Redrawn from Drake RL, Vogl W, Mitchell AWM: Gray's Anatomy for Students, Philadelphia, Churchill Livingstone)*

on the dorsal side of the right and left lobes of the thyroid gland (Figure 4-2). The exact positions of the parathyroid glands are variable, and >10% of humans harbor a fifth parathyroid gland. The predominant parenchymal cell type in the parathyroid gland is the **principal** (also called **chief) cell.** These cells are the primary endocrine cell of the gland. With age, a larger mitochondria-rich, eosinophilic cell type, the **oxyphil cell,** appears. Although the oxyphil cell is not normally important to PTH secretion, PTH-over-producing tumors (i.e., primary hyperparathy-roidism) can be derived from both principal and oxyphil cells.

Structure, Synthesis and Secretion of PTH Secreted PTH is an 84-amino acid polypeptide. PTH is synthe-sized as a **prepro-PTH,** which is proteolytically processed to **pro-PTH** at the endoplasmic reticulum and then to PTH in the Golgi and secretory vesicles. Unlike proin-sulin, all intracellular pro-PTH is normally converted to PTH before secretion. PTH has a short half-life (<5 minutes) because it is proteolytically cleaved into biologically-inactive N-terminus and C-terminus fragments that are excreted by the kidney. Older assays of PTH detected both intact 1-84 PTH, but also

inactive C-terminus fragments, and therefore detected unreliably high levels of PTH—especially in patients with renal disease. Current assays utilize two antibod-ies which recognize epitopes from both ends of the molecule, thereby more accurately measuring the intact 1-84 form of PTH (Figure 4-3).

The primary signal that stimulates PTH secretion is low circulating Ca^{2+} levels (Figure 4-4). The extracel-lular Ca^{2+} concentration is sensed by the parathyroid principal cells through a **Ca^{2+}-sensing receptor (CaSR).** The CaSR is a member of the 7-transmembrane, G-protein–coupled receptor superfamily, which forms disulfide-linked dimers in the membrane of chief cells of the parathyroid glands. The CaSR is also expressed in calcitonin-producing C cells, renal tubules, and in several other tissues. In the parathyroid gland, increasing amounts of extracellular Ca^{2+} binds to the CaSR and activates incompletely understood downstream signaling pathways that repress PTH secretion. Thus, basal PTH secretion (i.e., PTH secre-tion in the absence of CaSR signaling) is high, but is inhibited by high extracellular Ca^{2+}-CaSR binding and signaling.

Although the CaSR binds to extracellular Ca^{2+} with relatively low affinity, the CaSR is extremely sensitive to *changes* in extracellular Ca^{2+}. A 0.1-mM drop in blood Ca^{2+} produces an increase in circulating PTH levels from basal (5% of maximum) to maximum levels (Figure 4-5). Thus, the CaSR regulates PTH output in response to subtle fluctuations in Ca^{2+} on a minute-to-minute basis. It should be noted that the

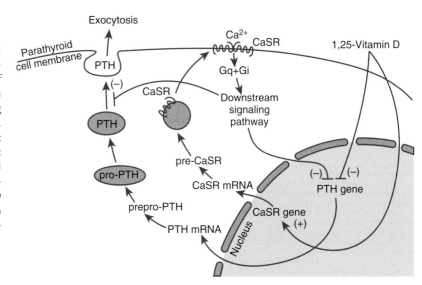

FIGURE 4-4 ■ Regulation of PTH gene expression and PTH secretion. The primary regulator of PTH is extracellular Ca^{2+}, which is sensed by the Ca^{2+}-sensing receptor (CaSR). The CaSR is a GPCR linked to Gq and Gi, but the downstream signaling that inhibits PTH secretion and PTH gene expression is poorly understood. 1,25-Dihydroxyvitamin D inhibits PTH gene expression directly, and indirectly by stimulating CaSR gene expression.

CaSR is also stimulated by high levels of magnesium, so that hypermagnesemia also inhibits PTH secretion.

Patients with **familial benign hypocalciuric hypercalcemia (FBHH)** or **neonatal severe hyperparathyroidism** are heterozygous or homozygous, respectively, for inactivating mutations of the CaSR. In these patients, the CaSR fails to appropriately inhibit PTH secretion in response to high levels of blood calcium. The CaSR also plays a direct role in Ca^{2+} reabsorption

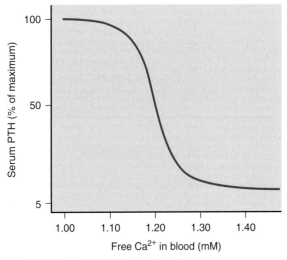

FIGURE 4-5 ■ Ca^{2+}/PTH secretion dose-response curve.

at the kidney. The **hypocalciuria** (i.e., inappropriately low Ca^{2+} excretion in the face of high circulating Ca^{2+} levels) in patients with FBHH is due to the lowered ability of the CaSR to monitor blood calcium and respond by increasing urinary Ca^{2+} excretion.

PTH production is also regulated at the level of gene transcription (see Figure 4-4). The prepro-PTH gene is repressed by a **calcium-response element** within the promoter of this gene. Thus, the signaling pathway that is activated by Ca^{2+} binding to the CaSR ultimately leads to repression of prepro-PTH gene expression and PTH synthesis. The prepro-PTH gene is also repressed by 1,25-dihydroxyvitamin D (acting through vitamin D-responsive elements—see later). The ability of 1,25-dihydroxyvitamin D to hold PTH gene expression in check is reinforced by the coordinated up-regulation of CaSR gene expression by positive vitamin D-responsive elements in the promoter of the CaSR gene (see Figure 4-4).

The PTH Receptor The PTH receptor is a 7-transmembrane, G-protein–linked membrane receptor. Because this receptor also binds PTHrP (see later), it is usually referred to as the **PTH/PTHrP receptor.** The PTH/PTHrP receptor is primarily coupled to a Gs signaling pathway that leads to increased cAMP, although it also is coupled to Gq/11-phospholipase C-dependent pathways. The PTH/PTHrP receptor is expressed on osteoblasts in bone and, in the proximal and distal tubules of the kidney, as the receptor for the systemic actions of PTH. However, the PTH/PTHrP receptor is also expressed in many developing structures in which PTHrP has an important paracrine function.

Vitamin D

Vitamin D is actually a prohormone, which must undergo two successive hydroxylations to become the active form, **1,25-dihydroxyvitamin D** (Figure 4-6). Vitamin D plays a critical role in Ca^{2+} absorption, and to a lesser extent Pi absorption, by the small intestine.

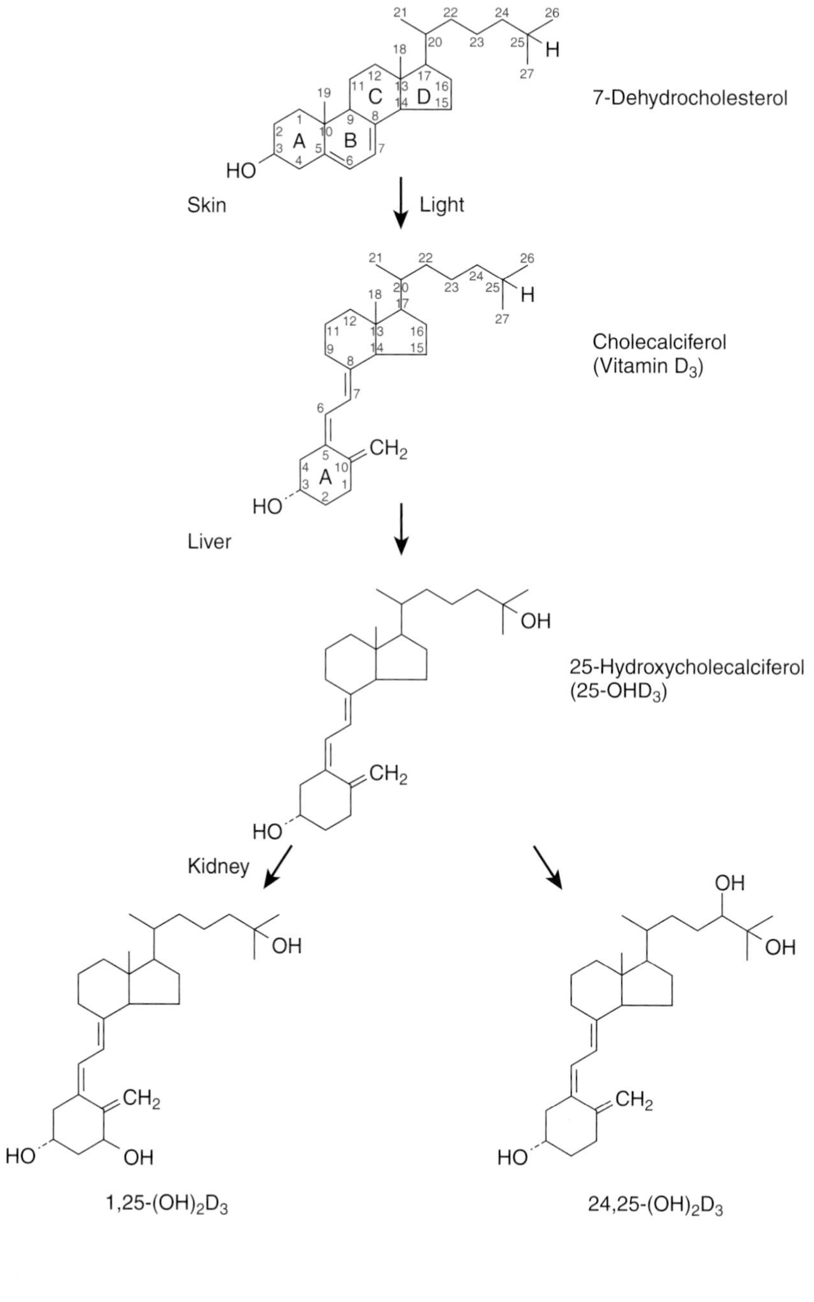

FIGURE 4-6 ■ Biosynthesis of 1,25-dihydroxyvitamin D.

Vitamin D also regulates aspects of bone remodeling and renal reabsorption of Ca^{2+} and Pi.

Structure, Synthesis, and Transport of Active Vitamin D Metabolites

Vitamin D_3 (also called **cholecalciferol**) is synthesized by ultraviolet light (UV B) conversion of 7-dehydrocholesterol in the more basal layers of the skin (Figure 4-7). UV radiation opens up the B ring of cholesterol, generating previtamin D_3, which then undergoes a temperature-dependent isomerization into D_3. Vitamin D_3 is therefore referred to as a **secosteroid,** which is a class of steroids in which one of the cholesterol rings is opened. **Vitamin D_2** (a secosteroid, also called **ergocalciferol**) is the form produced in plants. Vitamin D_3, and to a lesser extent D_2, are absorbed from the diet and are equally effective after conversion into active hydroxylated forms. The balance between UV-dependent, endogenously synthesized vitamin D_3, and absorption of dietary forms of vitamin D becomes important under certain situations.

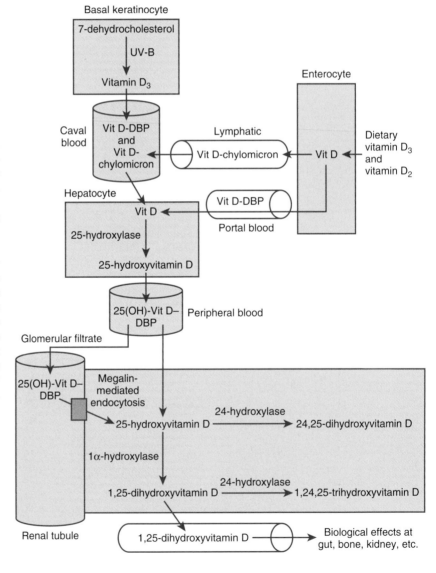

FIGURE 4-7 ■ Vitamin D metabolism. Vitamin D can be synthesized in the skin keratinocyte, or absorbed from the GI tract enterocyte. Vitamin D is transported to the liver hepatocyte, where it is hydroxylated at the 25 carbon. 25-Hydroxyvitamin D is carried in the blood by vitamin D binding protein (DBP) to the renal proximal tubules where it is hydroxylated at either the 1α position (activating) or the 24 position (inactivating). Note that 25-hydroxyvitamin D that exits into the glomerular filtrate can be recaptured by the apical membrane protein, megalin, which binds and internalizes DBP.

Individuals with higher epidermal melanin content and who live in higher latitudes convert less 7-dehydrocholesterol into vitamin D_3 and thus are more dependent on dietary sources of vitamin D. Dairy products are enriched in vitamin D_3, but not all individuals tolerate or enjoy dairy products. Institutionalized, sedentary elderly patients who stay indoors and avoid dairy products are particularly at risk for developing **vitamin D deficiency.**

D_3 is transported in the blood from the skin to the liver. Dietary D_3 and D_2 reach the liver directly via transport in the portal circulation and indirectly via chylomicrons (Figure 4-7). In the liver, D_2 and D_3 are hydroxylated at the 25-carbon position to yield **25-hydroxyvitamin D** (at this juncture, no distinction will be made between D_3 and D_2 metabolites, as they are equipotent). Hepatic vitamin D 25-hydroxylase is expressed at a relatively constant and high level, so that circulating levels of 25-hydroxyvitamin D largely reflect the amount of precursor available for 25-hydroxylation. Because the hydroxyl group at the 25 carbon represents the second hydroxyl group on the molecule (see Figure 4-6), 25-hydroxyvitamin D is also referred to as **calcife***diol.*

25-Hydroxyvitamin D is further hydroxylated in the mitochondria of the proximal tubules of the kidney at either the 1α-carbon or 24-carbon position (Figures 4-6 and 4-7). The 1α-hydroxylase (also called **CYP1α** in humans) generates **1,25-dihydroxyvitamin D** (also called **calcitriol**), which is the most active form of vitamin D. Hydroxylation at the 24 carbon position, generating **24,25-dihydroxyvitamin D** and **1,24,25-trihydroxyvitamin D,** represents an inactivation pathway.

Vitamin D and its metabolites circulate in the blood primarily bound to **vitamin D-binding protein (DBP).** DBP is serum glycoprotein of about 60 kDa molecular weight that is related to the albumin gene family and is synthesized by the liver. DBP binds >85% of 25-hydroxyvitamin D and 1,25-dihydroxyvitamin D. Because of binding to other proteins, only 0.4% of the active metabolite, 1,25-dihydroxyvitamin D, circulates as free steroid. DBP allows for the movement of the highly lipophilic molecules within the aqueous environment of the blood. Studies utilizing experimental mouse genetics indicate that DBP provides a reservoir of vitamin D metabolites that protects against vitamin D deficiency. The bound fractions of

vitamin D metabolites have a circulating half-life of several hours.

DBP may assist in the reuptake of the fraction of 25-hydroxyvitamin D that passes through the glomerular filter. DBP binds to 25-hydroxyvitamin D with high affinity, so that the significant amount of 25-hydroxyvitamin D that enters the glomerular lumen is complexed to DBP. The apical membranes of the proximal tubule cells express the protein, **megalin,** which is a member of the low-density lipoprotein receptor (LDL receptor) superfamily. Megalin functions to recapture a broad range of proteins from the glomerular filtrate. Megalin binds DBP, some of which is complexed with 25-hydroxyvitamin D, and internalizes the complex via receptor-mediated endocytosis (see Figure 4-7).

The renal 1α-hydroxylase represents a key target of regulation of vitamin D action (Figure 4-8). First of all, there is a product feedback loop—in which 1,25-dihydroxyvitamin D inhibits 1α-hydroxylase expression—and stimulates 24-hydroxylase expression. Ca^{2+} is also an important regulator of the renal 1α-hydroxylase. Low circulating levels of Ca^{2+} indirectly stimulate renal 1α-hydroxylase expression through increased PTH levels, whereas elevated Ca^{2+} inhibits 1α-hydroxylase activity directly through the CaSR in the proximal tubule. A low phosphate diet also stimulates renal 1α-hydroxylase activity in a PTH-independent manner. Some of the effect of a low-phosphate diet on renal 1α-hydroxylase activity is dependent on a functional pituitary gland, which may respond to hypophosphatemia by increased growth hormone secretion (see Chapter 5).

The Vitamin D Receptor 1,25-Dihydroxyvitamin D exerts its actions primarily through binding to the **nuclear vitamin D receptor (VDR).** The VDR is a 50-kDa protein, and is a member of the nuclear hormone receptor superfamily, which also includes steroid and thyroid hormone receptors, and metabolic receptors such as the PPARs (see Chapter 1). The VDR is a transcription factor and binds to DNA sequences (**vitamin D-responsive elements**) as a heterodimer with the retinoid X receptor (RXR). Thus, a primary action of 1,25-dihydroxyvitamin D is to regulate gene expression in its target tissues, including the small intestine, bone, kidneys, and parathyroid gland.

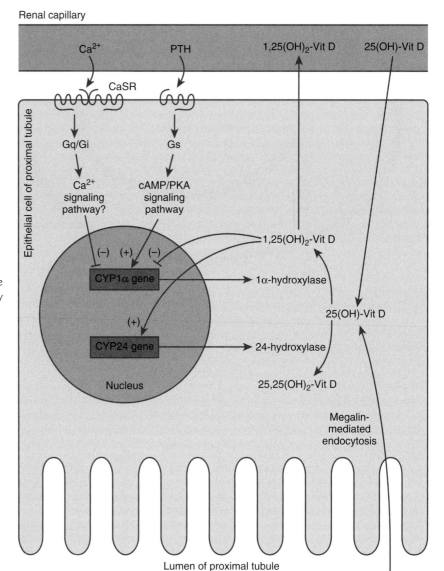

FIGURE 4-8 ■ Regulation of the renal Cyp1α gene expression by Ca^{2+} and hormones.

THE SMALL INTESTINE, BONE, AND KIDNEY DETERMINE Ca^{2+} AND Pi LEVELS

The general effects of PTH and 1,25-dihydroxyvitamin D on Ca^{2+} and Pi levels at the small intestine, bone, kidneys and parathyroid glands is summarized in Table 4-2.

Handling of Ca^{2+} and Pi by the Small Intestine

Dietary levels of calcium can vary, but in general, North Americans consume about 1.5 g of calcium per day. Of this, about 200 mg are absorbed by the proximal small intestine. Importantly, fractional absorption of calcium is stimulated by 1,25-dihydroxyvitamin D,

TABLE 4-2
Actions of PTH and 1,25-Dihydroxyvitamin D on Ca^{2+}/Pi Homeostasis

	SMALL INTESTINE	BONE	KIDNEY	PARATHYROID GLAND
PTH	No direct action	Promotes osteoblastic growth and survival Regulates M-CSF, RANKL, and OPG production by osteoblast Chronic high levels promote net Ca^{2+} and Pi release from bone	Stimulates 1a-hydroxylase activity Stimulates Ca^{2+} reabsorption by distal nephron by increasing. Inhibits Pi reabsorption by proximal nephron (represses NPT2a expression)	No direct action
1,25-dihydroxyvitamin D	Increases Ca^{2+} absorption by increasing TrpV channels, calbindin-D, and PMCA expression Marginally increases Pi absorption	Sensitizes osteoblasts to PTH Regulates osteoid production and calcification	Minimal actions on Ca^{2+} reabsorption Promotes Pi reabsorption by proximal nephron (stimulates NPT2a expression)	Directly inhibits PTH gene expression Directly stimulates CaSR gene expression

so that absorption can be made to be more efficient in the face of declining dietary calcium.

Ca^{2+} is absorbed from the duodenum and jejunum by both a Ca^{2+}- and hormonally-regulated, active-transport transcellular route, and by a passive, bulk-flow paracellular route. Little is known about whether the paracellular route is regulated. However, significant progress has been made in our understanding of the transcellular route (Figure 4-9). Ca^{2+} enters the transcellular route by gaining access to the intestinal enterocytes through the apical membrane. The movement of Ca^{2+} from the lumen of the GI tract into the enterocyte, which is favored both by concentration and electrochemical gradients, is facilitated by apical **epithelial calcium channels,** called **TrpV5** and **TrpV6.** Once inside, Ca^{2+} ions bind to abundant cytoplasmic

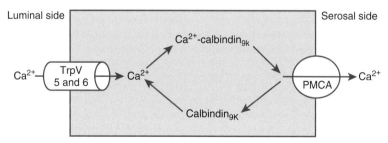

FIGURE 4-9 ■ Intestinal absorption of Ca^{2+} via the transcellular route. Ca^{2+} enters through the Ca^{2+} channel, TrpV5 or TrpV6, in the luminal membrane of the enterocyte. Ca^{2+} is then shuttled from the apical side of the cell to the basal side by the carrier protein, calbindin$_{9k}$. Ca^{2+} is then actively transported out of the basolateral side by the plasma membrane Ca^{2+} ATPase (PMCA), and calbindin$_{9k}$ recycles. 1,25-Dihydroxyvitamin D increases the expression of all of these proteins in the GI tract.

proteins called **calbindin-Ds,** specifically **calbindin-D_{9K}** in the human intestine. Calbindin-D_{9K} serves to maintain the low cytoplasmic free Ca^{2+} concentrations, thus preserving the favorable lumen-to-enterocyte concentration gradient during a meal. Calbindin-D_{9K} may also play a role in apical-to-basolateral shuttling of Ca^{2+}. Ca^{2+} is actively transported across the basolateral membrane against an electrochemical and concentration gradient by the **plasma membrane calcium ATPase (PMCA).** The **sodium/calcium exchanger (NCX)** may also contribute to the active transport of Ca^{2+} out of the enterocytes. 1,25-Dihydroxyvitamin D stimulates the expression of all of the components (i.e., TrpV channels, calbindin-D_{9K}, and PMCA) involved in Ca^{2+} uptake by the small intestine. PTH affects Ca^{2+} absorption at the gut indirectly by stimulating renal 1α-hydroxylase activity.

The fraction of phosphate absorbed by the jejunum remains relatively constant at about 70% and is under minor hormonal control by 1,25-dihydroxyvitamin D. The limiting process in transcellular Pi absorption is transport across the apical brush border, which is carried out by an isoform (NPT2b) of the **sodium/Pi co-transporter, NPT2.**

Handling of Ca^{2+} and Pi by Bone

Bone represents a massive and dynamic extracellular deposit of proteins and minerals (mainly Ca^{2+} and Pi). Once maximal bone mass has been achieved in the adult individual, the skeleton is constantly remodeled through the concerted activities of the resident bone cell types. The processes of **bone accretion** and **bone resorption** are in balance in a healthy, physically active and appropriately nourished individual. Of the approximately 1 kg of calcium immobilized in bone, about 500 mg of Ca^{2+} (i.e., 0.05% of skeletal calcium) is mobilized from and deposited into bone each day. However, the process of bone remodeling can be modulated in order to provide a net gain or loss of Ca^{2+} and Pi to the blood, and is responsive to physical activity (or lack thereof), diet, age, and hormonal regulation. Because the integrity of bone is absolutely dependent on Ca^{2+} and Pi, chronic dysregulation of Ca^{2+} and Pi levels, and/or of the hormones that regulate Ca^{2+} and Pi, lead to pathological changes in bone.

The Histophysiology of Adult Bone

The biogenesis, growth, and remodeling of bone is a complex process, and will not be fully explained here. The key features required to understand the role of adult bone in the hormonal regulation of calcium/phosphate metabolism are discussed subsequently.

Most of the bone (about 75%) is **compact, cortical bone** that makes up the outer surfaces of long and flat bones (Figure 4-10). The inner core of bones is composed of interconnecting spicules whose orientation becomes organized by stress forces. This bone is called **cancellous** (or **trabecular**) bone, and although it makes up only 25% of total bone mass, its surface area is several-fold greater than that of cortical bone. The greater surface area means that trabecular bone is much more accessible to bone cells, and thus more dynamic in its turnover.

In the adult, bone remodeling involves (1) the destruction of preformed bone, with the release of Ca^{2+}, Pi, and hydrolyzed fragments of the proteinaceous matrix (called **osteoid**) into the blood; and (2) new synthesis of osteoid at the site of resorption, and subsequent calcification of the osteoid, primarily with Ca^{2+} and Pi from the blood. Bone remodeling occurs continually in about 2 million discrete sites involving subpopulations of bone cells called **basic multicellular units.**

The cells involved in bone remodeling fall into two major classes: cells that promote the formation of bone **(osteoblasts),** and cells that promote the resorption of bone **(osteoclasts).** It should be emphasized, however, that the process of bone remodeling is a highly integrated process, and that osteoblasts also play a primary role in the initiation and regulation of bone resorption (Figure 4-11). Osteoblasts develop from mesodermally-derived stromal cells that have the potential to differentiate into muscle, adipose, cartilage and bone (i.e., osteoblasts) cells. Several paracrine and endocrine factors modulate the osteoblast differentiation program, which is dependent on the expression of bone-specific transcription factors. For example, the transcription factor Runx2 is essential for osteoblast differentiation and is mutated in patients with **cleidocranial dysplasia,** which is a congenital syndrome characterized by multiple defects in bone formation.

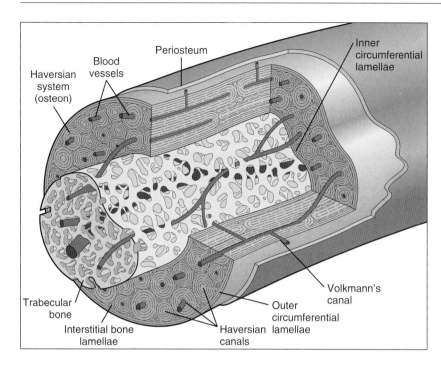

FIGURE 4-10 ■ Diagram of a typical long bone shaft showing compact, cortical bone around the perimeter and cancellous, trabecular bone in the center. *(From Stevens A, Lowe J: Human histology, ed 3, Philadelphia, 2005, Mosby.)*

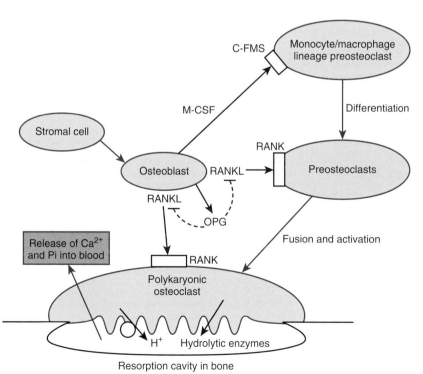

FIGURE 4-11 ■ Osteoblast regulation of osteoclast differentiation and function.

Osteoblasts express factors that induce osteoclast differentiation from cells of the monocyte/macrophage lineage and fully activate osteoclast function (see Figure 4-11). Osteoblasts release **monocyte-colony stimulating factor (M-CSF)**, which is a secreted cytokine that binds to its receptor, **c-Fms**, on osteoclast precursor cells. M-CSF induces the earliest differentiative processes that lead to osteoclast precursors. M-CSF also acts in concert with another factor, **RANKL** (named for *receptor activator of NF-κB ligand*), to promote osteoclastogenesis. RANKL can exist as a 40- to 45- kDa protein on the cell membrane of osteoblasts and as a soluble 31- kDa form. RANKL binds to its receptor, **RANK**, on osteoclast precursor membranes. RANK is structurally related to the receptor for **tumor necrosis factor-α (TNF-α)**, and signals through NF-κB-related pathways to induce osteoclastogenesis. This process involves the clustering and fusion of several osteoclast precursors, giving rise to a fused, polykaryonic osteoclast. The perimeter of the osteoclast membrane facing the bone adheres tightly to the bone, essentially sealing off the area of osteoclast-bone contact (see Figure 4-11). The osteoclast cell membrane facing the bone transforms into a **ruffled membrane**, from which enzymes (e.g., cathepsin K) and HCl are secreted. The acidic enzyme-rich microenvironment proceeds to dissolve the calcified crystals and ultimately hydrolyses type I collagen and other osteoid components. After about 2 weeks, osteoclasts receive a different signal from neighboring osteoblasts. This signal is **osteoprotegerin (OPG)**, which acts as a soluble decoy receptor for RANKL (see Figure 4-11). Consequently, the pro-osteoclastic signal from osteoblasts is terminated.

During a reversal phase, osteoclasts are then recruited to adjacent sites of bone, which extends the resorption cavity—also called the **cutting cone**—further into the bone. Alternatively, some osteoclasts may undergo apoptosis. Adjacent osteoblasts migrate into the resorbed area (now vacated by osteoclasts) and begin to lay down osteoid. Some of the components in osteoid (e.g., osteocalcin and alkaline phosphatase) promote its calcification. This process removes Ca^{2+} and Pi from the blood and deposits them first as calcium phosphate crystals. Later, bicarbonate and hydroxide ions are incorporated into the calcium phosphate to form **hydroxyapatite crystals.**

The bone is laid down in organized layers, called **lamellae,** starting from the perimeter of the resorption cavity and progressing inward. In the fully repaired region, multiple concentric lamellae surround a central **Haversian canal** or groove housing a nutritive capillary (see Figure 4-10). This area of bone accretion is also called the **closing cone.** As the osteoblasts become surrounded by and entrapped within bone, they become **osteocytes** that sit within small spaces, called **Haversian lacunae.** Osteocytes remain interconnected through cell processes that run within canaliculi and form communicating junctions with adjacent cell processes. The new concentric layers of bone, along with the interconnected osteocytes and the central canal, are referred to collectively as an **osteon.** The exact function(s) of osteocytes is unclear, although evidence exists for a role of osteocytes in the sensing of mechanical stress in bones.

The importance of the RANK/RANKL/osteoprotegerin system is made evident by mutations in the human genes for RANK and osteoprotegerin that are associated with bone deformities. Loss of RANKL in mice causes **osteopetrosis** (i.e., excessive bone density) because of the loss of osteoclasts. Conversely, loss of osteoprotegerin causes **osteoporosis** (reduced bone density) because of a high number of overly active osteoclasts. Furthermore, our current understanding of bone regulation is based on how hormones, cytokines, and other factors alter the balance between RANKL and on osteoprotegerin and on how they regulate the differentiation, survival, and apoptosis of osteoblasts versus osteoclasts.

As a calciotropic hormone, PTH is a primary endocrine regulator of bone remodeling in adults. The PTH/PTHrP receptor is expressed on osteoblasts, but not on osteoclasts. Therefore, PTH directly stimulates osteoblastic activity and stimulates osteoclastic activity indirectly through osteoblast-derived paracrine factors (i.e., M-CSF, RANKL). Intermittent administration of low doses of PTH promotes osteoblast survival and bone anabolic functions and increases bone density and reduces the risk of fracture in humans. In contrast, sustained elevated levels of PTH shift the balance to a relative increase in osteoclast activity, thereby increasing bone turnover and reducing bone density.

Regulation of bone remodeling by PTH requires normal levels of 1,25-dihydroxyvitamin D. In vitamin

D-deficient individuals, the Ca^{2+}-PTH secretion curve is shifted to the right. Thus, normal Ca^{2+} levels are less effective in suppressing PTH secretion, and elevated PTH levels and increased bone turnover result. The vitamin D receptor is expressed in osteoblasts, and normal 1,25-dihydroxyvitamin D levels are also required for coordination of osteoid production with its calcification. In vitamin D-deficient individuals, osteoid is not properly calcified and the bone is weak. In children, this leads to **rickets,** in which growth of long bones is abnormal and the weakened bones lead to bowing of extremities and collapse of the rib cage (see p. 101). In adults, vitamin D deficiency leads to **osteomalacia,** which is characterized by poorly calcified osteoid associated with pain, increased risk of fracture, and vertebral collapse (see p. 101).

Handling of Ca^{2+} and Pi by the Kidneys

The kidneys filter a large amount of Ca^{2+} (about 10 g) each day, but most of the filtered Ca^{2+} is reabsorbed by the nephron. Renal excretion typically accounts for the loss of about 200 mg of Ca^{2+}/day, which is counterbalanced by net intestinal absorption of about 200 mg/day. In the proximal tubule, most of the Ca^{2+} is reabsorbed by a passive, paracellular pathway. As in the duodenum, transcellular Ca^{2+} transport also exists and involves the constitutive expression of apical epithelial calcium channels (Trp-V5 and Trp-V6), intracellular Ca^{2+}-binding proteins (calbindins), and active Ca^{2+} extrusion (by PMCA and NCX) at the basolateral membrane. In contrast to the proximal nephron, Ca^{2+} uptake by the thick ascending limb of the loop of Henle and the distal convoluted tubule occurs solely via the transcellular route. This active reabsorption of Ca^{2+} by the distal nephron is stimulated by PTH (Figure 4-12).

As discussed, intestinal absorption of phosphate is largely proportional to the amount of phosphate in the diet and is only slightly regulated by 1,25-dihydroxyvitamin D. This leaves the kidney with an important role in the regulation of circulating phosphate levels. Phosphate is mostly reabsorbed by the proximal convoluted tubule via a hormonally-regulated transcellular route. As in the small intestine, phosphate enters the apical surface of the proximal tubules in a rate-limiting manner via a sodium-phosphate co-transporter (NPT). In contrast to the NPT isoform expressed in the intestine (NPT2b), the kidney expresses an additional isoform, NPT2a, which is under strong hormonal regulation. PTH downregulates NPT2a expression on the apical membranes of proximal renal tubule cells, thereby increasing phosphate excretion (see Figure 4-12). In contrast, 1,25-dihydroxyvitamin D increases NPT2 gene expression in the proximal tubules.

Integrated Physiologic Regulation of Ca^{2+}/Pi Metabolism: Response of PTH and 1,25-Dihydroxyvitamin D to a Hypocalcemic Challenge

The integrated response of PTH and 1,25-dihydroxyvitamin D to a hypocalcemic challenge is shown in Figures 4-13 and 4-14. Low blood Ca^{2+}, as detected by the CaSR on the parathyroid chief cells, stimulates PTH secretion. In the kidney, PTH rapidly increases Ca^{2+} levels by increasing fractional reabsorption of Ca^{2+} in the distal renal tubules. The renal effects of PTH on Ca^{2+} reabsorption are reinforced by Ca^{2+} levels as sensed by the CaSR, and to a lesser extent, by 1,25-dihydroxyvitamin D. PTH also inhibits the activity of the sodium-dependent phosphate transporter (NPT-2), thereby increasing Pi excretion. The relative loss of phosphate serves to increase free, ionized Ca^{2+} in the blood. At the bone, PTH stimulates osteoblasts to secrete RANKL, which, in turn, rapidly increases osteoclast activity, leading to increased bone resorption and the release of Ca^{2+} and Pi into the blood.

In a slower phase of the response to hypocalcemia, PTH and low Ca^{2+} directly stimulate 1α-hydroxylase (CYP1α) expression in the proximal renal tubule, thereby increasing 1,25-dihydroxyvitamin D levels. In the small intestine, 1,25-dihydroxyvitamin D supports adequate Ca^{2+} levels in the long-term by stimulating Ca^{2+} absorption. These effects occur over hours and days, and involve increasing the expression of TRPV5 and TRPV6 calcium channels, $calbindin_{9k}$, and PMCA.1,25-dihydroxyvitamin D also stimulates osteoblast release of RANKL, thereby amplifying the effect of PTH.

1,25-Dihydroxyvitamin D, and CaSR, play key roles in a negative feedback. Thus, elevated PTH stimulates 1,25-dihydroxyvitamin D production, which then

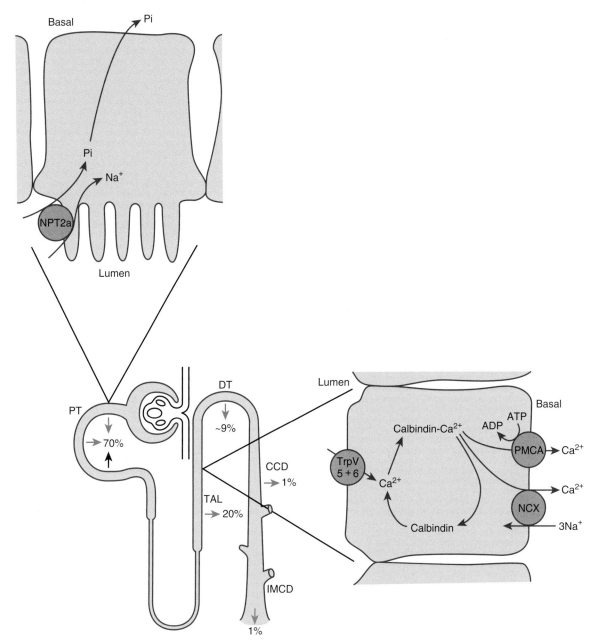

FIGURE 4-12 ■ Handling of Ca^{2+} and Pi by the distal nephron and proximal nephron, respectively. PTH stimulates Ca^{2+} reabsorption by the distal nephron and inhibits Pi reabsorption at the proximal tubule. *(Diagram of the nephron and the transport pattern of Ca^{2+} along the nephron is from Koeppen BM, Stanton BA: Renal physiology, ed 3, St. Louis, 2001, Mosby.)*

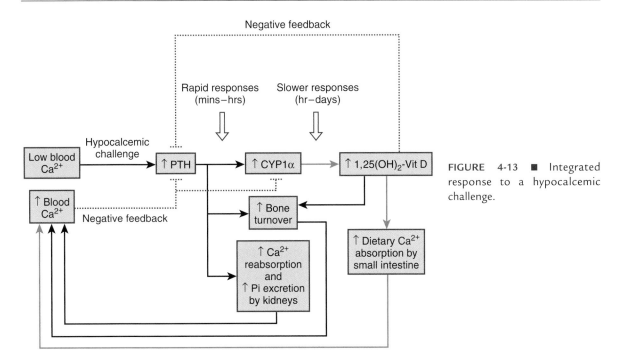

FIGURE 4-13 ■ Integrated response to a hypocalcemic challenge.

inhibits PTH gene expression directly, and indirectly by upregulating the CaSR. 1,25-Dihydroxyvitamin D also represses renal 1α-hydroxylase activity, while increasing 24-hydroxylase activity. As blood Ca^{2+} levels rise back to normal levels, they shut off PTH secretion and 1α-hydroxylase

Pharmacologic Hormonal Regulation of Calcium and Phosphate: Calcitonin

The primary actions of **calcitonin** are on bone and kidney. Calcitonin lowers serum calcium and phosphate levels, primarily by inhibiting bone resorption, in many species of animals. However, although human calcitonin can lower serum calcium and phosphate levels in humans, it takes high doses to show this effect. There are no definitive complications from calcitonin deficiency or excess in humans. For this reason, it is unlikely that calcitonin has an important physiologic role in humans. Medical interest in calcitonin stems from the fact that potent forms of calcitonin can be used therapeutically in the treatment of bone disorders. Calcitonin is also a useful histochemical marker of medullary thyroid cancer.

Parafollicular C Cells The cells that produce calcitonin are called the **parafollicular C cells.** These cells are derived from the ultimobranchial bodies and become incorporated and interspersed among the thyroid follicles as the thyroglossal duct migrates caudally. Parafollicular C cells do not invade the thyroid epithelium and thus are not in contact with the follicular colloid (see Chapter 6).

Structure, Synthesis, and Secretion of Calcitonin Calcitonin is a 32-amino acid polypeptide. Because there is minimal species variation, calcitonins from other species are biologically active in humans. In fact, salmon calcitonin is about 20 times more potent in humans than human calcitonin. Normal serum calcitonin levels are about 10 to 50 pg/ml, and its half-life in circulation is less than 1 hour. Because the primary site of inactivation is the kidney, serum calcitonin levels are often elevated in renal failure. Alternative splicing of the calcitonin gene in other tissues can produce **calcitonin gene–related peptide (CGRP),** which is a potent vasodilator and positive cardiac inotrope. The secretion of calcitonin is primarily regulated by the same CaSR that regulates PTH secretion. However, elevated extracellular

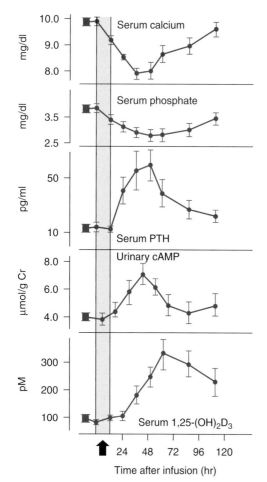

FIGURE 4-14 ■ Response of parathormone-calciferol axis to hypocalcemia. Eight patients with Paget's disease received mithramycin (25 μg/kg) by infusion (*shaded band*). Note that response of serum 1,25-$(OH)_2D_3$ lags 12 to 24 hours behind changes in serum parathormone (PTH) and urinary cyclic adenosine monophosphate (cAMP). (*Redrawn from Bilezikian JP, et al: N Engl J Med, 299:437, 1978.*)

Ca^{2+} levels stimulate the synthesis and secretion of calcitonin.

The Calcitonin Receptor The **calcitonin receptor** is closely related to the secretin and PTH/PTHrP receptors. It is a 7-transmembrane, gas-coupled receptor that acts primarily through cAMP-dependent signaling pathways. In contrast to the PTH/PTHrP receptor,

the calcitonin receptor is expressed in osteoclasts. Calcitonin acts rapidly and directly on osteoclasts to suppress bone resorption. **Paget's disease** is characterized by excessive bone turnover that is driven by large, bizarre osteoclasts (see p. 101). Because these osteoclasts retain the calcitonin receptor, active forms of calcitonin can be used to suppress aberrant osteoclastic activity in patients with this disease. The calcitonin receptor is also expressed in the nephron, where calcitonin inhibits phosphate and calcium reabsorption.

Hormonal Regulation of Calcium and Phosphate: Regulators Overexpressed by Cancers

Parathyroid Hormone-Related Peptide (PTHrP) This is a peptide paracrine factor that shows limited structural similarity to PTH, but nevertheless binds to and signals through the PTH/PTHrP receptor. PTHrP is expressed in several developing tissues, including the growth plate of bones and in the mammary glands. PTHrP is not regulated by circulating calcium and normally does not play a role in Ca^{2+}/Pi homeostasis in the adult. However, certain neoplasias can secrete high levels of PTHrP, which then produces symptoms of hyperparathyroidism (see later).

Fibroblast Growth Factor 23 (FGF23) This is an approximately 30-kDa peptide that is normally expressed at low levels in several tissues and that promotes phosphate excretion. FGF23 is inactivated by a protease that cleaves FGF23 into N-terminus and C-terminus peptides. One protease which appears to process FGF23 appears to be **PHEX** (for phosphate-regulating gene with homologies to endopeptidases on the X chromosome). PHEX is mutated in **X-linked hypophosphatemia,** characterized by renal phosphate wasting, rickets, osteomalacia, and inappropriate low/normal levels of 1,25-dihydroxyvitamin D. Current evidence indicates that when PHEX is mutated, FGF23 levels increase and inhibit both phosphate reabsorption and 1α-hydroxylase in the proximal renal tubules. Increased expression of FGF23 has been linked to patients with **autosomal-recessive hypophosphatemic rickets** and **tumor-induced rickets/ osteomalacia.**

Regulation of Ca^{2+}/Pi Metabolism by Immune/Inflammatory Cells

It is interesting to note that the RANKL/RANK/osteoprotegerin signaling system is similar to TNF receptor/NF-κB signaling pathways used in cells involved in the immune system and in inflammation. This link is further stressed by the fact that activated T cells express high levels of RANKL in response to stimulation by the cytokines, TNF-α, and several interleukins. Thus, inflammatory bone diseases (e.g., rheumatoid arthritis) are associated with increased RANKL/osteoprotegerin ratios in the vicinity of the inflammatory site, with subsequent erosions of bone and osteoporosis.

RANKL is also overproduced by cells associated with several malignant bone diseases (e.g., multiple myeloma, skeletal metastatic breast cancer). As noted earlier, some malignant cells also overexpress PTHrP, which induces RANKL expression in neighboring osteoblasts. Thus, several malignancies are associated with bone damage and hypercalcemia. The 1α-hydroxylase enzyme is expressed by monocytes and peripheral macrophages. In the autoimmune disease of sarcoidosis, overactive macrophages produce high levels of 1,25-dihydroxyvitamin D, resulting in hypercalcemia.

Regulation of Ca2+/Pi Metabolism by Gonadal and Adrenal Steroid Hormones

Gonadal and **adrenal steroid hormones** have profound effects on calcium and phosphate metabolism and skeletal health. **Estradiol-17β** (E_2; see Chapter 9) has a bone anabolic and calciotropic effect at several sites. E_2 stimulates intestinal calcium absorption and renal tubular calcium reabsorption. E_2 is also one of the most potent regulators of osteoblast and osteoclast function. Estrogen promotes survival of osteoblasts and apoptosis of osteoclasts, thereby favoring bone formation over resorption. In postmenopausal women, estrogen deficiency results in an initial phase of rapid bone loss that lasts about 5 years, followed by a second phase of slower bone loss. During the second phase, the individual is chronically challenged with hypocalcemia due to inefficient calcium absorption and renal calcium wasting. This can result in secondary hyperparathyroidism, which further exacerbates bone loss. Exercise and high levels of dietary calcium with supplemental vitamin D can prevent postmenopausal osteoporosis. **Androgens** also have bone anabolic and calciotropic effects, although some of these effects are due to the peripheral conversion of testosterone to E_2 (see Chapter 8).

In contrast to gonadal steroids, the **adrenal glucocorticoids** (e.g., **cortisol**) promote bone resorption and renal calcium wasting, and inhibits intestinal calcium absorption. Patients treated with high levels of a glucocorticoid (e.g., as an anti-inflammatory and immunosuppressive drug) can suffer glucocorticoid-induced osteoporosis.

PATHOLOGIC DISORDERS OF CALCIUM AND PHOSPHATE BALANCE

Hyperparathyroidism (Primary)

Primary hyperparathyroidism is caused by excessive production of PTH by the parathyroid glands. It is frequently caused by a single adenoma confined to one of the parathyroid glands. A common cause of parathyroid adenoma is the overexpression of the PRAD1 gene (parathyroid adenomatosis gene), which encodes the cell cycle regulator, cyclin D1.

Patients with primary hyperparathyroidism have high serum calcium levels and, in most cases, low serum phosphate levels. Hypercalcemia is a result of bone demineralization, increased GI calcium absorption (mediated by 1,25-dihydroxyvitamin D), and increased renal calcium reabsorption. The major symptoms of the disorder are directly related to increased bone resorption, hypercalcemia, and hypercalciuria (Figure 4-15). High serum calcium levels decrease neuromuscular excitability. People with hyperparathyroidism often show psychologic disorders, particularly depression, that may be associated with increased serum calcium levels (Box 4-1). Other neurologic symptoms include fatigue, mental confusion, and, at very high levels (greater than 15 mg/dl), coma. Hypercalcemia can cause cardiac arrest. Hypercalcemia can result in peptic ulcer formation because calcium increases gastrin secretion (see Chapter 2). Kidney stones (nephrolithiasis) are common because hypercalcemia eventually leads to

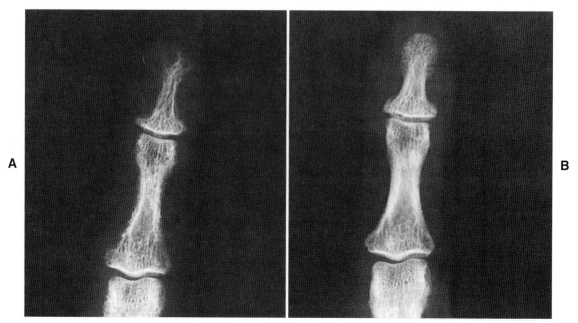

FIGURE 4-15 ■ Primary hyperparathyroidism. X-ray films of middle and distal phalanges of index finger show subperiosteal bone resorption of shafts and tip of distal phalanx (**A**). Second x-ray film was taken when bone had healed after treatment by removal of parathyroid hematoma (**B**). *(From Besser GM, Thorner MO: Clinical endocrinology, London, 1994, Mosby-Wolfe.)*

hypercalciuria and increased phosphate clearance leads to phosphaturia. The high urinary calcium and phosphate concentrations increase the tendency for precipitation of calcium-phosphate salts in the soft tissues of the kidney. When serum calcium levels exceed about 13 mg/dl with a normal phosphate level, the calcium phosphate **solubility product** is exceeded.

> ### BOX 4-1
> ### SYMPTOMS OF HYPERPARATHYROIDISM
>
> Kidney stones
> Osteoporosis
> Gastrointestinal disturbances, peptic ulcers, nausea, constipation
> Muscle weakness, decreased muscle tone
> Depression, lethargy, fatigue, mental confusion
> Polyuria
> High serum phosphate concentration; low serum calcium concentration

At this level, insoluble calcium phosphate salts form, which results in calcification of soft tissues such as blood vessels, skin, lungs, and joints.

People with hyperparathyroidism have evidence of increased bone turnover, such as elevated levels of serum alkaline phosphatase and osteocalcin, which indicate high osteoblastic activity, and increased urinary hydroxyproline levels, which indicate high bone resorptive activity. Hydroxyproline is an amino acid characteristically found in type I collagen. When the collagen is degraded, urinary hydroxyproline excretion increases. Although hyperparathyroidism will eventually cause **osteoporosis** (bone loss involving both osteoid and mineral), it is not necessarily the presenting symptom. However, bone demineralization is apparent. These individuals frequently exhibit **hyperchloremic acidosis.** They also show high urinary cAMP levels (Figure 4-16). Some people with hyperparathyroidism have the bone disorder **osteitis fibrosa cystica,** which is characterized by bone pain, multiple bone cysts, a tendency for pathologic fractures of long bones, and histologic abnormalities of the bone.

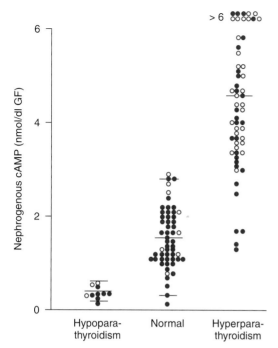

FIGURE 4-16 ■ Nephrogenous cyclic adenosine monophosphate (cAMP), expressed as function of glomerular filtration rate in control subjects and patients with primary hypoparathyroidism and hyperparathyroidism. *Open circles,* patients with renal impairment; *closed circles,* subjects with normal renal function; *long horizontal bars,* mean values; *short bars,* ±2 SD. GF, glomerular filtrate. *(Redrawn from Broadus AD, et al: J Clin Invest 60:77, 1977.)*

Pseudohypoparathyroidism

Pseudohypoparathyroidism is a rare familial disorder characterized by tissue resistance to PTH. In many instances, the problem is thought to originate with the PTH receptor. Often there is a decrease in levels of the guanine nucleotide-binding protein, Gs. Individuals with pseudohypoparathyroidism demonstrate increased PTH secretion and low serum calcium levels, sometimes associated with congenital defects of the skeleton, including shortened metacarpal and metatarsal bones.

Hypoparathyroidism

Hypoparathyroidism is associated with low serum calcium levels and high serum phosphate levels. The hypocalcemia results from both a PTH and a 1,25-dihydroxyvitamin D deficiency. Consequently, there is a decrease in bone calcium mobilization by both osteoclastic resorption and osteocytic osteolysis. Because 1,25-dihydroxyvitamin D is deficient, GI absorption of calcium is impaired. The PTH deficiency decreases renal calcium reabsorption, thereby decreasing fractional calcium reabsorption. Although fractional calcium reabsorption decreases, the urinary calcium level is generally low. Urinary cAMP concentration also decreases (see Figure 4-16). Alkalosis occurs because bicarbonate excretion decreases; this further lowers the free calcium level in serum. Although the serum calcium level is low, bone demineralization is usually not a problem because of the high serum phosphate level. Hypocalcemia increases neuromuscular excitability, increasing the possibility of tetany and even convulsions. Hypocalcemia alters cardiac function. It can produce a first-degree heart block. The low serum calcium level decreases myocardial contractility.

The most prominent symptom of hypoparathyroidism is increased neuromuscular excitability (Box 4-2). Low serum calcium concentrations decrease the neuromuscular threshold. This can be manifested as repetitive responses to a single stimulus and as spontaneous neuromuscular discharge. The increased neuromuscular excitability can result in tingling in the fingers or toes (paresthesia), muscle cramps, or even tetany. Laryngeal spasms can be fatal. Sometimes the serum calcium level is not low enough to produce overt tetany, but a latent tetany can be demonstrated by inflating a blood pressure cuff on the arm to a pressure greater than systolic pressure for

---

BOX 4-2
SYMPTOMS OF HYPOPARATHYROIDISM

Tetany, convulsions, paresthesias, muscle cramps
Decreased myocardial contractility
First-degree heart block
Central nervous system problems, including irritability and psychosis
Intestinal malabsorption
Low serum calcium concentration; high serum phosphate concentration

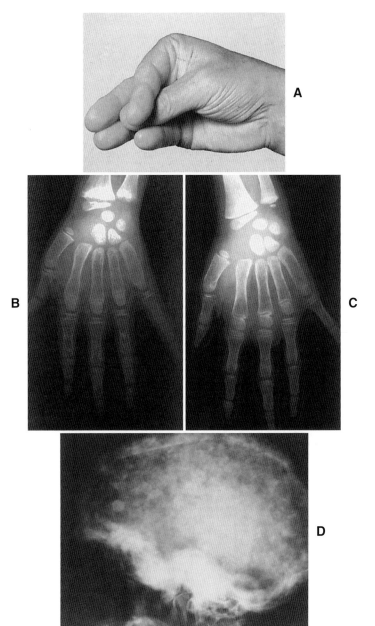

FIGURE 4-17 ■ **A,** Position of hand in hypocalcemic tetany. **B,** X-ray film of left hand of 9-year-old boy with rickets caused by malnutrition. He would eat only potato chips. All of bony structures are osteopenic. Note widening of space between provisional zone of calcification and epiphysis of left radius. **C,** After 2 months of forced feedings, rickets has subsided. Note decreased width of space between provisional zone of calcification and epiphysis of radius and increased bone calcification. **D,** X-ray film of skull of patient with Paget's disease. Thickness of skull is increased and sclerotic changes are seen scattered throughout skull, consistent with healing phase of Paget's disease. (*A from Hall R, Evered DC: Color atlas of endocrinology, ed 2, London, 1990, Mosby-Wolfe; **B** to **D** courtesy Dr. C. Joe.*)

2 minutes. The resultant oxygen deficiency precipitates overt tetany as demonstrated by **carpal-pedal spasms.** This is called **Trousseau's sign** (Figure 4-17 A). Another test is to tap the facial nerve, which evokes facial muscle spasms (**Chvostek's sign**).

Treatment of hypoparathyroidism is difficult because of the lack of readily available effective human PTH. The disorder is frequently treated with a high-calcium diet, vitamin D, and occasionally thiazide diuretics to decrease renal calcium clearance.

Thiazide diuretics increase calcium reabsorption in the thick ascending limb of the loop of Henle. Acute hypocalcemia can be treated with intravascular calcium gluconate infusion.

Hypomagnesemia resulting from either severe malabsorption or chronic alcoholism can cause hypoparathyroidism. Hypomagnesemia impairs the secretion of PTH and decreases the biological response to PTH.

Vitamin D Deficiency

Vitamin D deficiency produces hypocalcemia and hypomagnesemia and decreases GI absorption of calcium and phosphate. The drop in the serum calcium level stimulates PTH secretion, which stimulates renal phosphate clearance, thereby aggravating the serum phosphate loss. Since the level of the calcium phosphate product in serum, and hence in body fluids, is low, bone mineralization is impaired and demineralization is increased. This leads to osteomalacia in adults or rickets in children. The secondary elevation in PTH can produce osteoporosis. Rickets and osteomalacia are disorders in which bone mineralization is defective. Osteoid is formed, but it does not mineralize adequately. If the calcium phosphate product level or the pH in bone fluid bathing the osteoid is low, demineralization rather than mineralization is favored. Rickets is caused by a vitamin D deficiency before skeletal maturation; it involves problems in not only the bone but also in the cartilage of the growth plate (see Figure 4-17B and C). *Osteomalacia* is the term used when inadequate bone mineralization occurs after skeletal growth is complete and the epiphyses have closed.

Paget's Disease

Paget's disease results in bone deformities. It is characterized by an increase in bone resorption followed by an increase in bone formation. The new bone is generally abnormal and often irregular. Serum alkaline phosphatase and osteocalcin levels are increased, as are those of urinary hydroxyproline. Pain, bone deformation, and bone weakness can occur (see Figure 4-17D).

Bone Problems of Renal Failure (Renal Osteodystrophy)

Approximately 0.9 g, or more than 50% of dietary phosphate, is normally lost in the urine in 1 day. Consequently, the kidneys serve as the major excretory route for phosphate. As renal function, and hence phosphate clearance, decreases, the serum phosphate concentration rises. The increase in serum phosphate concentration will lower serum calcium levels by exceeding the solubility product and hence increasing calcium-phosphate precipitation. A drop in the serum calcium level is an effective stimulus for PTH, and serum PTH levels also rise (Figure 4-18). In addition, vitamin D activation by 1α-hydroxylase occurs in the renal proximal tubules. In kidney failure, vitamin D activation is impaired, which decreases GI absorption of calcium and phosphate. This results in a further drop in the serum calcium level and aggravates the

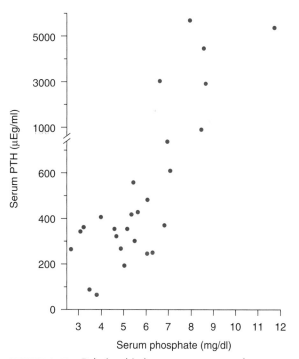

FIGURE 4-18 ■ Relationship between serum parathormone (PTH) level and serum phosphate level in patients with renal failure. *(Redrawn from Bordier PF, Marie PF, Arnaud CD: Kidney Int 7[suppl 2]:102, 1975.)*

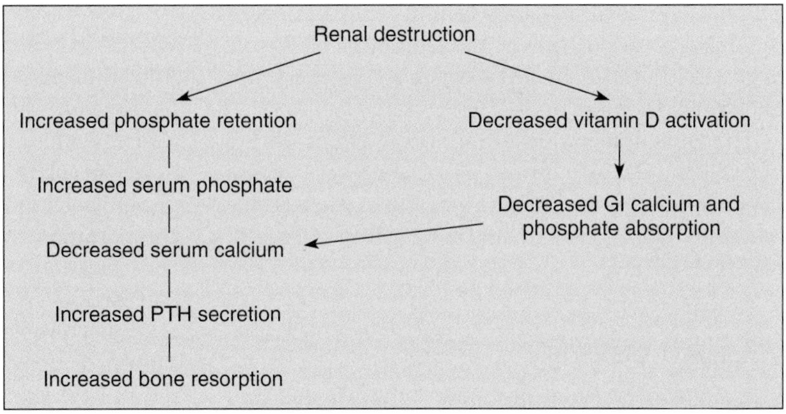

FIGURE 4-19 ■ The physiologic basis of bone loss in renal failure. PTH, parathormone; GI, gastrointestinal.

preexisting problem with excess PTH secretion. The result is to stimulate bone resorption and demineralization. As bone demineralization occurs, it will aggravate the hyperphosphatemia because the renal mechanisms of counteracting the hyperphosphatemia are now defective. Figure 4-19 shows the effect of renal impairment on phosphate, calcium, vitamin D, and PTH.

SUMMARY

1. Serum calcium levels are a function of the rate calcium enters from GI absorption and bone demineralization and leaves through bone mineralization, GI excretion, and renal excretion. Serum calcium levels are normally maintained within a narrow range.

2. Serum phosphate levels are determined by the rate phosphate enters from GI absorption, soft tissue efflux, and bone demineralization and leaves through GI excretion, soft tissue influx, bone mineralization, and renal excretion. Serum phosphate levels normally fluctuate over a relatively wide range.

3. The major physiologic hormones regulating serum calcium and phosphate levels are parathyroid hormone (PTH) and 1,25-dihydroxyvitamin D (calcitriol). Calcitonin is an important pharmacologic regulator of calcium and phosphate.

4. PTH is an 84-amino acid peptide whose expression is regulated by serum Ca^{2+} through the Ca^{2+}-sensing receptor (CaSR) and 1,25-dihydroxyvitamin D. PTH is made by the principal cells of the parathyroid glands. PTH binds to the PTH/PTHrP receptor,

which is primarily coupled to a Gs/cAMP/PKA pathway.

5. Vitamin D can be synthesized from 7-dehydrocholesterol in skin in the presence of ultraviolet light. It is hydroxylated to 25-hydroxycholecalciferol (calcifidiol) in the liver and activated by renal 1α-hydroxylase to 1,25-dihydroxycholecalciferol (calcitriol). PTH stimulates the renal 1α-hydroxylase activity, whereas 1,25-dihydroxyvitamin D negatively feeds back on the enzyme. 1,25-Dihydroxyvitamin D binds to a nuclear vitamin D receptor (VDR), which regulates specific gene expression.

6. 1,25-Dihydroxyvitamin D strongly promotes intestinal Ca^{2+} absorption, and weakly increases Pi absorption. PTH has little, if any, direct effect at the intestine.

7. Osteoblasts are bone-forming cells that are of mesenchymal origin. They synthesize bone matrix and produce an environment that promotes bone mineralization. Osteocytes are osteoblasts that have become entrapped in bone. Osteoclasts are large, multinucleate cells derived from hematopoietic

stem cells. Mature, activated osteoclasts secrete enzymes and acid that resorb bone.

8. The flux of Ca^{2+} and Pi into and out of bone is determined by the relative activities of osteoblasts versus osteoclasts, which exists as basic multicellular units at about 2 million sites within bone. Bone resorption is initiated by osteoblasts, which recruit and activate monocyte/macrophage-lineage cells to become mature polykaryonic osteoclasts. This occurs through the expression of M-CSF and RANKL by osteoblasts, which bind to their receptors, C-FMS and RANK, respectively, on osteoclasts. Bone repair is initiated by the release of osteoprotegerin (OPG) from osteoblasts, which acts as a soluble decoy for RANKL. This causes osteoclasts to stop bone resorption and either move to a new resorption site or undergo apoptosis. Osteoblasts then secrete osteoid, which undergoes calcification. As osteoblasts secrete osteoid in a lamellar, outside-in, configuration, they reform osteons.

9. The PTH/PTHrP receptor is expressed on the osteoblast, not the osteoclast. PTH promotes osteoblast differentiation, proliferation, and survival; intermittent administration of PTH promotes bone formation. PTH also increases M-CSF and RANKL expression by osteoblasts, and a chronic high level of PTH shifts the balance in favor of bone resorption.

10. 1,25-Dihydroxyvitamin D acts through the VDR on osteoblasts to increase osteoblast differentiation, promote secretion of normal osteoid components, and sensitize osteoblasts to PTH.

11. PTH increases the fractional reabsorption of calcium at the distal nephron. However, because the filtered load of calcium increases, renal excretion of calcium typically increases after PTH administration. PTH decreases renal Pi and bicarbonate reabsorption. 1,25-Dihydroxyvitamin D increases both Ca^{2+} and Pi reabsorption by the kidney.

12. Calcitonin acts on osteoclasts to inhibit their bone-resorptive function and on the kidney to inhibit Ca^{2+} reabsorption. Although active analogs of calcitonin are a useful pharmacologic agent for the treatment of imbalances in Ca^{2+} homeostasis (e.g., Paget's disease), endogenous human calcitonin does not play an important role in Ca^{2+}/Pi homeostasis.

13. Other factors that regulate Ca^{2+} and/or Pi levels, either physiologically or pathophysiologically, include PTHrP, FGF23, gonadal steroids, and adrenal steroids.

14. Patients with hyperparathyroidism typically have hypercalcemia, hypophosphatemia, hyperchloremia, and acidosis. They are prone to kidney stones because of hypercalciuria and hyperphosphaturia.

15. Patients with hypoparathyroidism typically have hypocalcemia, hyperphosphatemia, hypochloremia, and alkalosis. They may show symptoms of increased neuromuscular excitability such as paresthesias, muscle cramps, and tetany.

16. Children with a vitamin D deficiency are prone to develop rickets, whereas adults with a vitamin D deficiency develop osteomalacia. The vitamin D deficiency results in decreased GI absorption of calcium, phosphate, and magnesium.

KEY WORDS AND CONCEPTS

- 1,25-Dihydroxyvitamin D
- Calcitriol
- Parathyroid hormone (PTH)
- Hypocalcemia
- Hypercalcemia
- Inorganic phosphate (Pi)
- Hyperphosphatemia
- Calciotropic hormones
- Parathyroid glands
- Principal (chief) cell
- Oxyphil cell
- Prepro-PTH
- Pro-PTH
- Ca^{2+}-sensing receptor (CaSR)
- Familial benign hypocalciuric hypercalcemia (FBHH)
- Neonatal severe hyperparathyroidism
- Calcium response element
- PTH/PTHrP receptor
- 1,25-dihydroxyvitamin D
- Cholecalciferol
- Vitamin D-binding protein (DBP)
- Nuclear vitamin D–receptor (VDR)

- Vitamin D responsive elements
- Calcium channels
- TrpV5
- TrpV6
- Calbindin-Ds
- Calbindin-D$_{9K}$
- Plasma membrane calcium ATPase (PMCA)
- Sodium/calcium exchanger (NCX)
- Sodium/Pi co-transporter, NPT2
- Compact cortical bone
- Cancellous (trabecular) bone
- Osteoid
- Basic multicellular units
- Osteoblasts
- Osteoclasts
- Cleidocranial dysplasia
- Monocyte colony–stimulating factor
- Cacitonin gene–related peptide (CGRP)
- Parafollicular C cells
- Paget's disease
- Parathyroid hormone–related peptide (PTHrP)
- Fibroblast growth factor 23 (FGF23)
- X-linked hypophosphatemia
- Autosomal-recessive hypophosphatemic rickets
- Tumor-induced rickets/osteomalacia
- Gonadal/adrenal steroid hormones
- Estradiol-17β
- Adrenal corticoids (cortisol)
- Solubility product
- Osteoporosis
- Hyperchloremic acidosis
- Osteitis fibrosa cystica
- Carpal-pedal spasms
- Trousseau's sign
- Chvostek's sign

SELF-STUDY PROBLEMS

1. How would the loss of 1,25-dihydroxyvitamin D directly and indirectly alter PTH secretion?
2. What is the relation between osteoblasts and bone resorption?
3. Why does unregulated overproduction of PTHrP (e.g., produced by a tumor) cause hypercalcemia?
4. What would be the effect of overproduction of osteoprotegerin on bone density?

5. How does vitamin D deficiency affect Pi levels? Why?
6. Although PTH increases renal calcium reabsorption, excess PTH typically increases urinary calcium excretion. Why does this occur?
7. Why would long-acting forms of calcitonin be useful in the treatment of Paget's disease?
8. What is the physiologic basis for cardiac arrest in hyperparathyroidism?
9. What is the physiologic basis for polyuria and nocturia in hyperparathyroidism?
10. Why would hyperchloremic acidosis develop in people with hyperparathyroidism?
11. Why would urinary cAMP increase after PTH administration?
12. Why are the urinary calcium level and fractional reabsorption of calcium typically low in hypoparathyroidism?
13. Why would the alkalosis produced by hypoparathyroidism decrease serum free calcium levels?
14. Why does the low serum calcium level produced by hypoparathyroidism decrease myocardial contractility?
15. What is indicated when serum alkaline phosphatase, hydroxyproline, and osteocalcin levels increase?

BIBLIOGRAPHY

Bouillon RS, Van Cromphaut, Carmeliet G: Intestinal calcium absorption: molecular vitamin D-mediated mechanisms, *J Cell Biochem* 88(2):332-339, 2003.

Boyle WJ, Simonet WS, Lacey DL: Osteoclast differentiation and activation, *Nature* 423(6937):337-342, 2003.

Chen RA, Goodman WG: Role of the calcium-sensing receptor in parathyroid gland physiology, *Am J Physiol Renal Physiol* 286(6):F1005-1011, 2004.

Christakos SP, Dhawan, Lin Y et al: New insights into the mechanisms of vitamin D action, *J Cell Biochem* 88(4):695-705, 2003.

Fukagawa M, Kazama JJ, Kurokawa K: Renal osteodystrophy and secondary hyperparathyroidism, *Nephrol Dial Transplant* 17 Suppl 10:2-5, 2002.

Goodman WG, Juppner H, Salusky IB, Sherrad DJ: Parathyroid hormone (PTH), PTH-derived peptides, and new PTH assays in renal osteodystrophy, *Kidney Int* 63(1):1-11, 2003.

Harada SG, Rodan GA: Control of osteoblast function and regulation of bone mass, *Nature* 423(6937):349-355, 2003.

Hewison M, Zehnder D, Bland R, Stewart FM: 1-Alpha-hydroxylase and the action of vitamin D, *J Mol Endocrinol* 25(2):141-148, 2000.

Hofbauer LC, Schoppet M: Clinical implications of the osteoprotegerin/RANKL/RANK system for bone and vascular diseases, *JAMA* 292(4):490-495, 2004.

Khosla S: Minireview: the OPG/RANKL/RANK system, *Endocrinology* 142(12):5050-5055, 2001.

Murray TM, Rao LG, Divieti P, Bringhurst FR: Parathyroid hormone secretion and action: evidence for discrete receptors for the carboxyl-terminal region and related biological actions of carboxyl-terminal ligands, *Endocr Rev* 26(1):78-113, 2005.

Nykjaer A, Dragun D, Walther P et al: An endocytic pathway essential for renal uptake and activation of the steroid 25-(OH) vitamin D3, *Cell* 96(4):507-515, 1999.

Omdahl JL, Morris HA, May BK: Hydroxylase enzymes of the vitamin D pathway: expression, function, and regulation, *Annu Rev Nutr* 22:139-166, 2002.

Schiavi SC, Kumar R: The phosphatonin pathway: new insights in phosphate homeostasis, *Kidney Int* 65(1):1-14, 2004.

Takeda E, Yamamoto H, Nashiki K: Inorganic phosphate homeostasis and the role of dietary phosphorus, *J Cell Mol Med* 8(2):191-200, 2004.

White P, Cooke N: The multifunctional properties and characteristics of vitamin D-binding protein, *Trends Endocrinol Metab* 11(8):320-327, 2000.

RECOMMENDED READING

For more information on the handling of Ca^{2+} and Pi by the small intestine, please see Johnson L: *Gastrointestinal physiology*, ed 7, Philadelphia 2007, Mosby.

For more information on the handling of Ca^{2+} and Pi by the kidney, please see Koeppen BM & Stanton BA: Renal Physiology, ed 4, 2007, Mosby.

5

THE HYPOTHALAMUS-PITUITARY COMPLEX

OBJECTIVES

1. The embryology and anatomy of the pituitary gland will be discussed.

2. The function of the neurohypophysis will be discussed, including the synthesis, regulation, and function of two neurohormones—antidiuretic hormone (ADH; also called vasopressin) and oxytocin.

3. The neurovascular connection between the hypothalamus and the adenohypophysis will be discussed.

4. The concept of an endocrine axis will be developed.

5. The cytology of the adenohypophysis will be described, along with the structure and function of the six hormones produced by the adenohypophysis.

6. Growth hormone and prolactin have significant direct effects on nonendocrine organs, and these will be discussed.

7. Some forms of pituitary pathophysiology will be presented.

The **pituitary gland** (also called the **hypophysis**) is a small (about 0.5 g in weight) yet complex endocrine structure at the base of the forebrain (Figure 5-1A and B). It is composed of an epithelial component, called the **adenohypophysis,** and a neural structure, called the **neurohypophysis.** The adenohypophysis is composed of five cell types that secrete six hormones. The neurohypophysis acts as a site of release of multiple neurohormones. All endocrine functions of the pituitary gland are regulated by the hypothalamus and by negative and positive feedback loops.

EMBRYOLOGY AND ANATOMY

Microscopic examination of the pituitary reveals two distinct types of tissues: epithelial and neural (Figure 5-1C and D). This dual nature of the gland is best understood by reviewing its development.

During development, a caudal extension of the primitive forebrain (i.e., the diencephalon) grows toward the roof of the primitive oral cavity (Figure 5-2). This neural down growth, called the **infundibulum,** secretes factors that induce the epithelium of the roof of the oral cavity to extend cranially toward the base of the developing brain. This extension of the oral ectoderm is called **Rathke's pouch.** As Rathke's pouch moves upward, the following events occur:

1. Rathke's pouch loses its contact with the oral cavity, and, by doing so, becomes a ductless, endocrine structure. Remnants of Rathke's pouch may persist, and can give rise to **craniopharyngiomas.**

2. Rathke's pouch comes into direct contact with the infundibulum. The cells on the side of the pouch lumen facing the infundibulum give rise to the **pars intermedia** in the fetus. These cells die in the adult human. The cells on the side of the pouch

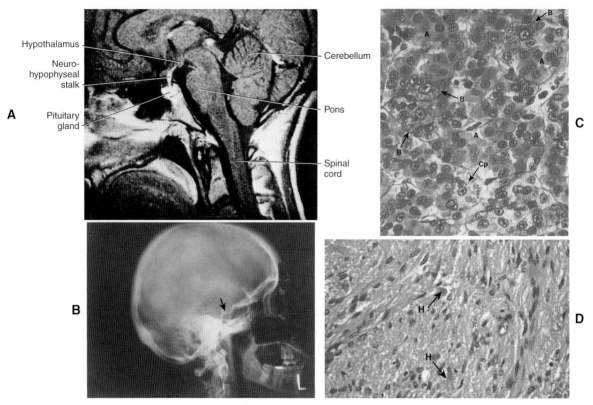

FIGURE 5-1 ■ **A,** Magnetic resonance image of the head shows the proximity of the hypothalamus and pituitary gland and their connection by a neurohypophyseal (pituitary) stalk. **B,** Pituitary gland is located in the sella turcica (*arrow*). *(**A,** Courtesy of Steven Weiner, MD. From Berne RM, Levy MN, Koeppen BM, Stanton BA: Physiology, ed 5, St. Louis, 2004, Mosby; **B,** Courtesy Dr. C. Joe.)* **C.** Histology of pars distalis. B, basophil; A, acidophil; Cp, chromophobe **D.** Histology of pars nervosa. H, Herring bodies. **C+D** from Wheater's Functional Histology, 5 ed; Young B, Lowe JS, Stevens A, Heath JW 2006, Churchill Livingstone.

lumen facing away from the infundibulum expand considerably and give rise to the **pars distalis.** The pars distalis makes up almost all of the adenohypophysis in the adult and is also referred to as the **anterior lobe of the pituitary** (or simply the **anterior pituitary**). A third division of Rathke's pouch develops into the **pars tuberalis** and is composed of a thin layer of cells that wrap around the infundibular stalk at its superior end. To summarize, the adenohypophysis (i.e., the epithelial pituitary) develops from epithelial cells (the oral ectoderm) and is composed of the pars distalis, a thin layer

called the pars tuberalis and the pars intermedia, which is lost in adult humans.

3. The infundibular process expands at its lower end to give rise to a structure called the **pars nervosa.** The pars nervosa is also called the **posterior lobe of the pituitary** (or simply, the **posterior pituitary**). At the superior end of the infundibulum, a funnel-shaped swelling develops called the **median eminence.** The rest of the infundibulum, which extends from the medium eminence down to the pars nervosa, is called the **infundibulum.** To summarize, the neurohypophysis develops from a down

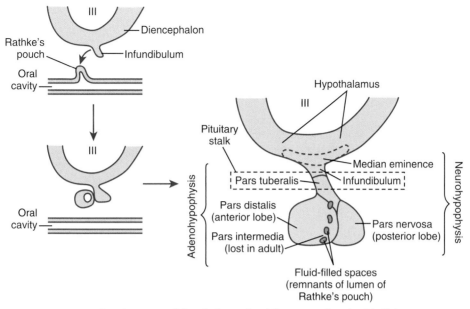

FIGURE 5-2 ■ Development of the pituitary gland from neural and epithelial sources.

growth of neural tissue at the base of the dien-cephalon (corresponding to the hypothalamus in the adult), and gives rise to the pars nervosa, the infundibulum, and the median eminence. The infundibulum and the pars tuberalis make up the **pituitary stalk**.

With development, the pituitary gland becomes encased in the sphenoid bone in a structure called the **sella turcica** (see Figure 5-1). The pituitary stalk emerges superiorly out of the sella turcica in the vicin-ity of the optic nerves and optic chiasm. Generally, cancers of the pituitary have only one way to expand, which is up into the brain and against the optic nerves. Thus, any increase in the size of the pituitary is often associated with dizziness and/or vision problems. The sella turcica is sealed off from the brain by a membrane called the **diaphragma sellae.** Defective development of the diaphragma sellae can allow cere-brospinal fluid to enter the sellar cavity and encroach on developing pituitary tissue. This can give rise to "**empty sella syndrome,**" which represents a reduc-tion of pituitary tissue (but not always pituitary func-tion) within the sella turcica.

THE NEUROHYPOPHYSIS

The pars nervosa is a **neurovascular** structure that is the site of release of neurohormones adjacent to a rich bed of fenestrated capillaries. The peptide hormones that are released are ADH and oxytocin. The cell bodies of the neurons that project to the pars nervosa are located in the **supraoptic nuclei (SON)** and **paraventricular nuclei (PVN)** of the **hypothalamus** (in this context, a "nucleus" refers to a collection of neuronal cell bodies residing within the CNS—a "ganglion" is a collection of neuronal cell bodies residing outside the CNS). The cells bodies of these neurons are described as **magnocellular** (i.e., large cell bodies), and are equipped with enough biosynthetic capacity to produce a short-lived peptide hormone that is released into and diluted by the peripheral circulation. The magnocellular neurons project axons down the infundibular stalk as the **hypothalamohypophyseal tracts.** These axons terminate in the pars nervosa (Figure 5-3). In addition to axonal processes and termini from the SON and PVN, there are glial-like supportive cells called **pituicytes.** As is typical of endocrine organs, the posterior pituitary is extensively vascularized

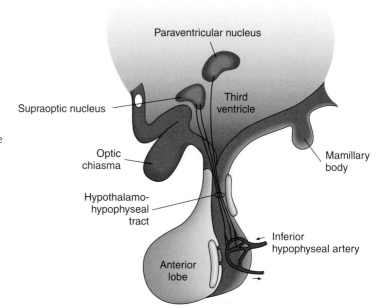

FIGURE 5-3 ■ Axonal projections from the PVN and SON to the pars nervosa.

and the capillaries are fenestrated, thereby facilitating diffusion of hormones into the vasculature.

Synthesis of ADH (Vasopressin) and Oxytocin

ADH and oxytocin are nonapeptides (nine amino acids) and are similar in structure—differing in only two amino acids (Figure 5-4). They have limited overlapping activity. ADH (vasopressin) and oxytocin are synthesized as preprohormones. Each prohormone harbors the structure of oxytocin or ADH, each of which is composed of 9 amino acids and a co-secreted peptide called either **neurophysin I** (associated with ADH) or **neurophysin II** (associated with oxytocin). These preprohormones are called **preprovasophysin** and **prepro-oxyphysin.** The N-signal peptide is cleaved as the peptide is transported into the endoplasmic reticulum. The prohormone is packaged in the endoplasmic reticulum and Golgi in a membrane-bound secretory granule in the cell bodies within the SON and PVN (Figure 5-5). The secretory granules are conveyed intra-axonally through a "fast" (i.e., mm/hr) ATP-dependent transport mechanism down the infundibular stalk to the axonal termini in the pars nervosa. During transit of the secretory granule, the prohormones are proteolytically cleaved, producing equimolar amounts of hormone and neurophysin. Secretory granules containing fully processed peptides are stored in the axonal termini. Axonal swellings due

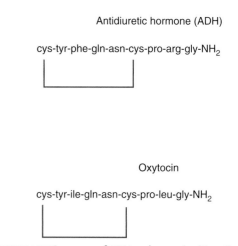

FIGURE 5-4 ■ Structure of ADH and oxytocin. (*From Berne RM, Levy MN, Koeppen BM, Stanton BA: Physiology, ed 5, St. Louis, 2004, Mosby.*)

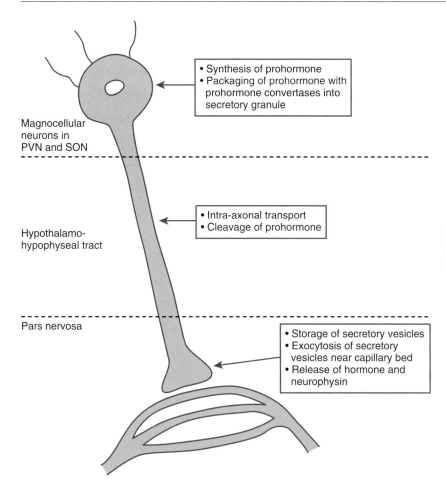

Magnocellular
neurons in
PVN and SON

• Synthesis of prohormone
• Packaging of prohormone with
  prohormone convertases into
  secretory granule

Hypothalamo-
hypophyseal tract

• Intra-axonal transport
• Cleavage of prohormone

Pars nervosa

• Storage of secretory vesicles
• Exocytosis of secretory
  vesicles near capillary bed
• Release of hormone and
  neurophysin

FIGURE 5-5 ■ Intra-axonal transport and processing of preprova-sophysin and prepro-oxyphysin.

to the storage of secretory granules can be observed by light microscopy with certain stains and are termed **Herring bodies** (Figure 5-1D).

ADH and oxytocin are released at the pars nervosa in response to stimuli that are primarily detected at the cell body and its dendrites in the SON and PVN of the hypothalamus. The stimuli are primarily in the form of neurotransmitters released from hypothalamic interneurons. On sufficient stimulus, the neurons will depolarize and propagate an action potential down the axon. At the axonal termini, the action potential increases intracellular Ca^{2+} and results in a stimulus-secretion response, with the exocytosis of ADH or oxytocin, along with neurophysins, into the extracellular fluid of the pars nervosa (see Figure 5-5). Both hormones and neurophysins gain access to the

peripheral circulation, and both can be measured in the blood.

There is no known biological function for circulating neurophysins. However, several mutations in familial diabetes insipidus (in which ADH production is deficient) have been mapped to mutations within the neurophysin structure, suggesting that the sequence and structure of the neurophysin portion is important for the correct processing of the prohormone.

Because posterior pituitary hormones are synthesized in the hypothalamus rather than the pituitary, hypophysectomy (pituitary removal) does not necessarily permanently disrupt synthesis and secretion of these hormones. Immediately after hypophysectomy, secretion of the hormones decreases. However, over a period of weeks, the severed proximal end of the tract will show histologic modification and pituicytes will form around the neuron terminals. Secretory vacuoles are visible and secretion of hormone resumes from this proximal end. Secretion of hormone can actually potentially return to normal levels. In contrast, a lesion higher up on the pituitary stalk can lead to loss of the neuronal cell bodies in the PVN and SON.

Antidiuretic Hormone

Actions of ADH The primary functions of ADH in humans are the maintenance of normal osmolality of body fluids and maintenance of normal blood volume. The primary target cells of the ADH are the cells lining the distal renal tubule and the principal cells of the collecting ducts in the kidney. ADH binds to the **vasopressin 2 (V2) receptor** on the basal side of renal cells (Figure 5-6). The V2 receptor is a GPCR linked to Gs-cAMP-PKA pathway. Signaling from the V2 receptor induces the insertion of vesicles containing the water channel protein, called **aquaporin 2,** into the apical membrane of the principal cells, thereby increasing water permeability of this membrane. ADH also increases the gene expression and new synthesis of aquaporin 2. As the basolateral side of the target cells constitutively expresses aquaporins 3 and 4, the ADH-induced increase in apical membrane aquaporin 2 enhances the transepithelial flow of water from the lumen toward the renal interstitium* Therefore, in the presence of ADH, urine flow decreases (**antidiuresis**) and urine osmolality approaches that of the medullary epithelium (about 1200 mOsm/kg). In the absence of ADH, urine flow increases (**diuresis**) and urine osmolality decreases.

ADH increases mesangial cell contraction, which lowers the filtration coefficient of the glomerular membrane and therefore decreases the glomerular filtration rate. This action will further decrease the volume of urine flow. ADH inhibits renin release, a response that could be beneficial in compensation for an increase in extracellular fluid osmolality.

*See Koeppen BM, Stanton BA: *Renal physiology,* ed 4. Mosby Monograph Series, Philadelphia, 2007, Mosby.

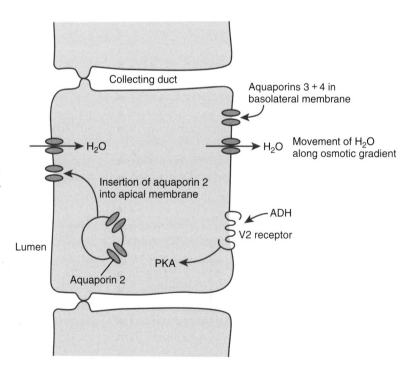

FIGURE 5-6 ■ Mechanism of ADH action on the kidney to promote water retention (i.e., antidiuresis).

Collecting duct

Aquaporins 3 + 4 in basolateral membrane

H_2O

H_2O Movement of H_2O along osmotic gradient

Insertion of aquaporin 2 into apical membrane

ADH

V2 receptor

Lumen

PKA

Aquaporin 2

As part of its role in the defense against the cardio-vascular consequences of severe volume depletion, ADH levels increase to supraphysiologic levels (i.e., increase by greater than 100-fold) during vasodilatory shock. At these levels, ADH binds to the V1 receptor on vascular smooth muscle. The V1 receptor is coupled to a Gq-phospholipase C–intracellular Ca^{2+} signaling pathway, which increases vascular smooth muscle contraction. Thus, the vasopressive actions of ADH become important during early states of vasodilatory shock.

Regulation of ADH Secretion ADH is released in response to increased extracellular fluid osmolality, or decreased blood volume and pressure. Osmoreceptive neurons, probably in the hypothalamus or circumven-tricular organs, innervate the magnocellular neurons of the PVN and SON. These osmoreceptive neurons respond to changes in extracellular fluid osmolality by shrinkage or swelling. Thus, increased osmolarity indirectly stimulates the magnocellular cells and action potential frequency increases in the neuronal axons constituting the hypothalamohypophyseal tract, with a resultant increase in posterior pituitary ADH release. Because the actual stimulus is cellular dehy-dration, the response to the hyperosmolality depends on the nature of the solutes. Solutes such as sodium, sucrose, and mannitol that do not readily enter the osmoreceptor cells are effective stimulators, whereas urea, to which the cells are more permeable, has about one third the potency of sodium. These effects may be demonstrated with the following relationship:

$$\uparrow ECF\ osmolality \rightarrow \uparrow ADH \rightarrow \uparrow Renal$$
$$water\ reabsorption \rightarrow \downarrow ECF\ osmolality$$

The regulatory system is sensitive to serum osmolality changes in the range of between 280 and 295 mOsm/kg (Figure 5-7). Within this range, a rise in as little as 1% in serum osmolality will stimulate a measurable increase in ADH secretion.

ADH release can also be stimulated by a drop in effective blood volume. The receptors for this stimulus are the cardiovascular volume receptors, including low-pressure receptors in the atria of the heart, great veins, and pulmonary vasculature and high-pressure receptors in the aortic arch and carotid sinus barore-ceptors (Figure 5-8). Although all of these volume

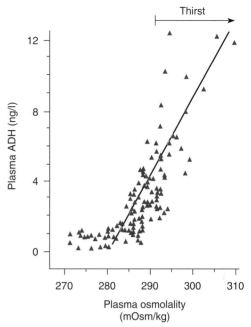

FIGURE 5-7 ■ Relation between plasma osmolality and plasma ADH. *(Redrawn from Wilson JD, Foster DW, Kronenberg HM, Larsen PR, editors: Williams' textbook of endocrinology, ed 9, Philadelphia, 1998, WB Saunders.)*

receptors are capable of regulating ADH secretion, the predominant regulator appears to be the atrial volume receptors. The sensitivity of the system to volume change is low at small volume changes. However, volume change does become a significant stimulus when circulating blood volume decreases 8% to 10% or more (Figure 5-9). This becomes the only mechanism of ADH stimulation during hemorrhage. A decrease in effective blood volume increases the sensitivity of ADH secretion to an increase in extracellular fluid osmolality.

Relationship Between Osmotic and Volume Stimuli Vascular volume influences the sensitivity of the system to osmotic stimuli. At lower vascular volumes, the system becomes more sensitive to a rise in serum osmolality (Figure 5-10). In turn, as vascular volume increases, the sensitivity of ADH release to osmotic stimuli decreases.

Other Factors Altering ADH Secretion Several drugs, including barbiturates, nicotine, and opiates, increase

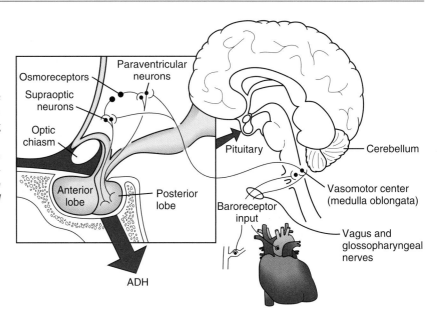

FIGURE 5-8 ■ Anatomy of the hypothalamus and pituitary gland (midsagittal section) depicting the pathways for ADH secretion. The *closed box* illustrates an expanded view of the hypothalamus and pituitary gland. *(From Koeppen BM, Stanton BA: Renal physiology, ed 3. St. Louis, 2001, Mosby.)*

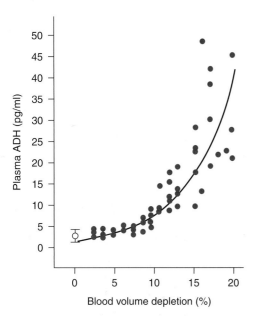

FIGURE 5-9 ■ Relation between blood volume and plasma antidiuretic hormone (ADH). *(Redrawn from Greenspan FS, Strewler GJ: Basic and clinical endocrinology, ed 5, Norwalk, Conn, 1997, Appleton & Lange.)*

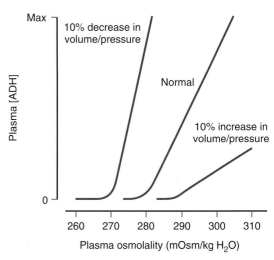

FIGURE 5-10 ■ Interaction between osmotic and hemodynamic stimuli for ADH secretion. With decreased blood volume and pressure, the osmotic set-point is shifted to lower plasma osmolality values and the slope in increased. *(From Koeppen BM, Stanton BA: Renal physiology, ed 3. St. Louis, 2001, Mosby.)*

ADH secretion. Alcohol is an effective suppressor of ADH secretion. For this reason, consumption of alcoholic beverages can lead to dehydration rather than volume expansion. Nausea increases ADH secretion, affording a protective effect against imminent volume loss due to vomiting. The hormones, atrial natriuretic peptide (ANP) and cortisol (see Chapter 7) inhibit ADH secretion.

Regulation of Thirst The regulation of thirst and drinking behavior is an important component of body fluid balance regulation. Thirst is regulated by many of the same factors that regulate ADH secretion. Increased serum osmolality, decreased vascular volume, and ADH secretion are effective stimuli for thirst. The osmoreceptors regulating thirst involve medial hypothalamic regions that approximate the osmoreceptors regulating ADH secretion. Angiotensin II is also thought to play a major role in the regulation of thirst. There are many components to the regulation of drinking, which include, in humans, chemical factors, social factors, and pharyngeal and gastrointestinal factors.

Degradation ADH is predominantly destroyed by proteolysis in the kidney and liver. The circulating half-life of ADH is approximately 15 to 20 minutes.

Pathologic Conditions Involving Antidiuretic Hormone A deficiency in ADH production results in **diabetes insipidus** (DI). People with DI are unable to concentrate urine normally and, therefore, excrete a large volume of urine. These individuals can have urinary flow rates as high as 25 liters/day. Thirst increases as a result of the dehydration caused by the high urinary flow. Diabetes insipidus differs from osmotic diuresis in that in the former, the urinary osmolality (or specific gravity) is much lower than plasma, whereas in the latter the urinary osmolality approaches that of plasma.

Neurogenic (Pituitary-Hypothalamic) Diabetes Insipidus Neurogenic DI is due to mutations in the preprovasophysin gene or to destruction of either the hypothalamus (e.g., by hypothalamic tumors) or the pars nervosa (e.g., by metastatic disease). People with neurogenic diabetes insipidus have a high urine volume and a low urinary osmolality (Table 5-1) and high plasma osmolality with inappropriately low ADH levels (Figure 5-11). If fluids are withheld, these patients continue to produce an excessive urinary volume and a dilute urine. If ADH is administered to people with this condition, they respond with a decrease in urinary volume and an increase in urinary osmolality.

Nephrogenic Diabetes Insipidus Those with nephrogenic DI have normal ADH production but lack a normal renal ADH response. The two primary defects in congenital nephrogenic DI are mutations in the V2 receptor and aquaporin 2. Acquired nephrogenic DI can occur from disruption of renal architecture with washout of the medullary gradient or by certain drugs (e.g., lithium) that impair the signaling pathway from the V2 receptor. Blood ADH levels are normal or elevated in patients with nephrogenic DI (see Figure 5-11) and administration of exogenous ADH analogs does not decrease the urinary flow rate.

TABLE 5-1			
Analysis of Various Types of Diabetes Insipidus			
	NEUROGENIC	NEPHROGENIC	PSYCHOGENIC
Plasma osmolality	↑	↑	↓
Urine osmolality	↓	↓	↓
Plasma ADH	Low	Normal to high	Low
Urine osmolality after mild water deprivation	No change	No change	↑
Plasma ADH after water deprivation	No change	↑	↑
Urine osmolality after administration of ADH	↑	No change	↑

ADH, antidiuretic hormone.

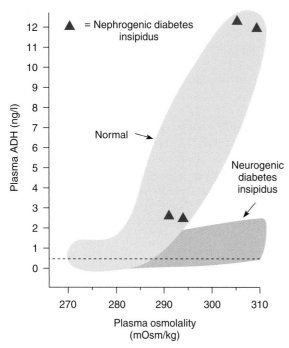

FIGURE 5-11 ■ Relation between antidiuretic hormone (ADH) 1 levels and serum osmolality in normal patients, those with neurogenic diabetes insipidus, and those with nephrogenic diabetes insipidus. *(Modified from Robertson GL, et al: J Clin Invest 52:2340, 1973; and Robertson GL: Ann Rev Med 25:315, 1974. Reprinted, with permission, from the Annual Review of Medicine, 1974 by Annual Reviews Volume 25 www.AnnualReviews.org.)*

Psychogenic Diabetes Insipidus Those with psychogenic DI are compulsive water drinkers. If water is withheld, the ADH secretion increases and urinary flow decreases while osmolality increases. Individuals with this disorder respond to treatment with ADH.

Syndrome of Inappropriate Secretion of Antidiuretic Hormone Many disorders can produce inappropriately high ADH concentrations relative to plasma osmolality. Some neoplasms produce ADH and release it into plasma. This is particularly common with pulmonary carcinomas, but it can occur in other types of tumors, including nonmalignant tumors. In addition, there are many other causes of the syndrome of inappropriate secretion of antidiuretic hormone (SIADH). Pulmonary tuberculosis is often associated with SIADH, as are

trauma, anesthesia, and pain. In SIADH, falling serum osmolality does not inhibit ADH secretion because control of ADH secretion is no longer linked to the normal regulatory mechanisms.

If the person with SIADH has a normal water consumption, water is retained because of the inappropriately high ADH levels. The resultant increase in blood volume and hence blood pressure increases renal glomerular filtration and therefore increases the loss of sodium in the urine. The hypervolemia stimulates release of **atrial natriuretic peptide (ANP),** which promotes renal sodium loss. The person consequently becomes hyponatremic (low blood sodium) and has a low serum osmolality. The urine osmolality is inappropriately high (the free water clearance decreases). If water is restricted in an individual with this condition, serum sodium and osmolality will return to normal.

Oxytocin

The nonapeptide oxytocin is structurally similar to ADH, and there is some overlap in biological activity. Although the major actions of oxytocin are on uterine motility and milk release, many other biological actions have been proposed.

Oxytocin and Uterine Motility Oxytocin stimulates contraction of the uterine myometrium. The magnitude of the oxytocin action depends on the phase of the menstrual cycle. Estrogens increase the uterine response to oxytocin and progestins decrease the response. Although uterine responsiveness to oxytocin increases around the time of parturition, oxytocin is not thought to be a factor initiating labor. Oxytocin secretion does not increase until after labor has begun. Once labor begins, the stretching of the vagina and cervix stimulates oxytocin release, which facilitates labor. This is referred to as a **neuroendocrine reflex,** which in this case has a **positive feedback** nature. Whereas negative feedback loops confer stability, positive feedback loops confer instability—that is, "something has to give." In the case of labor, increasing labor contractions stimulate the cervix and vagina, stimulating more oxytocin, increasing labor contractions, and so on. The pregnancy becomes unstable and is terminated by the delivery of the baby. Although oxytocin is not thought to be a factor initiating labor in

METABOLIC ACTIONS OF GROWTH HORMONE

Carbohydrates
Increases blood glucose
Decreases peripheral insulin sensitivity
Increases hepatic output of glucose
Administration results in increased serum insulin levels

Proteins
Increases tissue amino acid uptake
Increases incorporation into proteins
Decreases urea production
Produces positive nitrogen balance

Lipids
Is lipolytic
Can be ketogenic after long-term administration, particularly if insulin is deficient

Insulin-like Growth Factor
Stimulates IGF production
Stimulates growth
Is mitogenic

normal deliveries, oxytocin administration can initiate labor and it is used therapeutically to induce labor and decrease postpartum uterine bleeding. Women with diabetes insipidus and the accompanying oxytocin deficiency are capable of a relatively normal labor.

Sexual intercourse can stimulate oxytocin release in both men and women. Although the exact role of oxytocin in men is not entirely understood, the increased release of oxytocin during intercourse in women may aid in sperm transport in the female reproductive tract by stimulating uterine motility (see Chapter 10).

Oxytocin and Milk "Let-Down" Oxytocin stimulates contraction of the myoepithelial cells surrounding the mammary gland alveoli. Contraction of these cells expels milk from deep in the mammary gland into the larger ducts and sinuses of the gland, where it can be removed more readily by the suckling infant. This process is referred to as **milk ejection** or **let-down of milk.** The release of oxytocin is mediated by a neuroendocrine reflex. Suckling or tactile stimulation activates

sensory receptors located in the nipple and areola of the breast. These sensory fibers ultimately stimulate the hypothalamic magnocellular neurons. Stimulation of the magnicellular cells results in an increase in the frequency of transmission of action potentials along the axons from these cells extending to the pars nervosa, which increases oxytocin secretion. ADH secretion and oxytocin secretion are independently controlled. This reflex can be triggered through a conditioned response; the sight or sound of the hungry infant is adequate to stimulate oxytocin secretion (see Chapter 10). Oxytocin secretion can be blocked by pain, fear, or stress. Other actions of oxytocin are sodium retention and antidiuresis.

Metabolism Like ADH, oxytocin circulates unbound. It has a relatively short $t_{1/2}$ of 3 to 5 minutes. Its degradation occurs primarily in the liver and kidney. However, it can also be degraded in other tissues, including the mammary glands and uterus.

Pathologic Conditions Involving Oxytocin No known pathologic problems are associated with excess levels of oxytocin. Although a deficiency of oxytocin does not cause major problems, it can prolong labor and produce lactational difficulties as a result of poor milk ejection in some women.

THE ADENOHYPOPHYSIS

Because the pars distalis makes up most of the adenohypophysis in the adult human, the terms "adenohypophysis," "pars distalis" and "anterior pituitary" are often used synonymously. The pars distalis is composed of five endocrine cell types that produce six hormones (Table 5-2). Because of tinctorial characteristics of the cell types, the corticotropes, thyrotropes, and gonadotropes are referred to as pituitary **basophils,** whereas the somatotropes and lactotropes are referred to as pituitary **acidophils** (Figure 5-1C). All but one of these hormones are part of an endocrine axis.

The Endocrine Axes

A major part of the endocrine system is organized into **endocrine axes** (Figure 5-12), which contain three levels of hormonal output: The highest level of hormonal

TABLE 5-2
Endocrine Cell Types of the Adenohypophysis

CELL TYPE	CORTICOTROPE	THYROTROPE	GONADOTROPE	SOMATOTROPE	LACTOTROPE
Primary hypothalamic regulation	Corticotropin-releasing hormone (CRH) (41-aa peptide) stimulatory	Thyrotropin-releasing hormone (TRH) (tripeptide) stimulatory	Gonadotropin-releasing hormone (GnRH) (decapeptide) stimulatory	Growth hormone-releasing hormone (GHRH) (44-aa peptide) stimulatory & Somatostatin (tetradecapeptide) inhibitory	Dopamine (catecholamine) inhibitory Prolactin (PRL) releasing factor (stimulatory)
Tropic hormone secreted	Adrenocorticotropic Hormone(ACTH) (39-aa peptide)	Thyroid-stimulating hormone (TSH) (glycoprotein hormone)	Follicle-stimulating hormone & luteinizing hormone (FSH & LH) (glycoprotein hormone)	Growth hormone (GH) (ca. 22-kDa protein)	Prolactin (ca. 23-kDa protein)
Receptor	MC2R (Gs-linked GPCR)	TSH receptor (Gs-linked GPCR)	FSH & LH receptors (Gs-linked GPCRs)	GH receptor (JAK/STAT-linked cytokine receptor)	PRL receptor (JAK/STAT-linked cytokine receptor)
Target endocrine gland	Zona fasciculata and zona reticularis of the adrenal cortex	Thyroid epithelium	Ovary (theca & granulosa*) Testis (Leydig & Sertoli)	Liver (but also direct actions—especially in terms of metabolic effects)	No endocrine target organ—not part of an endocrine axis
Peripheral hormone involved in negative feedback	Cortisol	Triiodothyronine (T3)	Estrogen[†], progesterone, testosterone, inhibin[‡]	IGF-I	None

*Both follicular and luteinized thecal and granulosa cells.
[†]Estrogen can also have a positive feedback in women.
[‡]Inhibin selectively inhibits FSH release from the gonadotrope.
IGF-1, Insulin-like growth factor-1.

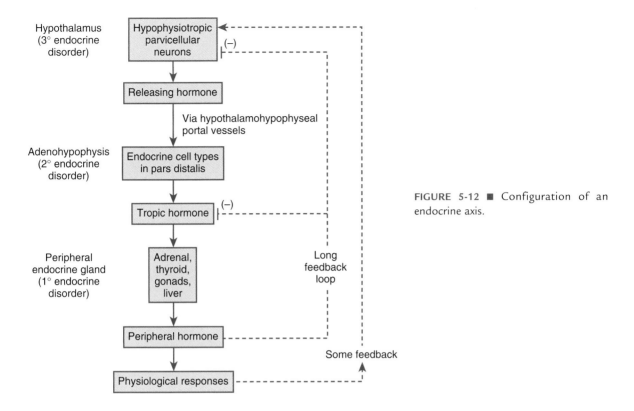

Hypothalamus (3° endocrine disorder)

Hypophysiotropic parvicellular neurons

(−)

Releasing hormone

Via hypothalamohypophyseal portal vessels

Adenohypophysis (2° endocrine disorder)

Endocrine cell types in pars distalis

Tropic hormone   (−)

Peripheral endocrine gland (1° endocrine disorder)

Adrenal, thyroid, gonads, liver

Long feedback loop

Peripheral hormone

Some feedback

Physiological responses

FIGURE 5-12 ■ Configuration of an endocrine axis.

output is actually neurohormonal, and is made up of several hypothalamic nuclei, collectively referred to as the **hypophysiotropic** region of the hypothalamus that regulate the adenohypophysis. These nuclei are distinguished from the magnocellular neurons of the PVN and SON that project to the pars nervosa in that they have small, **parvicellular,** neuronal cell bodies that project axons to the median eminence. Parvicellular neurons release neurohormones called **releasing hormones** at the median eminence (Figure 5-13). The median eminence is like the pars nervosa in that it represents another neurovascular organ. Releasing hormones secreted from axonal endings at the median eminence enter a primary plexus of fenestrated capillaries. Hypothalamic-releasing hormones are then conveyed from the median eminence to a second capillary plexus located in the pars distalis by the **hypothalamohypophyseal portal vessels** (a "portal" vessel is defined as a vessel that begins and ends in capillaries without going through the heart). With one exception (see later) all releasing hormones are short-lived

peptides (see Table 5-2), and reach significant levels only in the "private" portal system between the hypothalamus and the pituitary gland. At the secondary capillary plexus, the releasing hormones diffuse out of the vasculature and bind to their specific receptors on specific cell types within the pars distalis. The neurovascular link (i.e., the pituitary stalk) between the hypothalamus and pituitary is somewhat fragile and can be disrupted by physical trauma, surgery, or hypothalamic disease. Damage to the stalk and subsequent functional isolation of the anterior pituitary results in the decline of all anterior pituitary tropic hormones except PRL (see later).

The cells of the adenohypophysis make up the intermediate level of an endocrine axis. The pars distalis secretes protein hormones that are referred to as **tropic hormones—ACTH, TSH, FSH, LH, GH, and PRL** (see Table 5-2). With a few exceptions, tropic hormones bind their receptors on peripheral endocrine glands. Because of this arrangement, pituitary tropic hormones generally do not *directly* regulate physiologic responses.

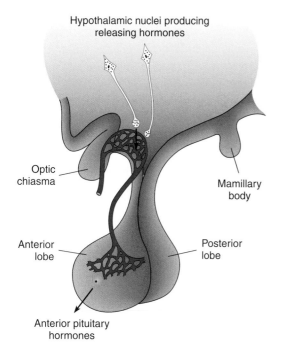

Hypothalamic nuclei producing
releasing hormones

Optic
chiasma

Mamillary
body

Anterior
lobe

Posterior
lobe

Anterior pituitary
hormones

FIGURE 5-13 ■ Hypophyseotropic hormones are secreted into hypophyseal portal circulation and then transported to anterior pituitary. *(Modified from Tyrrell JB, et al: Hypothalamus and pituitary. In Greenspan FS, Strewler GJ, editors: Basic and clinical endocrinology, ed 5, Norwalk, Conn, 1997, Appleton & Lange.)*

The third level involves the **peripheral endocrine organs,** which include the **thyroid gland,** the **adrenal cortex,** the **ovary,** the **testis,** and the **liver.** These peripheral endocrine glands are stimulated by pituitary tropic hormones to secrete **thyroid hormone, cortisol, estrogen, progesterone, testosterone,** and **insulin-like growth factor (IGF)-I.** Thus, we refer to the following endocrine axes: hypothalamus-pituitary-adrenal axis, hypothalamus-pituitary-thyroid axis, hypothalamus-pituitary-ovary axis, hypothalamus-pituitary-testis axis, and hypothalamus-pituitary-liver axis. These axes, through the peripheral hormones they regulate, have a broad range of effects on growth, metabolism, homeostasis and reproduction, as will be discussed in the Chapters 6, 7, 8, and 9. The endocrine axes have the following important features:

1. The activity of a specific axis is normally maintained at a **set-point** (which in truth is a range of activity).

The set-point is determined primarily by the integration of hypothalamic stimulation and peripheral hormone negative feedback. Importantly, the negative feedback is not exerted primarily by the physiologic responses regulated by a specific endocrine axis, but from the peripheral hormone acting on the pituitary and hypothalamus (see Figure 5-12). Thus, if the level of a peripheral hormone drops, the secretion of hypothalamic-releasing hormones and pituitary tropic hormones will increase. As the level of peripheral hormone rises, the hypothalamus and pituitary will decrease secretion owing to negative feedback. Although some nonendocrine physiologic parameters (e.g., acute hypoglycemia) can regulate some endocrine axes, the axes function semiautonomously with respect to the physiologic changes they produce. This configuration means that a peripheral hormone (e.g., thyroid hormone) can evolve to regulate multiple organ systems, without those organ systems exerting competing negative feedback regulation on the hormone. Clinically, this partial autonomy means that multiple aspects of a patient's physiology are at the mercy of whatever derangements exist within a specific axis.

2. Hypothalamic hypophysiotropic neurons often secrete in a **pulsatile** manner and are entrained to daily and seasonal rhythms through CNS inputs. Additionally, hypothalamic nuclei receive various neuronal inputs from higher and lower levels of the brain. These can be short term (e.g., various stresses/infections) or long term (e.g., onset of reproductive function at puberty). Thus, the inclusion of the hypothalamus in an endocrine axis allows for the integration of a considerable amount of information in determining and/or changing the set-point of that axis. Clinically, this means that a broad range of complex, neurogenic states can alter pituitary function. **Psychosocial dwarfism** is a striking example of this, in which children who are abused and/or under intense emotional stress have lower growth rates due to decreased growth hormone secretion by the pituitary gland.

3. The loss of a peripheral hormone (e.g., thyroid hormone) may be due to a defect at the level of the peripheral endocrine gland (e.g., thyroid), the pituitary gland, or the hypothalamus, which are referred to as **primary, secondary, and tertiary endocrine disorders,** respectively (see Figure 5-12).

A thorough understanding of the feedback relationships within an axis allows the physician to determine where the defect lies. Primary endocrine deficiencies tend to be the most severe because they often involve complete absence of the peripheral hormone. Disorders can also be due to excessive secretion at the primary, secondary, or tertiary level of an axis. This is usually due to a hormone-producing tumor (e.g., Cushing's disease is due to an ACTH-producing pituitary tumor).

The Endocrine Function of the Adenohypophysis

The adenohypophysis comprises the following endocrine cell types: **corticotropes, thyrotropes, gonadotropes, somatotropes,** and **lactotropes.** Each cell type is discussed subsequently in the context of hormonal production and action, hypothalamic regulation, and feedback regulation.

The Corticotrope

Corticotropes stimulate (i.e., are "tropic to") the adrenal cortex, as part of the **hypothalamus-pituitary-adrenal (HPA) axis.** Corticotropes produce the hormone, **adrenocorticotropic hormone (ACTH;** also called **corticotropin**), which stimulates two zones of the adrenal cortex (see Chapter 7).

ACTH is a 39-amino acid peptide that is synthesized as part of a larger prohormone, **pro-opiomelanocortin (POMC).** In fact. corticotropes are also referred to as **POMC cells.** POMC harbors the peptide sequence for ACTH, α- and β–melanocyte–stimulating hormones (MSH), endorphins (endogenous opioids) and enkephalins (Figure 5-14). However, the human corticotrope expresses only the prohormone convertases capable of producing ACTH as the sole active hormone secreted from these cells in humans. The other fragments that are cleaved out of POMC and secreted by the corticotropes are the N-terminal fragment and β-lipotropic hormone (β-LPH). Neither of these latter two fragments appears to play a physiologic role in humans.

ACTH circulates as an unbound hormone, and has a short half-life of about 10 minutes. ACTH binds to the **melanocortin-2 receptor (MC2R)** on cells in the adrenal cortex (Figure 5-15). MC2R is a GPCR coupled to Gs/cAMP/PKA signaling pathway. ACTH acutely increases cortisol and adrenal androgen production, but also increases expression of steroidogenic enzyme genes, and in the long term, promotes growth and survival of two zones of the adrenal cortex (see Chapter 7). At supraphysiologic levels (e.g., Cushing's disease), ACTH causes darkening of light-colored skin.

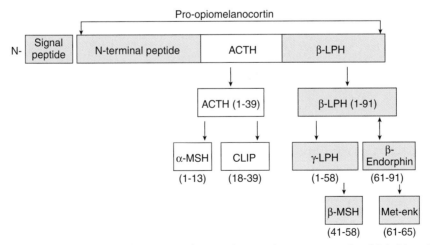

FIGURE 5-14 ■ Original gene transcript of pro-opiomelanocortin contains structures of multiple bioactive compounds. Note that ACTH is the only bioactive peptide released by the human corticotrope. ACTH, adrenocorticotropic hormone; β-LPH, β-lipotrophic hormone; α-MSH, α-melanocyte-stimulating hormone; CLIP, corticotropin-like intermediate peptide; γ-LPH, γ-lipotrophic hormone; β-MSH, β-melanocyte-stimulating hormone; Met-enk, metenkephalin.

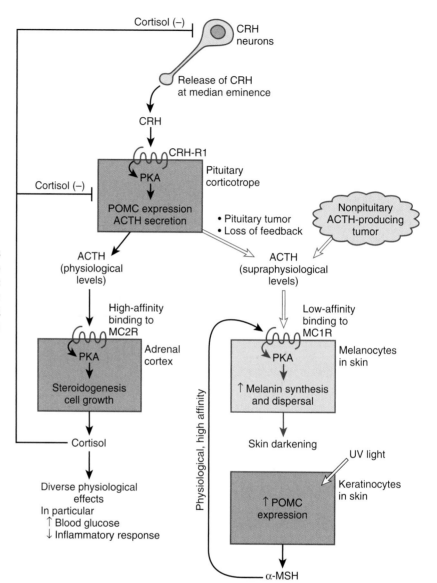

FIGURE 5-15 ■ Normal levels of ACTH act on the MC2R to increase cortisol. Supraphysiologic levels of ACTH act on both the MC2R and the MC1R on melanocytes, causing skin darkening.

Normally, keratinocytes express the POMC gene, but secrete α-MSH instead of ACTH. Keratinocytes secrete α-MSH in response to ultraviolet light, and α-MSH acts as a paracrine factor on neighboring melanocytes to darken the skin. α-MSH binds to the MC1R on melanocytes. However, at high levels, ACTH can also cross-react with the MC1R receptor on skin melanocytes (see Figure 5-15). Thus, darkening of skin is one indicator of excessive ACTH levels.

ACTH is under stimulatory control by the hypothalamus. A subset of parvicellular hypothalamic neurons expresses the peptide, **procorticotropin releasing hormone (pro-CRH).** Pro-CRH is processed to an amidated 41 amino acid peptide, **CRH.** CRH binds to the CRH receptor, **CRH-R1,** on corticotropes. CRH-R1 is a GPCR linked to a Gs/cAMP/PKA signaling pathway. CRH acutely stimulates ACTH secretion, and increases transcription of the POMC gene. The parvicellular

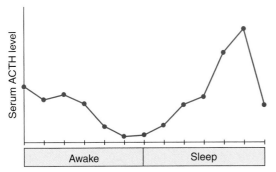

FIGURE 5-16 ■ Diurnal pattern for serum adrenocorticotropic hormone (ACTH).

neurons that express CRH also coexpress ADH. ADH binds to V3 receptors on corticotropes. The V3 receptor is GPCR linked to a Gq/phospholipase C signaling pathway. ADH potentiates the action of CRH on corticotropes.

ACTH secretion shows a pronounced diurnal pattern, with a peak in early morning and a valley in late afternoon (Figure 5-16). In addition, secretion of CRH, and hence secretion of ACTH, is pulsatile. There are multiple regulators of the hypothalamic-pituitary-adrenal (HPA) axis, and many of them are mediated through the central nervous system (Figure 5-17). Many types of stress, both neurogenic (e.g., fear) and

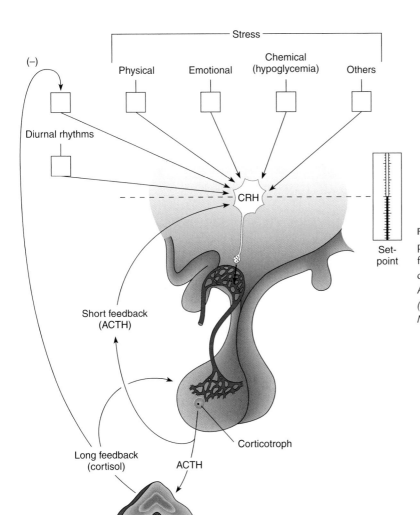

FIGURE 5-17 ■ Hypothalamic-pituitary-adrenal axis illustrating factors regulating secretion of corticotropin-releasing hormone (CRH). ACTH, adrenocorticotropic hormone. (Modified from Gwinup G, Johnson B: Metabolism 24:777, 1975.)

systemic (e.g., infection) stimulate ACTH secretion. The stress effects are mediated through CRH and vasopressin and the central nervous system. The response to many forms of severe stress can persist despite negative feedback from high cortisol levels. This means that the hypothalamus has the ability to reset the "set-point" of the HPA axis in response to stress. Severe, chronic depression can cause such a resetting of the HPA axis due to hypersecretion of CRH, and is, in fact, a factor in the development of **tertiary hypercortisolism.** Because cortisol has profound effects on the immune system (see Chapter 7), the HPA axis and the immune system are closely coupled, and cytokines—particularly interleukin-1 (IL-1), IL-2, and IL-6—stimulate the HPA axis.

Cortisol exerts a negative feedback on the pituitary, where it suppresses POMC gene expression and ACTH secretion, and on the hypothalamus, where it decreases pro-CRH gene expression and CRH release. As mentioned earlier, ACTH has a long-term effect on the growth and survival of adrenocortical cells. This means that long-term administration of exogenous corticosteroids will cause the adrenal cortex to atrophy because of the negative feedback of the exogenous hormone on ACTH secretion. In such a patient, termination of exogenous corticosteroid therapy must be gradual in order to allow the adrenal cortex to regain its normal functional capacity.

The Thyrotrope

Thyrotropes regulate thyroid function by secreting the hormone, thyroid stimulating hormone (TSH; also called thyrotropin), as part of the hypothalamus-pituitary-thyroid axis. TSH is one of three pituitary glycoprotein hormones that also include follicle-stimulating hormone (FSH) and luteinizing hormone (LH) (see later). TSH is a heterodimer composed of an α subunit, called a glycoprotein subunit (α-GSU), and a β subunit (β-TSH) (Figure 5-18). The α-GSU is common to TSH, FSH, and LH, whereas the β subunit is specific to the hormone (i.e., β-TSH, β-FSH, and β-LH are all unique). Glycosylation (in particular, terminal sialylation) of the subunits increases their stability in the circulation. The half-lives of TSH, FSH, and LH (and an LH-like placental glycoprotein hormone, human chorionic gonadotropin [hCG]) are relatively long, ranging from tens of minutes to several hours. Glycosylation also serves to increase the affinity and specificity of the hormones for their receptors.

TSH binds to the TSH receptor on thyroid epithelial cells (Figure 5-19). The TSH receptor is a GPCR linked to a Gs/cAMP/PKA signal transduction pathway. As discussed in Chapter 6, the production of thyroid hormones is a complex, multistep process. TSH stimulates essentially every aspect of thyroid function. TSH also has a strong tropic effect, stimulating hypertrophy, hyperplasia and survival of thyroid epithelial cells. Indeed, in geographical regions of low iodide availability (iodide is required for thyroid hormone synthesis), TSH levels become elevated because of reduced negative feedback. Elevated TSH levels can produce noticeable growth of the thyroid, causing a bulge in the neck, called a **goiter.**

The pituitary thyrotrope is stimulated by the releasing hormone, **thyrotropin-releasing hormone (TRH).** TRH is produced by a subset of parvicellular hypothalamic neurons. TRH is a tripeptide, with cyclization of a glutamine at its N-terminus (pyroGlu), and an amidated C-terminus (similar to the structure of

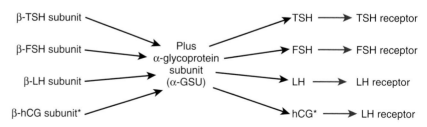

FIGURE 5-18 ■ Pituitary glycoprotein hormones. hCG is made by the placenta and binds to the LH receptor. FSH, follicle-stimulating hormone; hCG, human chorionic gonadotropin; LH, luteinizing hormone; TSH, thyroid-stimulating hormone.

β-TSH subunit
β-FSH subunit
β-LH subunit
β-hCG subunit*

Plus
α-glycoprotein subunit (α-GSU)

TSH → TSH receptor
FSH → FSH receptor
LH → LH receptor
hCG* → LH receptor

*hCG is human chorionic gonadotropin. hCG is made by the placenta, and binds to the LH receptor.

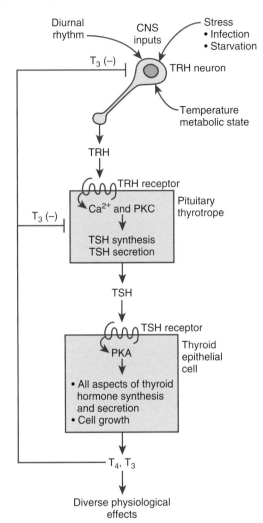

FIGURE 5-19 ■ Hypothalamus-pituitary-thyroid axis. TRH, thyrotropin-releasing hormone; TSH thyroid-stimulating hormone; PKC, protein kinase C; PKA, protein kinase A; T$_4$, tetraiodothyronine; T$_3$, triiodothyronine (active form of thyroid hormone).

lowest around dinnertime). TRH is regulated by various stresses, but unlike CRH, stresses inhibit TRH secretion. This includes physical stress, starvation, and infection. The active form of thyroid hormone, triiodothyronine (T$_3$), negatively feeds back on both pituitary thyrotropes and TRH-producing neurons. T$_3$ represses both β-TSH expression and the sensitivity of thyrotropes to TRH. T$_3$ also inhibits TRH production and secretion.

The Gonadotrope

The gonadotrope is a dual hormone producer in that the same cell secretes FSH and LH (also called gonadotropins). The gonadotrope regulates the function of gonads in both sexes. As such, the gonadotrope plays an integral role in the **hypothalamus-pituitary-testis axis** and the **hypothalamus-pituitary-ovary axis** (Figure 5-20).

As discussed earlier, FSH and LH are pituitary glycoprotein hormones composed of a common α-GSU dimerized with a unique β-FSH or β-LH subunit. Importantly, FSH and LH are segregated to a large degree into different secretory granules and are not co-secreted in equimolar amounts (in contrast to ADH and neurophysin, for example). This allows for the modulation of the ratio of FSH/LH secretion by the gonadotropes. FSH and LH bind to their respective receptors, which are both GPCRs primarily coupled to Gs/cAMP/PKA signaling pathways. The actions of FSH and LH on gonadal function are complex, especially in women, and will be discussed in detail in Chapters 8 and 9. In general, gonadotropins promote testosterone production in men and estrogen and progesterone secretion in women. FSH also increases the secretion of a TGF-β–related protein hormone, called inhibin, in both sexes.

FSH and LH secretion are regulated by one hypothalamic releasing hormone, **gonadotropin-releasing hormone** (**GnRH;** also called **LHRH**). GnRH is a 10 amino acid peptide produced by a subset of parvicellular hypothalamic GnRH neurons. GnRH is produced as a larger prohormone, and, as part of its processing to a decapeptide, is modified with a cyclized glutamine (pyroGlu) at its amino terminus, and an amidated carboxy terminus. During embryonic development, the GnRH neurons migrate to the

gastrin termini, Chapter 2). TRH is synthesized as a larger prohormone, which contains six copies of TRH within its sequence. TRH binds to the TRH receptor on the thyrotropes (see Figure 5-19). The TRH receptor is a GPCR linked to a Gq/phospholipase C signaling pathway. TRH neurons are regulated by numerous CNS-mediated stimuli. TRH is released according to a diurnal rhythm (highest during overnight hours,

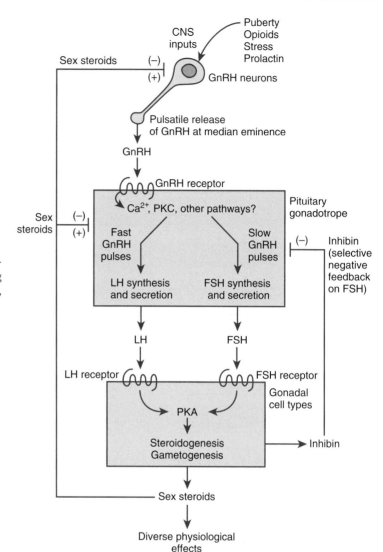

FIGURE 5-20 ■ Hypothalamus-pituitary-gonadal axis. GnRH, gonadotropin-releasing hormone; LH, luteinizing hormone; FSH, follicle-stimulating hormone.

mediobasal hypothalamus from the nasal placode. Patients with **Kallmann's syndrome** have **tertiary hypogonadotropic hypogonadism,** often associated with loss of sense of smell (anosmia). This is due to a mutation in the **KAL gene,** which results in the failure of the GnRH neuronal precursors to properly migrate to the hypothalamus and to establish a neurovascular link to the pars distalis.

GnRH binds to the GnRH receptor, which is a GPCR coupled primarily to a Gq/phospholipase C signaling pathway. GnRH is released in a pulsatile

manner, and both the pulsatile secretion and the frequency of the pulses have important effects on the gonadotrope. Continuous infusion of GnRH downregulates the GnRH receptor, resulting in a decrease in FSH and LH secretion. In contrast, pulsatile secretion does not desensitize the gonadotrope to GnRH and FSH and LH secretion is normal. At a frequency of 1 pulse per hour, GnRH preferentially increases LH secretion. At a slower frequency of 1 pulse per 3 hours, GnRH preferentially increases FSH secretion. The mechanism by which the frequency of GnRH secretion determines the ratio of FSH/LH levels in the blood is poorly understood, but may involve multiple signaling pathways linked to the GnRH receptor, leading to differential synthesis and/or glycosylation of FSH versus LH.

Gonadotropins increase sex steroid synthesis. In men, testosterone and estrogen negatively feed back at the level of the pituitary and the hypothalamus. Exogenous progesterone also inhibits gonadotropin function in men, and is being considered as a possible ingredient in a male contraceptive pill. Additionally, inhibin negatively feeds back selectively on FSH secretion in men and women. In women, progesterone and testosterone negatively feed back on gonadotropic function at the level of hypothalamus and pituitary. At low doses, estrogen also exerts a negative feedback on FSH and LH secretion. However, high estrogen levels (e.g., 500 pg/ml) maintained for 3 days causes a surge of LH and, to a lesser extent, FSH secretion (see Chapter 9). This positive feedback is observed at the hypothalamus and pituitary. At the hypothalamus, GnRH pulse amplitude and frequency increase. At the pituitary, high estrogen levels greatly increase the sensitivity of the gonadotrope to GnRH by increasing GnRH receptor levels and by enhancing postreceptor signaling pathway components.

The Somatotrope

The somatotropes produce **growth hormone** (**GH;** also called **somatotropin**). A major target of GH is the liver, where it stimulates the production of **insulin-like growth factor I (IGF-I).** Thus, the somatotrope is part of the hypothalamus-pituitary-liver axis (Figure 5-21). However, GH also has several direct actions at physiologic levels on non-endocrine organs.

GH is a 191-amino acid protein that is similar to **prolactin (PRL)** and **human placental lactogen (hPL),** and there is some overlap in activity among these hormones. Multiple forms of GH are seen in serum, thereby constituting a "family of hormones," with the 191-amino acid (22-kDa) form representing approximately 75% of the circulating GH. The GH receptor is a member of the cytokine/GH/PRL/erythropoietin receptor family and, as such, is linked to JAK/STAT signaling pathway (Chapter 1). Human GH can also act as an agonist for the PRL receptor. About 50% of the 22-kDa form of GH in serum is bound to the N-terminal portion (the extracellular domain) of the GH receptor, called **GH-binding protein (GHBP).** **Laron dwarfs,** who lack normal GH receptors but have normal GH secretion, do not have detectable binding protein in their serum. The exact biological significance of GHBP is not yet clear. GHBP reduces renal clearance and thus increases biological half-life of GH. The circulating $t_{1/2}$ for GH is only about 20 minutes. The liver and kidney are major sites of hormone degradation.

GH secretion is under dual control by the hypothalamus (see Figure 5-21). The hypothalamus predominantly stimulates growth hormone secretion via the peptide, **growth hormone–releasing hormone (GHRH). GHRH** is a member of the vasoactive intestinal peptide (VIP)/secretin/glucagon family, and is processed into a 44-amino acid peptide with an amidated C-terminus from a larger prohormone. GHRH binds to the GHRH receptor, which is coupled to a Gs/cAMP/PKA signaling pathways. GHRH enhances GH secretion and GH gene expression. The hypothalamus inhibits pituitary GH synthesis and release via the peptide, **somatostatin.** Somatostatin is a cyclic tetradecapeptide that is found in many locations in the body (see Chapter 2). Somatostatin in the anterior pituitary inhibits GH and TSH release. Somatostatin binds to the somatostatin receptor, which lowers cAMP through a Gi-linked signaling pathway.

GH secretion is also regulated by **ghrelin,** which is primarily produced by the stomach (see Chapter 2), but is also expressed in the hypothalamus. Ghrelin increases appetite and may serve as a signal to coordinate nutrient acquisition with growth.

The primary negative feedback on the somatotrope is exerted by IGF-I. GH stimulates IGF-I production by the liver and IGF-I then inhibits GH synthesis and secretion at the pituitary and hypothalamus by a classical "long" feedback loop. In addition, GH itself exerts negative feedback on GHRH release through a "short" feedback loop. GH also increases somatostatin release.

GH secretion, like that of ACTH, shows prominent diurnal rhythms, with peak secretion occurring in the early morning just before awakening (Figure 5-22). Its secretion is stimulated during deep, slow-wave sleep (stages III and IV). GH secretion is lowest during

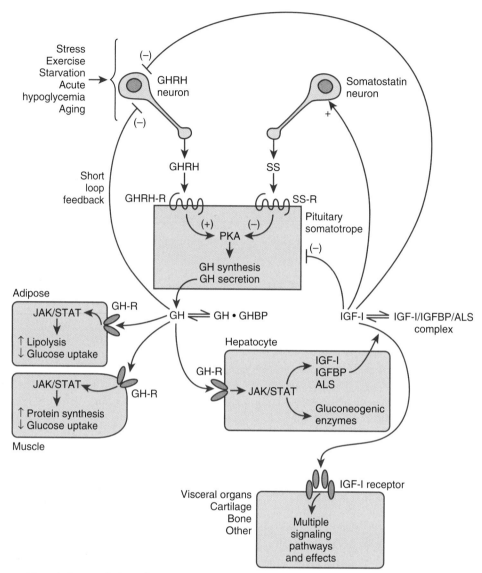

FIGURE 5-21 ■ Hypothalamus-pituitary-liver axis. GHRH, growth hormone-releasing hormone; SS, somatostatin; GHBP, growth hormone-binding protein; IGF-I, insulin-like growth factor-I; IGFBP, insulin-like growth factor-binding protein; ALS, acid labile subunit.

the day. This rhythm is entrained to sleep-wake patterns rather than light-dark patterns, so a phase shift occurs in people who work night shifts. As is typical of anterior pituitary hormones, GH secretion is pulsatile. The levels of GH in serum vary widely (0 to 30 ng/ml, with most values usually falling between 0 and 3). Because of this marked variation, serum GH values are of minimal clinical value unless the sampling time is known. Frequently, rather than measuring GH, the clinician measures insulin-like growth factor-I (IGF-I) because its secretion is regulated by GH and IGF-I has a relatively long circulating half-life that buffers pulsatile and diurnal changes in secretion.

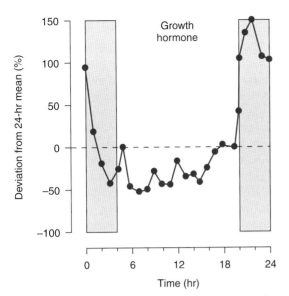

FIGURE 5-22 ■ Diurnal variation in serum growth hormone. (Redrawn from Krieger DT, Aschoff J: Endocrine and other biological rhythms. In DeGroot LJ, et al, editors: Endocrinology, vol 3, New York, 1979, Grune & Stratton.)

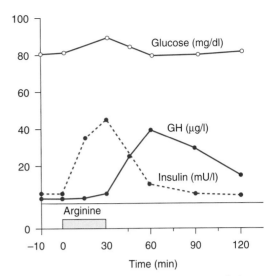

FIGURE 5-23 ■ Effect of intravenous arginine infusion on plasma growth hormone (GH), glucose, and insulin concentrations. (Redrawn from Wilson JD, Foster DW, editors: Williams' textbook of endocrinology, ed 8, Philadelphia, 1992, WB Saunders.)

GH secretion is also regulated by several different physiologic states (see Figure 5-21). GH is classified as one of the **stress hormones** and is increased by neurogenic and physical stress. As discussed later, GH promotes lipolysis, increases protein synthesis, and antagonizes the ability of insulin to reduce blood glucose. It is not surprising, therefore, that hypoglycemia is a stimulus for GH secretion and GH is classified as a **hyperglycemic hormone.** Although its secretion is not regulated by minor variations in serum glucose levels, its release is stimulated by falling glucose levels or by hypoglycemia. Falling blood glucose levels are such an effective stimulus that insulin-induced hypoglycemia is sometimes used as a provocative test of a person's ability to secrete GH. A rise in certain serum amino acids also serves as an effective stimulus for GH secretion. Arginine is one of these amino acids and the GH response to arginine infusion may be used to evaluate GH secretion (Figure 5-23). In contrast, an increase in blood glucose or free fatty acids inhibits GH secretion. Obesity also inhibits GH secretion, in part due to insulin resistance (relative hyperglycemia) and increased circulating free fatty acids. Conversely, exercise is an effective

stimulator of GH secretion. GH is also increased during starvation. Other hormonal regulators of GH include estrogen, androgens, and thyroid hormone, which enhance GH secretion; they have direct effects on IGF-I secretion and bone maturation as well.

Direct versus Indirect Actions of GH

Direct Actions of GH on Metabolism GH acts directly on the liver, muscle, and adipose tissue to regulate energy metabolism (see Box 5-1). It shifts metabolism to lipid use for energy, thereby conserving carbohydrates and proteins.

GH is a **protein anabolic hormone** that increases cellular amino acid uptake and incorporation into protein, and represses proteolysis. Consequently, it produces nitrogen retention (a positive nitrogen balance) and a decreased urea production. The muscle wasting that occurs concomitant with aging has been proposed to be caused, at least in part, by the decrease in GH secretion that occurs with aging.

GH is a **lipolytic hormone.** It activates hormone-sensitive lipase and therefore mobilizes neutral fats from adipose tissue. As a result, serum fatty acid levels rise after GH administration. More fats are used for energy production. Fatty acid uptake and oxidation increase in skeletal muscle and liver. GH can be ketogenic as a result of the increase in fatty acid oxidation (the ketogenic effect of GH is not seen when insulin levels are normal). If insulin is given along with GH, the lipolytic effects of GH are abolished.

GH alters carbohydrate metabolism. Many of its actions may be secondary to the increase in fat mobilization and oxidation. (An increase in serum free fatty acids inhibits glucose uptake in skeletal muscle and adipose tissue.) Following GH administration, blood glucose rises. The hyperglycemic effects of GH are mild and slower than those of glucagon and epinephrine. The increase in blood glucose results, in part, from decreased glucose uptake and use in skeletal muscle and adipose tissue. Liver glucose output increases and this is probably not a result of glycogenolysis. In fact, glycogen levels can rise after GH administration. However, the increase in fatty acid oxidation and, hence, the rise in liver acetyl coenzyme A (acetyl CoA) stimulate gluconeogenesis, followed by increased glucose production from substrates such as lactate and glycerol.

GH antagonizes the action of insulin at the post-receptor level in skeletal muscle and adipose tissue (but not the liver). **Hypophysectomy** (removal of the pituitary gland) can improve diabetic management because GH, like cortisol, decreases insulin sensitivity. Since GH produces **insulin insensitivity,** it is considered a **diabetogenic hormone.** When secreted in excess, GH can cause diabetes mellitus and the insulin level necessary to maintain normal metabolism increases; the excessive pancreatic insulin secretion resulting from the GH excess can cause damage to the pancreatic β cells. Normal levels of GH are required for normal pancreatic function and insulin secretion. In the absence of GH, insulin secretion declines.

Indirect Effects of GH on Growth GH promotes the growth of bones and visceral organs. GH administration increases skeletal and visceral growth; children without GH show growth stunting or dwarfism. If given in vivo, GH results in increased cartilage growth, long-bone length, and periosteal growth. Most of these are mediated by a group of hormones called **insulin-like**

growth factors (IGFs). These compounds were once called **somatomedins.**

Insulin-like Growth Factors The insulin-like growth factors (IGFs) are multifunctional hormones that regulate cellular proliferation, differentiation, and cellular metabolism. These protein hormones resemble insulin in structure and function. The two hormones in this family, IGF-I and IGF-II, are produced in many tissues and have autocrine, paracrine, and endocrine actions. IGF-I is the major form produced in most adult tissues and IGF-II is the major form produced in the fetus. Both compounds are structurally similar to proinsulin, with IGF-I having 42% structural homology with proinsulin. IGFs and insulin cross-react with each other's receptors, and IGFs in high concentration mimic the metabolic actions of insulin. Both IGF-I and IGF-II act through type-I IGF receptors, which are similar to insulin and EGF receptors and contain intrinsic tyrosine kinase. However, IGF-II also binds to the type II IGF/mannose-6-phosphate receptor. This receptor does not resemble the insulin receptor and does not have intrinsic tyrosine kinase. Binding to these receptors probably facilitates internalization and degradation of the growth factor. IGFs stimulate glucose and amino acid uptake and protein and DNA synthesis. They were initially called *somatomedins* because they mediate GH (somatotropin) action on cartilage and bone growth. IGFs have many other actions and GH is not the only regulator of IGF formation. Initially, IGFs were thought to be produced in the liver in response to a GH stimulus. It is now known that IGFs are produced in many tissues and many actions are autocrine or paracrine. The liver is probably the predominant source of circulation IGFs (see Figure 5-21).

Essentially all circulating IGFs are transported in serum bound to **insulin-like growth factor-binding proteins (IGFBPs).** IGFBPs bind to IGFs and then associate with another protein, called **acid labile subunit (ALS).** GH stimulates the hepatic production of IGF-I, IGFBPs, and ALS. The IGFBP/ALS/IGF-I complex mediates transport and bioavailability of the IGF-I. Although IGFBPs generally inhibit IGF action, they greatly increased the biological half-life of IGFs (up to 12 hours). **IGFBP proteases** degrade IGFBP, and probably play a role in locally generating free (i.e., active) IGFs. This is of interest in the context of IGF-responsive cancers (e.g., prostate cancer), which may over express one or more IGFBP proteases.

Although GH is an effective stimulator for IGF production, the correlation between GH and IGF-I is greater than the correlation between GH and IGF-II. During puberty, when GH levels increase, IGF-I levels increase in parallel. Insulin also stimulates IGF production and GH cannot stimulate IGF production in the absence of insulin. Starvation effectively inhibits IGF secretion, even when GH levels are high. PRL or hPL can increase IGF-II secretion in the fetus and IGF-II is considered a fetal growth regulator. Although GH is a primary stimulant for liver IGF production, parathormone (PTH) and estradiol are more effective stimuli for osteoblastic IGF-I production. Less is known about the control of bone IGF-II production.

IGFs have profound effects on bone and cartilage. They stimulate the growth of bones, cartilage, and soft tissue, and regulate essentially all aspects of the metabolism of the cartilage-forming cells, called chondrocytes. IGFs are mitogenic. Although appositional growth of long bones continues after closure of the epiphyses, growth in length ceases. IGFs stimulate osteoblast replication and collagen and bone matrix synthesis. Serum IGF levels correlate well with growth in children.

The metabolic actions of IGF mimic the metabolic actions of insulin and are opposed to GH in terms of lipid and carbohydrate metabolism. However, IGFs are probably not major regulators of intermediary metabolism in the body.

Role of Growth Hormone, Insulin-like Growth Factor, and Insulin in Starvation

When ample supplies of nutrients are available, the high serum amino acid levels stimulate GH and insulin secretion and the high serum glucose levels stimulate insulin secretion. The high serum GH, insulin, and nutrient supply stimulate IGF production and these conditions are appropriate for growth. However, if the diet is high in calories but low in amino acids, the conditions change. Whereas the high carbohydrate availability results in high insulin availability, the low serum amino acid levels inhibit GH and IGF production. These conditions allow dietary carbohydrates and fats to be used, but conditions are unfavorable for tissue growth. During fasting, when nutrient availability decreases, serum GH levels rise and serum insulin levels fall (because of hypoglycemia). IGF production is low and the conditions are not favorable for growth. Under these circumstances, the rise in GH secretion is beneficial because it promotes fat mobilization while minimizing tissue protein loss. In the absence of insulin, peripheral tissue glucose use decreases, thereby conserving glucose for essential tissues such as brain.

Pathologic Conditions Involving Growth Hormone

GH is necessary for growth before adulthood. Deficiencies can produce **dwarfism** and excesses can produce **gigantism.** Normal growth requires not only normal levels of GH but also normal levels of thyroid hormones and insulin.

Dwarfism If a GH deficiency occurs before puberty, growth is severely impaired (Figure 5-24). Individuals with this condition are relatively well proportioned and have normal intelligence. If the anterior pituitary deficiency is limited to GH, they can have a normal life span. They are sometimes "pudgy" because they lose GH-induced lipolysis. If they have **panhypopituitary dwarfism** (all anterior pituitary hormones are deficient), so that gonadotropins are deficient, they may not mature sexually and remain infertile. People with dwarfism show few metabolic abnormalities other than a tendency toward hypoglycemia, insulinopenia, and increased insulin sensitivity. There are multiple potential sites of impairment. GH secretion may be reduced, GH-stimulated IGF production may decrease, or IGF action may be deficient. **Laron dwarfs** are GH resistant because of a genetic defect in the expression of the GH receptor so that response to GH is impaired. Hence, although the serum GH levels are normal to high, they do not produce IGFs in response to GH. Treating patients afflicted by Laron dwarfism with GH will not correct the growth deficiency.

The **African pigmy** represents another example of abnormal growth. Individuals with this condition have normal serum GH levels, but they do not exhibit the normal rise in IGF that occurs at puberty.

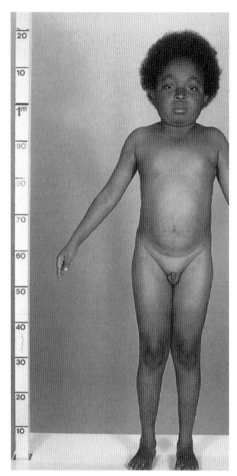

FIGURE 5-24 ■ A 17-year-old boy with GH deficiency associated with hypopituitarism. The patient has short stature for his age and underdeveloped genitalia. *(From Besser GM, Thorner MO: Clinical endocrinology, London, 1994, Mosby-Wolfe.)*

They also may have a partial defect in GH receptors because IGF-I levels do not rise normally after GH is administered. However, the IGF-II levels are normal. Unlike the Laron dwarfs, they do not totally lack the IGF response to GH.

Growth Hormone Deficiency in Adults GH deficiency in adults is only currently becoming recognized as a pathologic syndrome. If the GH deficiency occurs after the epiphyses close, growth is not impaired. A GH deficiency is one of many possible causes of hypoglycemia.

Recent studies have shown that extended deficiencies of GH lead to body composition changes. The percentage of the body weight that is fat increases, whereas the percentage that is protein decreases. In addition, muscle weakness and early exhaustion are symptoms of GH deficiency.

Because the muscle loss that occurs with aging may result from an age-related decline in GH production, GH is being used experimentally in elderly people to delay the physical decline associated with aging. The efficacy of this treatment in humans has not been established.

Growth Hormone Excess Before Puberty If there is excessive GH production before puberty, **gigantism** can result. Individuals with this condition can reach heights greater than 8 feet. The GH excess results in an increase in body weight as well as height. Many complications are associated with gigantism. These individuals frequently have glucose intolerance and hyperinsulinism. Overt clinical diabetes can develop, but ketoacidosis is rare. They have cardiovascular problems, including cardiac hypertrophy (all viscera increase in size); they are more susceptible to infections than normal; and they rarely live past their 20s. Hypersecretion of GH generally results from pituitary tumors; tumor growth eventually compresses other components of the anterior pituitary, decreasing secretion of other anterior pituitary hormones.

Figure 5-25 shows Robert Wadlow, the Alton Giant. At 1 year he weighed 62 pounds. His adult size was 8 feet, 11 inches and 475 pounds. Note the long extremities. The androgen deficiency secondary to the gonadotropin deficiency caused delayed puberty, resulting in late closure of the epiphyses.

Acromegaly If excessive GH is secreted after the epiphyses close, the long bones do not grow in length, but appositional growth occurs. Cartilage and membranous bones continue to grow and gross deformities can result. In addition, soft tissue growth increases and the abdomen protrudes as a result of visceral enlargement. Brain weight increases, with a resultant decrease in ventricular size. There is an increase in the growth of the nose, ears, and mandible—with the mandibular enlargement producing prognathism and widely spaced teeth. The calvarium thickens and the frontal sinuses enlarge, resulting in protrusion of the frontal

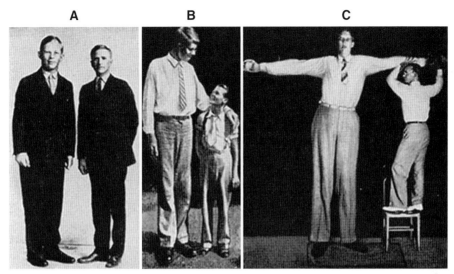

FIGURE 5-25 ■ A notable example of growth hormone excess was Robert Wadlow, later known as the "Alton Giant." Although he weighed only 9 pounds at birth, he grew rapidly and by 6 months of age he weighed 30 pounds. At 1 year of age he weighed 62 pounds. Growth continued throughout his life. Shortly before his death at age 22 from cellulitis of the feet, he was 8 feet, 11 inches tall and weighed 475 pounds.*(A and B, from Fadner F: Biography of Robert Wadlow, 1944, Bruce Humphreys. C, courtesy Dr. C.M. Charles and Dr. C.M. MacBryde.)*

ridge of the orbit of the eye. The characteristic enlargement of the hands and feet is the basis for the name **acromegaly** (*acro*, end or extremity; *megaly*, enlargement). The excessive bone and cartilage growth can produce carpal tunnel syndrome and joint problems. The voice deepens because of laryngeal growth. Acromegaly usually results from a functional tumor of the somatotropes. As it is generally slow in onset, patients typically do not seek medical help for 13 to 14 years. Unfortunately, by that time they typically have permanent physical deformities. People with gigantism eventually exhibit acromegaly if the condition is not corrected before puberty. A person with untreated acromegaly has a shortened life expectancy (Figure 5-26). Extended treatment of adults with GH results in changes in body composition, with the percentage of body protein increasing and the percentage of body fat decreasing.

The Lactotrope

The lactotrope produces the hormone, **prolactin (PRL),** which is a 199-amino acid single-chain protein.

The lactotrope differs from the other endocrine cell types of the adenohypophysis in two major ways:

1. The lactotrope is not part of an endocrine axis. This means that PRL acts directly on nonendocrine cells to induce physiologic changes.
2. The production and secretion of PRL is predominantly under inhibitory control by the hypothalamus. Thus, disruption of the pituitary stalk and the hypothalamohypophyseal portal vessels (e.g., due to surgery or physical trauma) results in an increase in PRL levels, but a decrease in ACTH, TSH, FSH, LH, and GH.

PRL circulates unbound to serum proteins and thus has a relatively short $t_{1/2}$ of about 20 minutes. As is typical of protein hormones, there is heterogeneity of circulating forms of PRL and the 199-amino acid form represents only 60% to 80% of the PRL measured by radioimmunoassays. Normal basal serum concentrations are similar in men and women.

PRL release is normally under tonic inhibition by the hypothalamus. This is exerted by dopaminergic tracts that secrete **dopamine** at the median eminence.

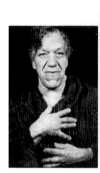
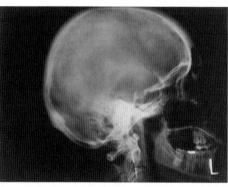
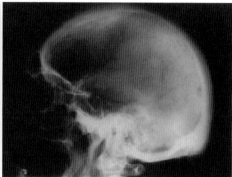

FIGURE 5-26 ■ Left, severe acromegaly. Middle, X-ray film of a normal skull. Right, X-ray film of skull of a woman with acromegaly that demonstrates effects of acromegaly on morphologic features of skull. Sella turcica is enlarged as a result of growth of pituitary adenoma. Skull is thicker than normal and protrusion of frontal ridge with enlargement of frontal sinuses is evident. (Left, from Clinical Pathological Conference, AM J Med 20:133, 1956; Middle and Right, courtesy of Dr. C. Joe.)

Dopamine binds to the **D$_2$ receptor,** which is linked to a Gi signaling pathway. There is also evidence for the existence of a **prolactin-releasing factor (PRF).** The exact nature of this compound is not known, although many factors, including TRH and hormones in the glucagon family (secretin, glucagon, VIP, and gastroin-hibitory peptide [GIP]) can stimulate PRL release.

Lactotropes increase in size and number during pregnancy. The human pituitary enlarges 2- to 3-fold in volume during pregnancy (Figure 5-27). The enlarged pituitary can cause vision problems because of pressure on the optic nerves. The increase in lac-totropes is due to stimulation by placental estrogen. Estrogen also directly increases PRL gene transcription and PRL secretion. Thus, PRL levels increase signifi-cantly during pregnancy and promote extensive lobu-loalveolar development of the breasts (see Chapter 10). After pregnancy and loss of placental estrogens, nurs-ing, and breast stimulation are strong stimuli for PRL synthesis and secretion. This response occurs within minutes and is mediated through a neurohormonal reflex. During the nursing period, PRL promotes the onset and maintenance of milk production by the breasts (see Chapter 10).

PRL is one of the many hormones released in response to *stress.* Surgery, fear, stimuli causing arousal, and exercise are all effective stimuli. As is the case with GH, sleep increases PRL secretion, and PRL has a pronounced sleep-associated diurnal rhythm (Figure 5-28). However, unlike GH, the sleep-associated PRL rise is not associated with a specific sleep phase.

Drugs that interfere with dopamine synthesis or action increase PRL secretion. Many commonly pre-scribed antihypertensive drugs and tricyclic antidepres-sant drugs are dopamine inhibitors. Bromocriptine is a dopamine agonist that can be used to inhibit PRL secretion. Somatostatin, TSH, and GH also inhibit PRL secretion.

The PRL receptor belongs to the cytokine/GH/PRL/erythropoietin receptor superfamily. Therefore, PRL acts through a JAK/STAT signaling pathway (Chapter 1).

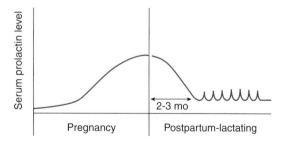

FIGURE 5-27 ■ Changes in serum prolactin levels in preg-nancy and during lactation.

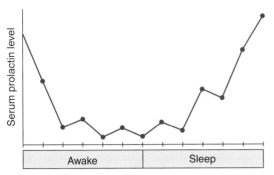

FIGURE 5-28 ■ Diurnal variation of serum prolactin levels.

At least 85 different actions have been proposed for PRL; which actions are seen often depends on the dose of hormone used and the species studied. In humans, the predominant physiologic role of PRL is the regulation of essentially every aspect of postnatal breast development and function. This is discussed in more detail in Chapter 10.

PRL has reproductive actions in many species, including humans. The primary action of PRL on reproduction in humans is repression of GnRH release. This accounts for **lactational amenorrhea,** which refers to cessation of menstrual periods in women who frequently and regularly nurse a baby. Pathophysiologically, excessive PRL secretion in humans inhibits reproductive function in both men and women. In the fetus, PRL and hPL have been proposed as growth stimulators through their effects on fetal IGF-II production. Hyperprolactinemia in humans produces glucose intolerance and hyperinsulinemia.

Pathologic Conditions Involving Prolactin

Hyperprolactinemia PRL-secreting tumors account for approximately 70% of all anterior pituitary tumors. Furthermore, many drugs interfere with dopamine production or action and hence increase PRL release. For these reasons, **hyperprolactinemia** is a common disorder in humans. Hyperprolactinemia in women is associated with oligomenorrhea or amenorrhea and infertility. GnRH release, the gonadotrope response to GnRH, and the ovarian response to LH all decrease. In the early stages of the pathologic condition,

PRL suppresses follicular maturation, leading to an inadequate corpus luteum and a short luteal phase. As the hyperprolactinemia persists, the preovulatory estrogen peak is lost, thereby lengthening the cycle and leading to oligomenorrhea and anovulatory cycles. Hyperprolactinemia can produce infertility in men. While breast enlargement can occur, true **gynecomastia** (inappropriate growth of breasts) and **galactorrhea** (inappropriate flow of milk) are rare.

The primary symptoms causing men and postmenopausal women with PRL-secreting tumors to seek medical attention may be those resulting from compression by the pituitary mass. These patients may experience severe headaches or visual disturbances that can include **bitemporal hemianopia** (defect in vision in the temporal half of the field of vision in both eyes). Both men and women may complain of decreased libido and signs of hypogonadism.

Prolactin Deficiency The only pathologic problem known to be associated with a deficiency in PRL secretion is the inability to initiate postpartum lactation.

Hypopituitarism

Panhypopituitarism There are many causes of hypopituitarism, which can involve either hypothalamic or pituitary problems. The deficiencies can be variable for the different anterior pituitary hormones. The symptoms of hypopituitarism are slow in onset and are reflected in deficiencies in the target organs of the anterior pituitary. Hypogonadism, hypothyroidism, hypoadrenalism, and growth impairment (in children) may be present. People with panhypopituitarism tend to have sallow complexions because of the ACTH deficiency and they become particularly sensitive to the actions of insulin because of the decreased secretion of the insulin antagonists, GH and cortisol. They are prone to develop hypoglycemia, particularly when stressed. Hypogonadism is manifested by amenorrhea in women, impotence in men, and loss of libido in both men and women. Some of the clinical manifestations of hypothyroidism are cold, dry skin, constipation, hoarseness, and bradycardia. The myxedema (nonpitting edema) associated with severe hypothyroidism is rare. Adrenal insufficiency caused by the ACTH deficiency can result in weakness, mild postural hypotension, hypoglycemia, and a loss in pubic and axillary hair. The only symptom associated with the PRL deficiency is the incapacity for postpartum lactation. Finely wrinkled skin is characteristic of a deficiency of both gonadotropin and GH. The GH deficiency can also lead to fasting hypoglycemia in adults and children. In children, growth is impaired and the relative increase in adipose tissue and decrease in muscle mass may produce a "chubby" appearance. The symptoms of the endocrine deficiencies are not as severe as they are in primary thyroid, adrenal, and gonadal deficiencies.

Pituitary Apoplexy Pituitary apoplexy results from acute infarction of the pituitary gland. There are multiple potential causes for hemorrhagic infarction of the pituitary, including tumor, trauma, bleeding disorder, and postpartum necrosis (**Sheehan's syndrome**). Sheehan's syndrome occurs when excessive blood is lost during and following delivery, resulting in ischemia of the enlarged pituitary of pregnancy. Damage to the pituitary can result in impaired secretion of some or all of the anterior pituitary hormones. The severity of the loss is variable and most individuals show relatively normal secretion of the posterior pituitary hormones.

Empty Sella Syndrome Empty sella syndrome occurs when the subarachnoid space extends into the sella turcica, thereby partially filling it with cerebrospinal fluid. This compresses the pituitary and enlarges the sella (Figure 5-29). The flattened pituitary may continue to function, sometimes even normally. There are many different causes of empty sella syndrome, which can be either congenital or acquired. It is relatively common and represents a major cause of sellar enlargement.

Growth

Normal growth is a complex process that requires normal endocrine function. There are definitive patterns for normal growth. The most rapid growth occurs during fetal development and the exact fetal growth regulators have not yet been well established. Although GH is not thought to regulate fetal growth, insulin, PRL, and hPL might be growth regulators. Postnatally, the most rapid growth occurs in the neonate. The next period of rapid growth occurs at puberty. It is during puberty that the rising estrogen levels act to stimulate closure of the epiphyses and hence cause the termination of long-bone growth.

The role of GH in growth regulation has been discussed. However, appropriate levels of thyroid hormones, insulin, and cortisol are also required for normal growth. The growth deficiencies associated with hypothyroidism are discussed in Chapter 6. Causes of retarded growth in children are listed in Box 5-2. In the absence of normal insulin levels, intermediary metabolism is impaired and IGF production decreases. Both of these hormones are important for normal growth. Whereas a cortisol deficiency is not typically associated with growth impairment, hypercortisolism is. Gonadal steroids are potent growth stimulators in puberty, but they also terminate long-bone growth by stimulating closure of the epiphyses. Growth is stunted if nutrition is not adequate. In either starvation or malnutrition, IGF-I production is low and growth is slowed.

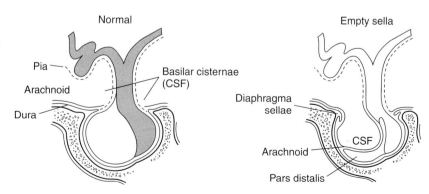

FIGURE 5-29 ■ Representation of normal relationship of meninges to pituitary gland (*left*) and findings in empty sella (*right*) as arachnoid membrane herniates through incompetent diaphragma sellae. CSF, cerebrospinal fluid. (*Redrawn from Jordan RM, Kendall JW, Kerber CW: Am J Med 62:569, 1977.*)

Another cause of growth impairment is **psychosocial growth retardation.** Infants who are not stimulated and nurtured or children developing in a hostile environment can demonstrate growth retardation. These children have an immature appearance and often have unusual eating and drinking habits. Pituitary function in these children is suppressed. However, when such children are removed from the poor environment, normal pituitary function resumes and growth resumes.

In many cases, deficient growth is merely a result of constitutional delay. This is not a pathologic condition but a genetic variation from the average. Chronic illnesses also impair growth. Genetic syndromes characterized by short stature such as Turner's syndrome (45,X gonadal dysgenesis) and skeletal dysplasias are not discussed in this section.

SUMMARY

1. The pituitary gland (also called the hypophysis) is derived from a neural structure (the infundibulum) and an epithelial structure (Rathke's pouch). The infundibulum develops into the neurohypophysis, which includes the median eminence, infundibular stalk, and pars nervosa. Rathke's pouch develops into the adenohypophysis, which includes the pars distalis, pars tuberalis, and the pars intermedia (the pars intermedia is lost in the adult human). The pituitary gland sits in a pocket of the sphenoid bone, called the sella turcica, at the base of the forebrain.

2. Magnocellular hypothalamic neurons in the paraventricular and supraoptic nuclei project axons down the infundibular stalk and terminate in the pars nervosa. The pars nervosa is a neurovascular organ, wherein neurohomones are released and diffuse into the vasculature.

3. Two neurohormones, antidiuretic hormone (ADH; also called vasopressin) and oxytocin are synthesized in the hypothalamus in the magnocellular neuronal cell bodies. ADH and oxytocin are transported intra-axonally down the hypothalamohypophyseal tracts to the pars nervosa. Stimuli perceived by the cell bodies and dendrites in the hypothalamus control the release of ADH and oxytocin at the pars nervosa.

4. The primary action of ADH is to promote water reuptake at the distal nephron and collecting duct. ADH also has vasopressive actions, which are important during vasodilatory shock.

5. Diabetes insipidus is a disease in which either there is deficient ADH (central DI) or deficient response to ADH at the kidney (nephrogenic DI). DI is associated with increased urine flow, dehydration, and increased thirst. The syndrome of inappropriate ADH secretion (SIADH) is characterized by high ADH levels, which increase volume and blood pressure and a low serum osmolarity.

6. Oxytocin acts on the breast to cause milk "letdown" during nursing and on the uterus to cause muscular contractions during labor.

7. The adenohypophysis secretes several tropic hormones, which are part of the endocrine axes. An endocrine axis includes the hypothalamus, the pituitary and a peripheral endocrine gland. The set-point of an axis is largely controlled by the negative feedback of the peripheral hormone on the pituitary and hypothalamus.

8. The adenohypophysis contains five endocrine cell types: corticotropes, thyrotropes, gonadotropes, somatotropes, and lactotropes. Corticotropes secrete ACTH, thyrotropes secrete TSH, gonadotropes secrete FSH and LH, somatotropes secrete GH and lactotropes secrete PRL.

9. The predominant control exerted by the hypothalamus on the anterior pituitary is mediated by releasing hormones. These small peptides are carried via the hypophyseal portal system to the anterior pituitary where they control synthesis and release of the pituitary hormones ACTH, TSH, FSH, LH, and GH. PRL is under predominantly inhibitory control by the hypothalamus through the catecholamine, dopamine.

10. GH stimulates growth primarily through the regulation of the growth-promoting hormones IGF-I and IGF-II. GH also has metabolic actions. It raises blood glucose by decreasing peripheral tissue utilization. It is protein anabolic and lipolytic.

11. The predominant action of PRL in humans is the initiation and maintenance of lactation.

12. Normal growth is a complex process that requires normal endocrine function. Consequently, growth deficiencies are associated with many endocrine disorders in children.

KEY WORDS AND CONCEPTS

- Pituitary gland
- Hypophysis
- Adenohypophysis
- Neurohypophysis
- Infundibulum
- Rathke's pouch
- Craniopharyngioma
- Pars intermedia
- Pars distalis
- Pars tuberalis
- Anterior pituitary
- Pars nervosa
- Posterior lobe of the pituitary
- Median eminence
- Infundibulum
- Sella turcica
- Diaphragma sellae
- Empty sella syndrome
- Supraoptic nucleus (SON)
- Paraventricular nucleus (PVN)
- Magnocellular neurons
- Hypothalamohypophyseal tract
- Pituicyte
- Neurophysin I
- Neurophysin II
- Preprovasophysin
- Preprooxyphysin
- Herring bodies
- Vasopressin 2 (V2) receptor
- Aquaporin 2
- Antidiuresis
- Antidiuretic hormone
- Diabetes insipidus
- Syndrome of inappropriate secretion of antidiuretic hormone (SIADH)
- Atrial natriuretic peptide (ANP)
- Oxytocin
- Neuroendocrine reflex
- Milk ejection (let-down)
- Positive feedback
- Basophils
- Acidophils
- Endocrine axes
- Hypophysiotropic region of the hypothalamus
- Parvicellular neurons
- Releasing hormones
- Hypothalamohypophyseal portal vessels
- Tropic hormones
- Peripheral endocrine organs
- Thyroid gland
- Adrenal cortex
- Ovary
- Testis
- Liver
- Thyroid hormone
- Cortisol
- Progesterone
- Testosterone
- Set-point
- Primary endocrine disorder
- Secondary endocrine disorder
- Tertiary endocrine disorder
- Psychosocial dwarfism
- Corticotrope
- Thyrotrope
- Gonadotrope

- Somatotrope
- Lactotrope
- Hypothalamus-pituitary-adrenal (HPA) axis
- Adrenocorticotropic hormone (ACTH)
- Pro-opiomelanocortin (POMC)
- Melanocortin-2 receptor (MC2R)
- Corticotropin-releasing hormone (CRH)
- Thyrotrope
- Tertiary hypercortisolism
- Thyroid-stimulating hormone (TSH)
- Thyrotropin
- Hypothalamus-pituitary-thyroid axis
- Pituitary glycoprotein hormone
- Alpha glycoprotein subunit (α-GSU)
- Gonadotrope
- Follicle-stimulating hormone (FSH)
- Luteinizing hormone (LH)
- Human chorionic gonadotropin (hCG)
- Thyrotropin-releasing hormone (TRH)
- Gonadotropin-releasing hormone (GnRH)
- Kallmann's syndrome
- Tertiary hypogonadotropic hypogonadism
- KAL gene
- Growth hormone (GH)
- Insulin-like growth factor I(IGF-I)
- Prolactin (PRL)
- Human placental lactogen (hPL)
- GH-binding protein (GHBP)
- Laron dwarfism
- Growth hormone-releasing hormone (GHRH)
- Somatostatin
- Ghrelin
- Stress hormones
- Hyperglycemic hormone
- Protein anabolic hormone
- Lipolytic hormone
- Diabetogenic hormone
- Hypophysectomy
- Somatomedin
- IGF-II
- IGF-binding proteins (IGFBPs)
- Acid labile subunit (ALS)
- IGFBP proteases
- Dwarfism
- Panhypopituitary dwarfism
- African pigmy

- Gigantism
- Acromegaly
- Dopamine
- Prolactin (PRL)
- Bitemporal hemianopia
- Prolactin-releasing factor (PRF)
- Lactational amenorrhea
- Panhypopituitarism
- Pituitary apoplexy
- Sheehan's syndrome
- Psychosocial growth retardation

SELF-STUDY PROBLEMS

1. Explain the origins of the neurohypophysis and adenohypophysis.
2. How is a portion of the neurohypophysis critical to the normal function of the adenohypophysis?
3. Which is ADH secretion more sensitive to: changes in volume or changes in osmolality?
4. Describe the production of ADH, both in terms of synthesis, processing, and secretion. Where do each of these occur?
5. How does SIADH result in hyponatremia?
6. How is psychogenic DI distinguished from neurogenic DI?
7. Name two proteins that are mutated in congenital nephrogenic DI.
8. How is oxytocin related to ADH?
9. Why are primary endocrine deficiencies typically more severe than secondary deficiencies?
10. Cushing's disease is hypercortisolism due to hypothalamic-independent excessive ACTH production by corticotropes. Is this a primary, secondary, or a tertiary endocrine disorder?
11. McCune-Albright syndrome is a genetically mosaic condition in which some cells express a Gs protein with an activating mutation. Explain why this can lead to excessive growth of somatotropes and high GH levels.
12. Why is GH referred to as a diabetogenic hormone?
13. How does stress (in any form) affect the secretion of the following: CRH, TRH, GnRH, and GHRH?
14. How is skin darkening related to primary hypocortisolism?

BIBLIOGRAPHY

Aimaretti GR, Baldelli, et al: IGFs and IGFBPs in adult growth hormone deficiency, *Endocr Dev* 9:76-88, 2005.

Cone RD, Low MJ, Elmquist JK, Cameron JL: Neuroendocrinology, In Larsen PR, Kronenberg HM, Melmed S, Polonsky K, editors: *Williams' textbook of endocrinology*, ed 10, Philadelphia, Saunders, 2003.

Cooper MS, Stewart PM: Diagnosis and treatment of ACTH deficiency, *Rev Endocr Metab Disord* 6:47-54, 2005.

Maghnie M: Diabetes insipidus, *Horm Res* 59 Suppl 1:42-54, 2003.

Melmed S, Kleinberg D: Anterior pituitary. In Larsen PR, Kronenberg HM, Melmed S, Polonsky K, editors: *Williams' textbook of endocrinology*, ed 10, Philadelphia, WB Saunders, 2003.

Nguyen MK, Nielsen S, et al: Molecular pathogenesis of nephrogenic diabetes insipidus, *Clin Exp Nephrol* 7:9-17, 2003.

Nishimura K, Takao T, et al: A case of anterior hypopituitarism showing recurrent pituitary mass associated with central diabetes insipidus, *Endocr J* 50:825-829, 2003.

Norrelund H: The metabolic role of growth hormone in humans with particular reference to fasting, *Growth Horm IGF Res* 15:95-122, 2005.

Robinson AG, Verbalis JG: Posterior pituitary gland. In Larsen PR, Kronenberg HM, Melmed S, Polonsky K, editors: *Williams' textbook of endocrinology*, ed 10, Philadelphia, WB Saunders, 2003.

Rizzoti K, Lovell-Badge R: Early development of the pituitary gland: induction and shaping of Rathke's pouch, *Rev Endocr Metab Disord* 6:161-72, 2005.

Verbalis JG: (2003). "Diabetes insipidus." *Rev Endocr Metab Disord* 4:177-85, 2003.

Woelfle J, Chia DJ, et al: Molecular physiology, pathology, and regulation of the growth hormone/insulin-like growth factor-I system, *Pediatr Nephrol* 20:295-302, 2005.

6

THE THYROID GLAND

OBJECTIVES

1. Explain the mechanism of synthesis of the thyroid hormones.

2. Describe the regulation of thyroid function and the actions of thyroid hormones.

3. Compare and contrast the functions of thyroxine and triiodothyronine.

4. Draw the regulatory feedback loop for the regulation of thyroid function.

5. Understand the etiology, major symptoms, and pathophysiology of the symptoms for Graves' disease, Hashimoto's thyroiditis, sporadic congenital hypothyroidism, and cretinism.

ANATOMY AND HISTOLOGY OF THE THYROID

The thyroid is a bilobed structure connected by an isthmus that extends across the ventral surface of the trachea below the larynx (Figure 6-1). As is common with endocrine glands, the thyroid has a sizable blood flow. In fact, when expressed on a tissue weight basis, its blood flow exceeds that of the kidney. In goiters, this flow can increase markedly, and this increased flow can produce an audible **bruit** over the gland. The gland is innervated by adrenergic fibers from the cervical ganglia and by cholinergic fibers from the vagus nerve. This autonomic innervation regulates blood flow (adrenergic increases blood flow; cholinergic decreases it). Some have proposed that there might also be some neuronal regulation of hormone synthesis and secretion (adrenergic increases hormone synthesis and secretion; cholinergic decreases it).

The gland contains follicles formed by epithelial cells called **follicular cells** (Figure 6-2). These cells are cuboidal in a normal gland, columnar in a highly stimulated gland, and squamous in an inactive gland. A clear viscous material called **colloid** is found in the lumen. Colloid is the glycoprotein **thyroglobulin (TG),** which contains the molecular structure of the thyroid hormones (see Figure 6-2). In the stroma around the follicles are the "light" or "C" cells that produce calcitonin. (Calcitonin is discussed in Chapter 4.)

THYROID HORMONES

The thyroid hormones are **iodothyronines,** compounds formed by coupling two iodinated tyrosine molecules in an ether linkage. The predominant hormones include the following:

1. **Thyroxine (T_4),** or 3,5,3',5'-tetraiodothyronine, constitutes about 90% of the thyroid hormone secreted by the gland.

2. **Triiodothyronine (T_3),** or 3,5,3'-triiodothyronine, constitutes about 9% of the hormone secreted from

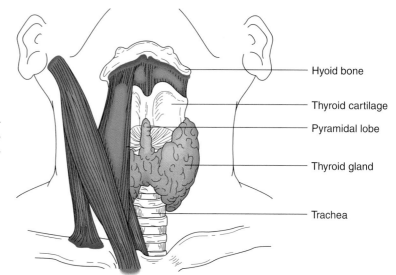

FIGURE 6-1 ■ Anatomy of thyroid. *(Redrawn from Greenspan FS, Strewler GJ, editors: Basic and clinical endocrinology, ed 5, Norwalk, Conn, 1997, Appleton & Lange.)*

- Hyoid bone
- Thyroid cartilage
- Pyramidal lobe
- Thyroid gland
- Trachea

the gland. T_4 is sometimes considered the prohormone for T_3.

3. **Reverse T_3** (rT_3), or 3,3′,5′-triiodothyronine, represents about 1% of the hormone secreted from the gland and is not thought to be biologically active.

When tyrosine molecules are iodinated, **monoiodotyrosine (MIT)** and **diiodotyrosine (DIT)** are formed (Figure 6-3). These **iodotyrosines** are not biologically active.

Synthesis of Thyroid Hormones

Iodide Transport Since iodine is a trace element, an effective mechanism is present for selectively trapping iodide in the thyroid follicular cell. Iodine is taken up as inorganic iodide; this active transport system is referred

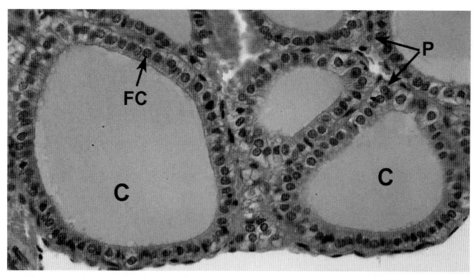

FIGURE 6-2 ■ Normal rat thyroid. Single layer of cuboidal epithelial cells (follicular cells [FC]) surround colloid (C). Parafollicular cells (P) produce calcitonin.

BOX 6-1

OVERVIEW

The thyroid hormones have widespread actions. They are a major regulator of the body's energy metabolism and regulate many aspects of development. Their actions include regulating neurologic, cardiovascular, musculoskeletal, and reproductive function.

to as the **iodide trap** (Figure 6-4). The effectiveness of iodide trapping is sometimes assessed by the thyroid/serum **(T/S) ratio.** The **T/S** iodine concentration is generally measured with radioactive iodide. The ability of the thyroid to accumulate iodide is remarkable; values as high as 400 have been reported. The normal T/S iodine concentration in a euthyroid person is approximately 30 (the iodide concentration in the follicular cell is 30 times the concentration in the serum). Iodide is concentrated against both its electrical and concentration gradients. The carrier, which is located in the basilar membrane (near extracellular fluids) of the follicular cell, is capable also of transporting other, strongly basic anions, and its affinities for perchlorate and for thiocyanate are actually greater than its affinity for iodide concentration. **Thyrotropin (thyroid-stimulating hormone [TSH])** regulates the T/S ratio for iodide. When the TSH levels drop after hypophysectomy, the T/S ratio drops. If TSH levels are high, as they are in secondary (pituitary) hyperthyroidism, the T/S ratio is high. The salivary glands, mammary glands, gastric mucosa, choroid plexus, placenta, skin, and ovaries are also capable of iodide accumulation. The thyroidal iodide trap is used clinically in several ways; the thyroid gland can be selectively destroyed by oral administration of radioactive iodide [^{131}I] because the isotope is accumulated in the gland, incorporated into TG, and retained there for a prolonged period of time. The beta emissions of the isotope destroy the follicular cells.

The thyroid may be scanned by administering radioactive iodide, allowing time for uptake, and then imaging the gland. Because the radioisotope pertechnetate (TcO_4^-) has a much shorter half-life ($t_{1/2}$) (6 hours) than ^{131}I (8 days), it is a safer isotope to use for this purpose. It is possible to use ^{123}I to measure the **radioactive iodide uptake (RAIU)** of the thyroid and hence, assess its ability to take up serum iodine (Figure 6-5).

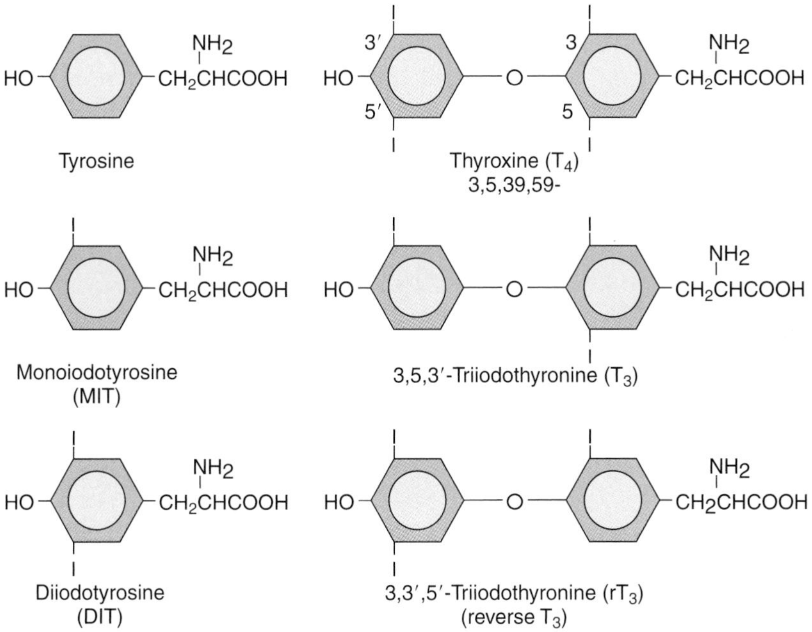

FIGURE 6-3 ■ Tyrosine and some of its iodinated derivatives.

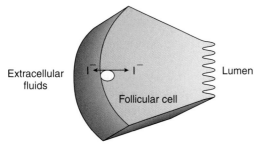

FIGURE 6-4 ■ Iodide (I⁻) is actively transported into follicular cell.

An actively functioning gland will have a faster uptake than a poorly functioning gland.

Thyroglobulin Synthesis TG is the precursor of all thyroid hormones. It is a large glycoprotein. The dimeric form has a molecular weight of approximately 660 kDa.

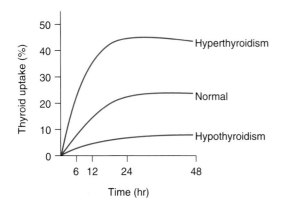

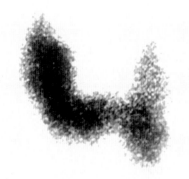

FIGURE 6-5 ■ **A,** Radioactive iodine uptake over 48 hours in patients with normal and abnormal thyroid function. **B,** Scan of thyroid gland after ¹²³I administration.

TG does not have an unusually high concentration of tyrosine molecules. In fact, this large molecule has only about 132 tyrosine residues. Approximately 20% of these residues are iodinated and only about 5% will be coupled to become the active thyroid hormones, T_4 and T_3. Like other proteins in the cell, TG is synthesized on the rough endoplasmic reticulum of the follicular cell and the glycosylation occurs in the Golgi apparatus. TG is then packaged in exocytotic vesicles and extruded into the lumen of the follicle (Figure 6-6).

Oxidation of Iodide Once within the follicular cell, the iodide is oxidized into an active intermediate. The reaction is catalyzed by **thyroid peroxidase (TPO);** hydrogen peroxide (H_2O_2) is the oxidizing agent. TPO is a membrane-bound enzyme found on the apical surface (near the lumen) of the follicular cell. The exact state of this active intermediate is not known. It could be the free radical of iodide. In the latter case, the reaction could be expressed as follows:

$$I^- + H_2O_2 \rightarrow 2\ HO^- + E - I \cdot (TPO)\ (Active\ iodide)$$

Where E = enzyme

Iodide must be oxidized before organification of iodine can occur.

Organification (Iodination) Iodination is also catalyzed by TPO. "Active iodide" is probably added to the tyrosyl residue after the incorporation of tyrosine into TG. Organification of the iodine produces MIT and DIT residues in the TG molecule.

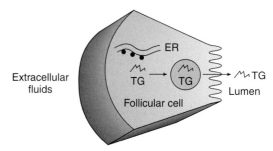

FIGURE 6-6 ■ Synthesis of thyroglobulin (TG). TG is synthesized on polyribosome of endoplasmic reticulum (ER), packaged in membrane-bound secretory vesicle in Golgi apparatus and secreted into lumen.

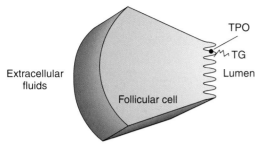

FIGURE 6-7 ■ Organification and coupling. Thyroid peroxidase (TPO) at apical surface of follicular cell catalyzes organification and coupling of thyroglobulin (TG).

Coupling Two DITs are coupled to form T_4, or one MIT and one DIT are coupled to form T_3. Such coupling occurs while the DIT and MIT are part of the TG molecule. Both intramolecular and intermolecular coupling occurs. TPO catalyzes this reaction also. TG contains only about three residues of T_4 or T_3 per molecule of TG. There is about 10 times more T_4 than T_3 in TG, and there is very little rT_3 (Figure 6-7).

Storage The thyroid hormones are stored as a part of the TG molecule in the lumen of the follicle. This TG is referred to as colloid.

Thyroid Hormone Secretion

TSH stimulates endocytosis of colloid droplets into the follicular cell (Figure 6-8). Pseudopodia from

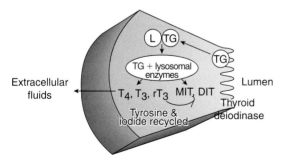

FIGURE 6-8 ■ Secretion of thyroid hormones. Thyroglobulin (TG) is endocytosed and merges with lysosome (L) that contains proteolytic enzymes that hydrolyze TG to release hormones. Iodinated tyrosines (MIT and DIT) are deiodinated by thyroid deiodinase.

the follicular cell engulf the droplet, forming a membrane-bound droplet in the interior of the follicular cell rather than in the lumen. This droplet then fuses with a lysosome to form a **phagosome** (**endosome**). The proteolytic enzymes (**proteases**) within the phagosome hydrolyze TG to the constituent amino acids and T_4, T_3, rT_3, and MIT and DIT. Because MIT and DIT are not biologically active, their secretion into plasma would be inefficient use of the scarce mineral iodine. However, the follicular cells contain **thyroid deiodinase,** which is specific for iodotyrosines and not iodothyronines. This enzyme releases iodine from these iodotyrosines so that it can be re-used in the iodination of new TG. The iodothyronines then leave the follicular cell. Although the exact mechanism for transporting the hormones out of the cell is not known, many investigators think it is by simple diffusion.

Extrathyroidal Pools There are large extrathyroidal pools of thyroid hormones. About one third of the body's T_4 is in the liver and kidney. The T_4 pool is larger (20 times greater than the T_3 pool) and slower in turnover (10% per day) than the T_3 pool (70% per day). Because the size of this pool is large relative to the secretion rate, it can serve to "buffer" acute changes in the hormone secretion rate. If thyroidal T_4 secretion doubles in a 24-hour period, it only increases serum T_4 levels approximately 5%. Because of this effect, T_4 may be administered orally once a day and serum hormone levels will not change appreciably over the 24-hour period. However, because the pool for T_3 is much smaller, serum concentrations would be more variable if T_3, rather than T_4, were administered. Although it was once thought that T_3 was the best form to use for treating hypothyroidism because it is the more potent form, T_4 is now considered the more appropriate compound for replacement therapy.

Wolff-Chaikoff Effect Excess iodine given to a person with a normal thyroid gland inhibits organification and hormone synthesis. This blockage is temporary, and "escape" generally occurs within several days despite continued high dietary iodine. Exactly how this effect occurs is not known.

Compounds Altering Thyroid Hormone Synthesis

Goitrogens are substances that can block thyroid hormone production and therefore produce goiters. The **thioureas,** like **propylthiouracil (PTU),** act at several points. They inhibit TPO and block oxidation of iodide and organification. They act also on the peripheral tissues to inhibit the 5'-monodeiodinase (D1), which converts T_4 to the more active compound T_3. Methimazole is another commonly used goitrogen. It inhibits organification but does not affect peripheral deiodination. Other compounds act as competitive inhibitors of iodide uptake. These include perchlorate and thiocyanate. The latter is found in cabbage and cassava.

Thyroid Hormone Transport

Protein Binding When thyroid hormones are secreted into the blood, they bind reversibly to serum carrier proteins. Bound and free hormones are in equilibrium; as the levels of free hormones change, the levels of bound hormones also change in accordance with the law of mass action. The protein with the highest affinity for T_4 and T_3 is **thyroxine-binding globulin (TBG)** (Box 6-2). Although the affinity is high, the capacity (quantity available) is low. This compound binds the largest portion of the circulating thyroid hormones. In fact, 77% of the bound T_4 is bound to TBG. The second highest quantity is bound to **transthyretin (TTR;** also called **thyroxine-binding prealbumin).** This compound's affinity for T_4 is less than that of TBG, and the quantity in the blood is higher (higher capacity). TTR does not effectively bind T_3. Albumin binds a small portion of the circulating thyroid hormones. Although the quantity of circulating albumin is high relative to the other two proteins (high capacity),

the affinity of albumins for thyroid hormones is relatively low. In addition, small amounts of thyroid hormones are found bound to sterol hormone-binding proteins and to serum lipoproteins. Many drugs, such as salicylates and phenytoin, decrease the binding affinity of TBG to thyroid hormones (Box 6-3).

Thyroid hormones have an exceptionally high binding affinity for these proteins. Serum T_4 is approximately 99.96% bound and 0.04% free (Figure 6-9).

BOX 6-3
FACTORS ALTERING SERUM TBG-BOUND HORMONE

Increased Thyroxine-Binding Globulin (TBG) Concentration
- High estrogen levels because of pregnancy or oral contraceptives

Decreased TBG Concentration
- Androgens, glucocorticoids
- Malnutrition

Drugs Decreasing Binding
- Phenytoin (Dilantin)
- Salicylates

BOX 6-2
PROTEIN BINDING OF THYROID HORMONE

$$T_4 + TBG \leftrightarrow [T_4 \cdot TBG]$$

$$K = [T4] [TBG]]/[T4 \cdot TBG]$$

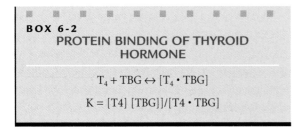

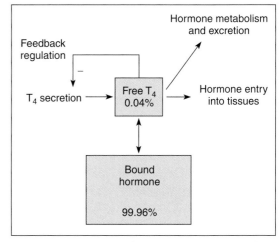

FIGURE 6-9 ■ Binding of T_4. Free serum T_4 is in equilibrium with bound hormone. Free form is generally considered to be the biologically active form.

Because T_3 has a lower affinity for these proteins, about 99.6% of serum T_3 is bound and 0.4% is free. These binding proteins play multiple roles. The theory has been questioned that only the free form of the hormone can enter cells and exert a biological effect. Because there is a simple equilibrium between bound and free forms of the hormone, the bound hormone serves as a reservoir for the hormone (a significant portion of the "nonthyroidal pool") and therefore buffers short-term changes in hormone secretion rate. This nonthyroidal pool is approximately 770 µg in adult humans. Homeostatic regulation of thyroid hormone levels controls the serum free T_4 (T_3) and not the total hormone. Because studies on patients with a complete TBG deficiency suggest that the patients are normal, what role do these binding proteins play? Thyroid hormones are only sparingly soluble in blood; hence, without the binding proteins, the quantity of hormone that could be transported in blood would be much smaller, providing less of a buffering effect against changes in glandular secretion. Furthermore, binding to the large proteins decreases renal filtration of thyroid hormones. Because protein binding may limit cellular transport of thyroid hormones, it decreases metabolic clearance of the hormones.

Standard radioimmunoassays (RIAs) of the thyroid hormones measure total T_4 (or T_3) and hence, measure both bound and free forms. However, it may be the free hormone that has the greatest clinical significance. Estrogens nonspecifically stimulate the synthesis of liver-binding proteins, including TBG. During pregnancy, TBG levels can increase to the extent that serum total T_4 is about twice what it is in the nonpregnant state. The pregnant woman is not clinically hyperthyroid and her free T_4 level remains within the upper normal range. Obviously, if physicians do not acknowledge the effect of estrogen on TBG levels, they could erroneously conclude that a pregnant woman is hyperthyroid.

There are other disorders or drugs that can alter binding protein levels or affinity. The clinician must be alert to this possibility and understand the significance of such changes. It is now possible to measure free T_4 and free T_3 levels by RIA, but the assays are not yet completely reliable under all of the conditions that can alter TBG levels.

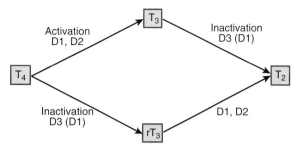

FIGURE 6-10 ■ The role of the major deiodinases (D1, D2, D3) in the activation and inactivation of thyroid hormones.

Metabolism of Thyroid Hormones

T_4 is the major secretory product of the thyroid. The predominant pathway for its metabolism is progressive deiodination (Figure 6-10). T_4 is initially deiodinated either in the outer ring to form the more potent compound T_3 [by the enzymes type 1 deiodinase (D1) or type 2 deiodinase (D2)], or deiodinated in the inner ring to form the inactive compound rT_3 primarily by type 3 deiodinase (D3), although D1 has some inner ring activity. This makes D3 the major T_4 and T_3 inactivating enzyme. D1 is located in the plasma membrane where it is thought to serve a major role in conversion of T_4 to T_3 *before* cellular entry. It is found in peripheral tissues such as liver and kidney and is responsible for the majority of the T_4 to T_3 conversion that occurs in the circulation. D2 is found primarily in pituitary gland, brain, and brown fat. It is an endoplasmic reticulum protein; it is thought to play a major role in regulating intracellular T_3 levels in these tissues. D3 is found primarily in placenta, brain, and skin and is located on the plasma membrane; it is more readily available to circulating T_4 and T_3. Because the thyroid secretes very little T_3, 80% of the circulating T_3 is produced by peripheral deiodination of T_4. Most of the circulating rT_3 is produced by peripheral deiodination of T_4. Because the initial monodeiodination of T_4 produces either a more potent compound or an inactive compound, this is an important step in determining the biological activity of the thyroid hormones.

During starvation and debilitating illnesses, the activity of D1 is decreased and hence, the production of T_3 is decreased. Because D1 is also the enzyme that deiodinates rT_3 to T_2, the levels of rT_3 in serum rise. Some scientists have proposed that this is an important control mechanism that decreases the basal metabolic rate under these circumstances. Other less important pathways for the thyroid hormone metabolism include (1) conjugation with sulfate or glucuronate and secretion in the bile; (2) decarboxylation and deamination to **triac** and **tetrac;** and (3) decarboxylation to T_3-**amine** or T_4-**amine.**

CONTROL OF THYROID FUNCTION

Thyroid-stimulating hormone (TSH) or thyrotropin is a glycoprotein hormone produced in the thyrotropes of the anterior pituitary. The hormone consists of two polypeptide chains. TSH stimulates growth and vascularity of the thyroid gland and the synthesis and secretion of the thyroid hormones. It affects every step in the pathway for hormone synthesis and secretion. It increases iodide uptake, oxidation of iodide, organification, and coupling. When TSH levels increase, the follicular cell becomes more columnar in shape, endocytosis of colloid increases, and TG proteolysis increases.

Control Mechanisms

TSH secretion is inhibited by high serum T_4 levels and to a lesser extent by T_3 levels (Figure 6-11). The actual control within the thyrotrope is a function of the intracellular T_3 levels; these levels are determined by the transport of T_4 into the cell from serum and the deiodination of this T_4 to T_3. Approximately 80% of pituitary intracellular T_3 comes from in situ deiodination of T_4 (D2), whereas 20% comes from serum T_3. For this reason, regulation of intracellular D2 levels can control the sensitivity of the pituitary to feedback inhibition. TSH secretion can be modulated by **thyrotropin-releasing hormone (TRH).** TRH increases the level of the set-point ("thermostat") for the regulatory feedback loop. This compound is a 3-amino acid peptide produced in the hypothalamus (and other regions of the brain) that acts on the pituitary to stimulate TSH synthesis and secretion.

The sensitivity of the pituitary to TRH depends on intrapituitary T_3 levels. When intracellular T_3 is high, there is down-regulation of TRH receptors and the pituitary response to TRH decreases. However, if serum T_4 levels are low, intracellular T_3 levels drop and

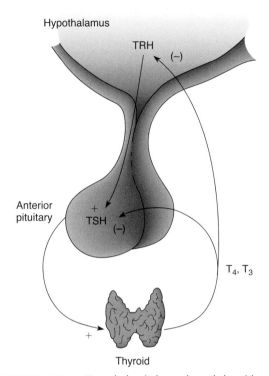

FIGURE 6-11 ■ Hypothalamic-hypophyseal-thyroid axis. Thyrotropin-releasing hormone (TRH) produced in hypothalamus reaches the thyrotropes by hypothalamic-hypophyseal portal system and enhances secretion of thyroid-stimulating hormone (TSH) by altering the set-point of T_3 inhibition of TSH secretion.

the concentration of thyrotrope TRH receptors increases. As a result of this change, the pituitary sensitivity to TRH stimulation increases. Clinical use has been made of this concept (Figure 6-12). After a bolus injection of TRH, serum TSH levels rise rapidly to reach a peak within 30 minutes in the normal person and then fall to basal levels within 3 hours. If the person is **hypothyroid,** basal serum TSH levels would be higher and the rise in serum TSH in response to the TRH would be greater. If the person has high serum T_4 levels, as in Graves' disease (thyroid hyperplasia not of pituitary or hypothalamic origin), the sensitivity of the pituitary to TRH can become so low that there is little or no TSH secretion in response to the TRH. If the patient has hypothalamic (tertiary) hypothyroidism, the pituitary can respond to TRH. However, it

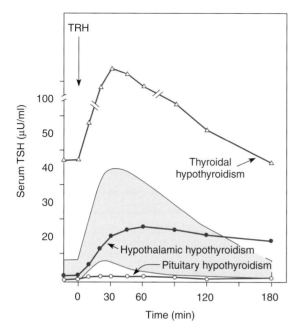

FIGURE 6-12 ■ TSH responses to thyrotropin-releasing hormone (TRH) in patients with primary, secondary, and tertiary hypothyroidism. The shaded area represents the normal range. *(Redrawn from Utiger RD: Tests of thyroregulatory mechanisms. In Werner SC, Ingbar SM, editors: The thyroid, ed 5, Philadelphia, 1986, Lippincott.)*

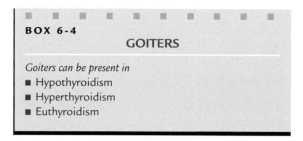

BOX 6-4

GOITERS

Goiters can be present in
- Hypothyroidism
- Hyperthyroidism
- Euthyroidism

relationship, the role of iodine availability and thyroid function is evaluated. If there is a dietary iodine deficiency, the synthesis of thyroid hormones could be decreased. As glandular T_4 (T_3) secretion decreases, pituitary TSH synthesis and secretion will increase (Figure 6-13). TSH stimulates growth and vascularity of the thyroid. Consequently, the gland will enlarge.

does not show the exaggerated response that would be expected in a hypothyroid person. This is probably because the pituitary has not been previously exposed to TRH regulation. The most common response is a rise in TSH secretion that is similar in magnitude to that of a euthyroid person, but the response is slower to develop and lasts longer. Although these tests were once used to distinguish hypothalamic from pituitary hypothyroidism, they often are unnecessary now because of the availability of ultrasensitive TSH assays.

Perturbations of Control System

A **goiter** is an enlargement of the thyroid gland; the size of the gland depends on the level of TSH stimulation. However, gland size does not indicate the level of thyroid function. It is possible to have a goiter and be **hypothyroid, euthyroid** (normal thyroid function), or **hyperthyroid** (Box 6-4). To demonstrate this

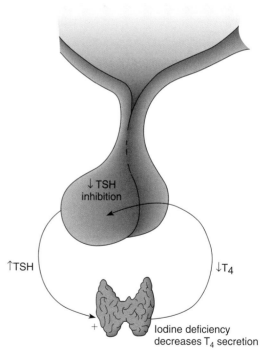

FIGURE 6-13 ■ Iodide deficiency decreases hormone synthesis, which can increase thyroid-stimulating hormone (TSH) secretion and hence, glandular growth.

However, TSH also stimulates the uptake of the remaining iodide and the synthesis and secretion of hormone. The T/S ratio increases as the "trapping" efficiency of the gland improves. If the iodine deficiency is not too great, the gland can compensate and return serum T_4 to normal levels. However, it took a hypertrophied gland to produce this compensation. Consequently, the patient has a goiter and yet is euthyroid. (In long-term iodine-deficient states, the thyroid becomes more sensitive to TSH and frequently serum TSH levels will be within the normal range but the gland will be enlarged.) If there is insufficient iodide availability, even with intense TSH stimulation, the patient will be hypothyroid and will have a goiter.

In **Graves' disease,** the thyroid is stimulated by abnormal immunoglobulins (**thyroid-stimulating antibodies [TSAb]),** which are not regulated by the hypothalamus-pituitary (Figure 6-14). The gland

hypertrophies because TSAb binds to the TSH receptors on the follicular cell and mimics the action of TSH. TSAb, like TSH, can stimulate the synthesis and secretion of T_4 (T_3); consequently, the person is hyperthyroid and has a goiter (see Figure 6-14). Serum TSH levels in these patients are low to nonmeasurable.

MECHANISMS OF HORMONE ACTION

Thyroid Hormone Receptors

Thyroid hormones enter the cell, most likely by plasma membrane transport systems and bind to high-affinity, low-capacity nuclear receptors (Figure 6-15) that are bound to the **thyroid-responsive element** of DNA. When the hormone binds to the ligand-binding domain of the DNA-bound receptor, the hormone-bound receptors can act as transcription factors to regulate gene transcription of certain mRNAs. There is considerable homology between the DNA-binding region of this receptor and those for estrogen and retinoic acid. There is some homology with those for glucocorticoid, mineralocorticoid, progesterone, and androgen receptors. These receptors function like hormone-dependent transcription factors. The affinity of the receptor for T_3 is approximately 10 times that for T_4.

Although most of the actions of thyroid hormones appear to be mediated by nuclear receptors, nongenomic actions have also been shown. Possible direct targets of thyroid hormone in the plasma membrane include the glucose transporters, calcium ATPase and adenylate cyclase. Thyroid hormones may act on mitochondria independent of any nuclear action and specific mitochondrial thyroid receptors have been proposed that could serve as mitochondrial transcription factors.

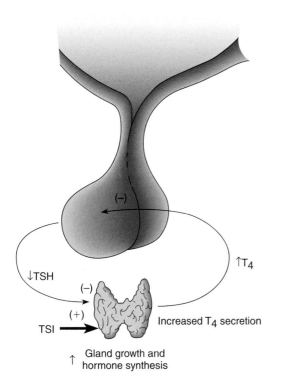

↓TSH
(−)
(+)
TSI
↑T_4
Increased T_4 secretion
↑ Gland growth and hormone synthesis

FIGURE 6-14 ■ Gland growth and function in Graves' disease are stimulated by thyroid-stimulating immunoglobulins (TSI). TSH, thyroid-stimulating hormone.

Thyroid-Stimulating Hormone Receptor

TSH receptors are present on the surface of the thyroid follicular cell (type 1). TSH predominantly acts on the thyroid follicular cell by stimulating cyclic adenosine monophosphate (cAMP) production. TSH receptors have been found on nonthyroidal tissues. Although adipocytes, lymphocytes, fibroblasts, and gonads have TSH receptors (type 2), the role of TSH receptors in

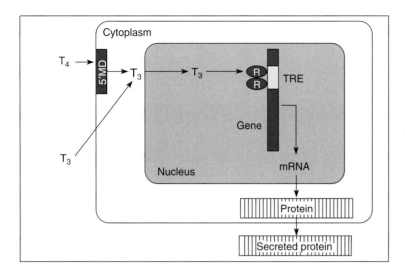

FIGURE 6-15 ■ Mechanisms of action of thyroid hormones. R, thyroid receptor; 5′MD, 5′-monodeiodinase; TRE, thyroid-responsive element.

these tissues is not yet known. However, TSH does stimulate adipocyte lipolysis. Furthermore, in Graves' disease—an autoimmune disease involving the TSH receptor—problems are sometimes seen with fibroblasts in the eye (resulting in *exophthalmos*) and the skin of the pretibial region *(pretibial myxedema)*. These problems could be mediated by nonthyroidal TSH receptors. TSH has enough structural similarity to human chorionic gonadotrophin (hCG) that there is some cross-reaction between hCG and TSH on the TSH receptor. Consequently, during the first trimester of pregnancy, when hCG levels are high, enlargement of the thyroid and increased thyroid hormone secretion are seen.

ACTIONS OF THYROID HORMONES

Maturational and Differentiational Effects

Thyroid hormones play a crucial role in amphibian metamorphosis. If a tadpole is given excess T_4, it undergoes metamorphosis prematurely and develops into a miniature frog. On the other hand, if thyroid function in the tadpole is blocked with propylthiouracil (PTU), the tadpole does not undergo metamorphosis. Thyroid hormones actually stimulate synthesis of the enzymes that dissolve the tadpole tail.

Thyroid hormones are also important for normal human maturation (Box 6-5). Bone maturation is delayed in hypothyroid children (Figure 6-16). These children often show delayed or absent puberty. Thyroid hormones play an important role in perinatal lung maturation and have been administered in utero to stimulate surfactant formation in high-risk infants.

Neurologic Effects

Thyroid hormones are necessary for normal fetal and neonatal brain development (Box 6-5). They regulate neuronal proliferation and differentiation, myelinogenesis, neuronal outgrowth, and synapse formation. There is a critical period of brain development that begins in utero and extends to approximately age 2 years during which a thyroid hormone deficiency results in

---

BOX 6-5
ACTIONS OF THYROID HORMONES

■ Maturation and differentiation
■ Neurologic function
■ Growth
■ Metabolism
■ Sympathetic nervous system function
■ Skeletal muscle
■ Cardiovascular system
■ Reproduction

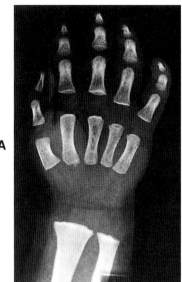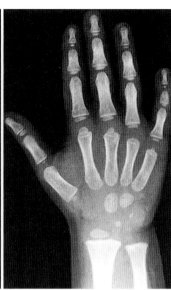

FIGURE 6-16 ■ X-ray films of hands of 3-year-old hypothyroid child **(A)** and normal child **(B)**. Note marked delay in bone development in hypothyroid child. *(From Besser GM, Thorner MO: Clinical endocrinology, London, 1994, Mosby-Wolfe.)*

A

B

structural and physiologic impairment. Thyroid hormone replacement subsequent to this period cannot reverse the damage caused by deficiency. Congenital hypothyroidism can result in severe and irreversible brain damage. Because infants with neonatal hypothyroidism (**sporadic congenital hypothyroidism**) who are not treated have severe neurologic impairment, a neonatal thyroid screening program was implemented in the United States. The incidence of sporadic congenital hypothyroidism is approximately 1:4000 to 1:5000 children. The disorder is not always visually apparent at birth. The mental retardation that could result without treatment is severe enough to warrant the cost of routine screening. It is important that the diagnosis be made and treatment initiated within the first month of birth, and most clinicians attempt to begin replacement therapy as soon as possible within that period. Some people have even attempted hormone replacement in utero.

Thyroid hormones also affect neurologic function subsequent to the critical period, but these changes can be reversed by correcting the thyroid disorder. Hypothyroid adults tend to be dull and lethargic and to have prolonged reflex times. Their thought processes and speech are slow. They often sleep excessively. Hypothyroidism can produce psychological disturbances, leading to **myxedema madness.** Patients who are hyperthyroid tend to be excitable, restless, and distractable; they have insomnia and a decreased reflex time.

Effects on Growth

Adequate thyroid hormone levels are necessary for normal growth (Box 6-5). Children with thyroid hormone deficiencies show stunted growth, which can be severe. When thyroid hormone levels are low, growth hormone and IGF secretion decline, which increases growth stunting. However, both thyroid hormones and growth hormone are essential for normal growth.

Metabolic Actions

Thyroid hormones control the **basal metabolic rate (BMR)** (Box 6-5). They are calorigenic and hence, increase oxygen consumption and heat production. This response has a long latent period in vivo. In fact, after serum thyroid hormone levels are increased, it takes approximately 10 days for the BMR to reach a maximal level. Before the advent of RIAs for thyroid hormones, the BMR was used as a clinical test for thyroid disorders. The BMR decreases in hypothyroidism and increases in hyperthyroidism. In hyperthyroidism, mitochondria increase in size and number. The complexity of their cristae increases—as does the concentration of the oxidative phosphorylation enzymes. Some tissues do not respond to T_4 with an increase in oxygen consumption (spleen, testis, and adult brain).

Thyroid hormones increase membrane Na^+-K^+ adenosine triphosphatase (ATPase) concentration and activity and increase membrane Na^+ and K^+ permeability. As much as 15% to 40% of the basal energy used in the cell is applied to maintaining this electrochemical gradient. Thyroid hormone increases the activity of Na^+-K^+ ATPase and hence, increases energy expenditure in resting cells. Thyroid hormone administration decreases the ratio of intracellular sodium to potassium concentration in liver, skeletal muscle, and heart. Thyroid hormones increase energy expenditure by increasing futile cycling because they frequently stimulate both anabolic and catabolic enzymes of the same pathways.

In general, thyroid hormones stimulate all metabolic pathways, both anabolic and catabolic (with some exceptions). They stimulate protein synthesis, but they also stimulate protein degradation. The actual effects are dose dependent. Moderate doses of T_4 are protein anabolic in a hypothyroid individual and these moderate doses decrease nitrogen excretion. However, high doses can lead to net protein catabolism and increased urinary nitrogen excretion. Thyroid hormones stimulate protein turnover. Whether the tissue concentrations of fats, protein, or glycogen change depends on the relative effects on anabolic and catabolic pathways. Thyroid hormones increase cellular uptake of amino acids and incorporation of these amino acids into protein. In hypothyroidism, protein synthesis decreases but so does its degradation. In actuality, the percentage of the body weight that is protein tends to decrease. In hyperthyroidism, both synthesis and degradation increase. Total protein concentration is not necessarily compromised with mild hyperthyroidism but, if the disturbance is excessive, there may not be adequate substrate available to maintain protein levels. The same can be said about fat and glycogen synthesis and degradation.

Thyroid hormones stimulate lipogenesis. However, they also are lipolytic and can increase hormone-sensitive lipase activity. In general, degradation is affected more than synthesis. Again, fat synthesis and degradation decrease in hypothyroidism. In this case, the percentage of fat in the body increases over time.

As expected, hyperthyroidism results in increased lipid synthesis and degradation. Total lipids decrease. Although the liver synthesis of triglycerides increases after thyroid hormone administration, triglyceride clearance from plasma increases because lipoprotein lipase concentration increases. Thyroid hormones can lower serum cholesterol in a euthyroid person, but the effects are transient. Although thyroid hormones increase cholesterol synthesis, they also increase availability of low-density lipoprotein (LDL) receptors and, therefore, more cholesterol (predominantly as LDL) is cleared from serum. Serum cholesterol levels increase in hypothyroidism.

Thyroid hormones affect essentially all aspects of carbohydrate metabolism. Blood glucose levels usually are normal in both hypothyroidism and hyperthyroidism. However, a hyperthyroid person often responds abnormally to a glucose tolerance test. After ingestion of the glucose load, blood glucose tends to rise more rapidly than normal. There are several proposals for this abnormality. Thyroid hormones increase the rate the gastrointestinal tract absorbs glucose, and the high hormone levels may increase both insulin resistance and insulin degradation. Glycogen metabolism also is altered in thyroid disorders. In hypothyroidism, liver synthesis and degradation decrease, but glycogen levels increase. With hyperthyroidism, glycogen synthesis and degradation increase, and as substrate availability is compromised, glycogen concentration decreases.

The clinician treating a patient with a thyroid disorder must consider the role of thyroid hormones in turnover within the body. If a patient is hypothyroid, the thyroid disorder may increase the half-lives of medications or hormones and the dosage may have to be decreased. Alternatively, if the patient is hyperthyroid, the dosage may have to be increased.

Actions Mimicking Sympathetic Nervous System Activity

Many actions of excessive thyroid hormone levels resemble those of increased sympathetic nervous system (SNS) activity (increased β-adrenergic receptor stimulation). These actions include increasing the heart rate and producing tremor and excessive sweating. The β-blocker propranolol relieves many of these symptoms without lowering serum T_4 levels. Hyperthyroidism does not increase serum catecholamines, but in some tissues it increases the β-receptor quantity, and in others it increases β-receptor affinity for catecholamines. It might also increase adenylyl cyclase sensitivity to β-adrenergic stimulation.

Actions on Skeletal Muscle

Thyroid hormones have direct actions on muscle. They increase both the content of the plasmalemma electrogenic Na^+-K^+ pump and increase the resting membrane potential. They also increase the rate and amount of calcium uptake in the sarcoplasmic reticulum, thereby increasing calcium availability on stimulation. They influence the isotype availability of myosin and increase myosin ATPase activity. The maximal shortening velocity can increase after thyroid hormone administration. Myopathies are common in both hypothyroidism and hyperthyroidism. In hypothyroidism, muscle stiffness and discomfort are common, and delayed muscle contraction and relaxation lead to slow movements. Muscle mass may increase but the mechanism is not understood. Muscle glycogenolysis is impaired and glycogen accumulates. Hyperthyroidism can result in muscle weakness, wasting, and fatigability. These problems are most apparent in the proximal muscles of the limbs and can lead to difficulties in climbing stairs. There are probably multiple causes of the myopathies in hyperthyroidism. Thyroid hormone excess can deplete proteins. Furthermore, thyroid hormones can inhibit phosphocreatine kinase and impair the ability of the muscle to phosphorylate creatine.

Actions on Cardiovascular System

Thyroid hormones increase the heart rate, myocardial contractility, and consequently the cardiac output. Although these effects can be mediated by potentiating the effects of SNS stimulation as discussed previously, the hormones also have direct actions on the myocardium. They increase actin and myosin concentration, the membrane Na^+-K^+ ATPase (the electrogenic pump) content, and myosin ATPase activity. In contrast to the effects on skeletal muscle, hyperthyroidism produces myocardial hypertrophy rather than atrophy. Thyroid hormone also acts directly as both a positive inotrope and chronotrope, independent of its action by potentiation of catecholamines. There is an increase in the rate of pressure development (dP/dt) and the maximum velocity of shortening (Vmax). Thyroid hormones also increase the velocity of relaxation by increasing expression of cardiac-specific slow sarcoplasmic reticulum calcium ATPase. Characteristic changes are sometimes seen in the electrocardiogram (ECG) of people with thyroid disorders. The ECG of a hypothyroid person may show inverted T waves (particularly in lead II) and low P, QRS, and T-wave amplitudes. The hyperthyroid person may show ECG changes indicative of left ventricular hypertrophy.

In hyperthyroidism, stroke volume, heart rate, and mean systolic ejection velocity increase, accompanied by decreased peripheral resistance. Peripheral resistance is decreased when thyroid hormone levels are high for two reasons: (1) thyroid hormones act directly on vascular smooth muscle to cause vasodilation; (2) the increased heat and metabolite production results in cutaneous vasodilation. People with hyperthyroidism have warm, moist skin. Because cardiac output increases and peripheral resistance decreases, the pulse pressure increases (Table 6-1).

Heart rate and stroke volume decrease in hypothyroidism and peripheral resistance is usually increased. Again, the effects on peripheral resistance reflect both the loss of cutaneous vasodilation and the loss of the direct action of thyroid hormones on vascular smooth muscle. The cutaneous vasoconstriction is responsible for the cold skin of patients with myxedema.

PATHOLOGIC CONDITIONS INVOLVING THE THYROID

Hypothyroidism

Children Hypothyroidism in children is different from hypothyroidism in adults because thyroid hormones are important for normal development and maturation. There are multiple causes of hypothyroidism in children. Dietary iodine deficiency beginning in utero impairs the ability of the thyroid to synthesize thyroid hormones and results in **endemic cretinism** (Figure 6-17). Although, technically, the term *cretinism* should be reserved for children with endemic iodine

TABLE 6-1		
Physiologic Action of Thyroid Hormones		
	HYPOTHYROID	**EUTHYROID**	**HYPERTHYROID**
Metabolic rate	Decreased BMR		Increased BMR
Proteins	↓ Synthesis, ↓ degradation, ↓ turnover (% BW as protein will ↓)	Protein anabolic	↑ Synthesis, ↑ degradation, ↑ turnover (catabolic if insufficient dietary protein)
Lipids	↓ Synthesis, ↓ degradation, ↓ turnover (% of BW as lipid increases), ↓ serum cholesterol	↑ Beta oxidation, ↑ lipolysis, ↑ lipogenesis	↑ Synthesis, ↑ degradation, ↑ turnover (% of BW as lipid decreases), ↓ serum cholesterol
Glucose	Normal	Normal	Normal serum glucose; abnormal glucose tolerance test
Glycogen	↓ Synthesis, ↓ degradation, ↓ turnover, glycogen accumulates		↑ Synthesis, ↑ degradation, ↑ turnover, glycogen is depleted
Actions with SNS			Excess mimics effects of ↑ β-adrenergic stimulation; can ↑ number and affinity of β-receptors and ↑ adenylyl cyclase sensitivity
Direct cardiovascular actions	↓ Amplitude of ECG waves	↑ HR, ↑ CO, ↑ contractility, ↑ pulse pressure, ↑ actin and myosin	↑ Amplitude of ECG waves

BMR, basal metabolic rate; BW, body weight; CO, cardiac output; ECG, electrocardiogram; HR, heart rate; SNS, sympathetic nervous system.

deficiency, the term is often loosely applied to all forms of hypothyroidism beginning at or before birth. For children whose hypothyroidism does not result from iodine deficiency, the term *sporadic congenital hypothyroidism* is more appropriate. There are multiple causes for sporadic congenital hypothyroidism, including thyroid agenesis or dysgenesis and thyroidal defects in hormone biosynthesis, such as organification defects. There are also rare cases of hereditary thyroid hormone resistance. Another cause of neonatal

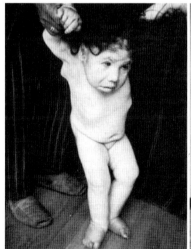
A

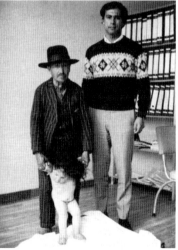
B

FIGURE 6-17 ■ **A,** A 28-year-old Ecuadoran woman with endemic cretinism. **B,** She is held by her father and accompanied by a normal-height Ecuadoran man. *(From Fierro-Benitez R, Ramirez I, Garces J, et al: Am J Clin Nutr 27:531, 1974.)*

hypothyroidism is the transfer of thyroid-blocking antibodies across the placenta from a mother with autoimmune thyroid disease.

The symptoms of hypothyroidism in newborns can include respiratory distress syndrome, poor feeding, hoarse cry, umbilical hernia, and retarded bone age. Because visible symptoms are not always obvious, routine neonatal thyroid screening is essential to detect the disorder and to begin replacement therapy early enough to prevent mental retardation.

Untreated hypothyroidism in children results in mental retardation and growth stunting. These children may show delayed or absent sexual maturity. However, in a small percentage of cases, precocious puberty may occur. This is possible because the high serum TSH levels in congenital hypothyroidism result in some TSH binding to LH and FSH receptors (remember, all three of these hormones are from the same family of glycoprotein hormones); TSH then mimics the action of these gonadotropins. The developmental and maturational changes discussed earlier cannot be entirely reversed by subsequent replacement therapy.

Adults Common symptoms of hypothyroidism in adults are listed in Box 6-6. Hypothyroidism results in a decreased BMR, hypothermia, and cold intolerance. The skin tends to be dry and cool because of decreased sweating, decreased sebaceous gland secretion, and cutaneous vasoconstriction. Sweating decreases in response to lower heat production, and there is insufficient adenosine triphosphate (ATP) for normal sweat formation. These people tend to feel cold in a warm room (Figure 6-18).

There are neurologic symptoms as well. Adults with hypothyroidism tend to become dull and lethargic, their speech rate slows, and their reflex time is prolonged. They are prone to depression and will frequently sleep excessively. Resultant psychological problems can reach the level of frank psychosis; the term *myxedema madness* has been used to describe the psychiatric problems that can result.

The patients tend to demonstrate a generalized, nonpitting edema called **myxedema.** This myxedema results from the accumulation of **glycosaminoglycans (GAGs)** (mucopolysaccharides; primarily hyaluronic acid and chondroitin sulfate) in the interstitial

> **BOX 6-6**
> ### COMMON SYMPTOMS OF HYPOTHYROIDISM
>
> - Decreased basal metabolic rate
> - Weakness, fatigue, lethargy
> - Somnolence
> - Mental slowness
> - Muscle aches
> - Cold intolerance
> - Dry cold skin
> - Prolonged reflex times
> - Decreased sweating
> - Weight gain
> - Thick tongue
> - Myxedema
> - Goiter
> - Slow speech
> - Hoarseness
> - Amenorrhea
> - Psychosis
> - Electrocardiogram changes
> - Thin, brittle hair
> - Constipation

spaces—hence, fluid is retained. This swelling leads to the hoarseness frequently described in these people. The skin thickens and coarsens, facial features thicken, the tongue enlarges, and there is noticeable periorbital edema. Although the term *myxedema* is frequently used synonymously with hypothyroidism, its use is not appropriate because myxedema is a descriptive term for a specific type of nonpitting edema; it is also seen in pathologic disorders other than hypothyroidism. In fact, **pretibial myxedema** is a common occurrence in the hyperthyroidism of Graves' disease.

Because thyroid hormones regulate protein metabolism, it is not surprising that changes are seen in hair texture. There are changes in hair follicle function and the hair becomes thin, coarse, brittle, and lacks luster. The loss of the lateral one third of the eyebrows is common. Nail deformities are also noted frequently.

Gastrointestinal disturbances are common in thyroid disorders and hypothyroid people tend to have problems with constipation. Appetite and food consumption tend to decrease; however, BMR and

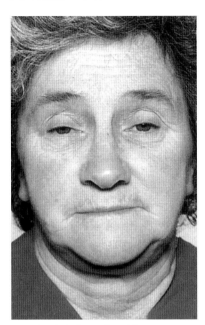

FIGURE 6-18 ■ Adult hypothyroidism. Note puffy face, puffy eyes, frowzy hair, and dull, apathetic appearance. *(From Hall R, Evered DC: Color atlas of endocrinology, ed 2, London, 1990, Mosby-Wolfe.)*

Causes of hypothyroidism are listed in Box 6-7. Many of the symptoms of hypothyroidism described for adults are also seen in children. Although most of the symptoms are reversed on correction of the thyroid disorder, developmental disturbances are often not entirely reversible with subsequent treatment.

Hyperthyroidism

Thyrotoxicosis results when tissues are exposed to excessive quantities of thyroid hormones. The most prevalent form of hyperthyroidism is Graves' disease. This is an autoimmune disorder in which T lymphocytes become sensitized to antigens within the thyroid gland and subsequently stimulate B lymphocytes to produce antibodies (IgGs) to these antigens. In most cases, antibodies are produced to thyroglobulin (TG), thyroid peroxidase (TPO), and the TSH receptor. The latter antibodies mimic the action of TSH on the thyroidal TSH receptors (serving as TSH agonists). They bind to the follicular cell membrane and stimulate cAMP production and hence, hormonogenesis and secretion. Like TSH, these antibodies stimulate the growth and vascularity of the thyroid gland.

Thyroid-related IgGs are a diverse group of antibodies directed against various different sites within the follicular cell membrane. Some appear to be cytotoxic, some stimulate cAMP, and some block the

therefore caloric use also decrease. Consequently, these individuals frequently gain weight.

Menstrual irregularities are common in both hypothyroidism and hyperthyroidism. Women with hypothyroidism find it difficult to become pregnant; when pregnancy occurs, the incidence of spontaneous abortion, stillbirths, and fetal impairment increases.

Cardiovascular signs occurring in hypothyroidism include bradycardia, decreased myocardial contractility, and hence, reduced cardiac output. The voltage of the deflections on the ECG is reduced and there may be pericardial effusion as a result of the interstitial edema. These people may have hypertension because of increased peripheral resistance at rest. Such changes result in decreased pulse pressure. Elevated serum cholesterol and triglyceride levels are common, as is the development of atherosclerosis. At one time, thyroid hormones were used to treat hyperlipemia in euthyroid people, but the effects were transient and the side effects were unacceptable.

action of TSH. Individuals with this disorder show an increased frequency of certain haplotypes: HLA-B8 and HLA-DR3 in whites, HLA-BW46 in Chinese, and HLA-BW35 in Japanese. There is strong familial predisposition for the disorder and women have 7 to 10 times the incidence of men. This antibody production is not related to the circulating levels of pituitary TSH secretion; hence, the feedback loop between the thyroid and the hypothalamus-pituitary is no longer regulating the thyroid. The high circulating T_4 and T_3 levels inhibit pituitary TSH synthesis and secretion.

The symptoms frequently seen in hypothyroidism are listed in Box 6-8. Because the antibodies can stimulate thyroid growth, a goiter is usually present. As expected, both the BMR and body heat production increase. Some symptoms of hyperthyroidism result, at least partially, from potentiated catecholamine actions. These include **lid retraction** (resulting in a "wide-eyed" stare), tachycardia, and tremor.

Eye changes (**exophthalmos**) are common in Graves' disease (Figure 6-19). The most common observations are lid lag (upper lid is slow to follow the movement of the gaze downward), upper lid retraction, stare, extraocular muscular weakness, diplopia,

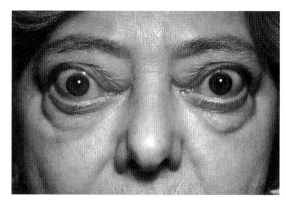

FIGURE 6-19 ■ Severe exophthalmos of Graves' disease. Note lid retraction, periorbital edema, and proptosis. *(From Hall R, Evered DC: Color atlas of endocrinology, ed 2, London, 1990, Mosby-Wolfe.)*

periorbital edema, and proptosis. Proptosis may become so severe that the eyelids cannot close and corneal ulceration results. Proptosis occurs because the retro-orbital contents increase. Both the retro-orbital connective tissue and the muscles are involved. The extraocular muscles can increase to 8 times their original volume. Muscle weakness is associated with the muscle enlargement. There is fibroblastic proliferation and GAGs accumulate in the retro-orbital tissues (Figure 6-20). The pathogenesis of this ophthalmopathy is not well understood. These ocular abnormalities are immunologically mediated. The ophthalmopathy is not caused by the high levels of serum T_4 and T_3, and correcting the hyperthyroidism does not necessarily prevent progression. The retro-orbital fibroblasts and adipocytes are targets of the autoimmune attack. TSH receptors associated with these cells may promote the T lymphocytes activated against the TSH receptor to infiltrate the orbit and skin. These activated cells then release cytokines such as interferon-γ, interleukin-1, and transforming growth factor-β. The cytokines stimulate fibroblasts to produce GAGs that accumulate and produce edema. Edema within the retro-orbital muscles and adipose tissue produces proptosis and extraocular muscle dysfunction.

Dermopathy (pretibial myxedema) may be associated with Graves' disease. Between 2% and 10% of the patients have myxedema in the pretibial area (pretibial myxedema) and/or feet. In these regions, the skin

---

■ ■ ■ ■ ■ ■ ■ ■ ■ ■ ■

BOX 6-8
SYMPTOMS OF HYPERTHYROIDISM

- Nervousness
- Heat intolerance
- Palpitations
- Muscle weakness
- Increased defecation frequency
- Increased appetite
- Moist, warm skin
- Bruit over thyroid
- Goiter
- Tremor
- Pretibial myxedema (Graves' disease)
- Fatigue
- Eye problems (Graves' disease)
  - Exophthalmos
  - Lid retraction
  - Extraocular muscle weakness
  - Eye irritation

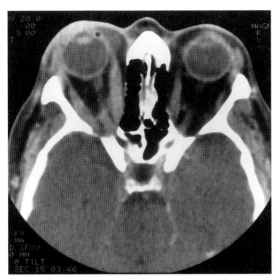

FIGURE 6-20 ■ CT scan of middle cranial fossa of woman with exophthalmos. Extraocular muscles are enlarged, and eyes protrude beyond rims of orbit. *(Courtesy Dr. C. Joe.)*

thickens and forms "pig-like" plaques. The edges of these plaques are well defined, and nodules are sometimes present. As with the myxedema of hypothyroidism, GAGs accumulate in the dermis. These regions itch and are sometimes painful. The pathologic basis of this dermopathy is thought to be an autoimmune disorder. T lymphocytes infiltrate the skin in the pretibial region, where fibroblasts have TSH receptors (type 2); these lymphocytes release cytokines that stimulate GAG production and subsequent edema. Other forms of hyperthyroidism include toxic multinodular goiter, toxic adenoma, and sometimes Hashimoto's thyroiditis.

Thyroiditis

Subacute thyroiditis is an acute inflammation of the thyroid that is probably the result of viral infection.

The symptoms generally include fever and tenderness of the gland. Symptoms of hyperthyroidism may be present, although the thyroidal status depends on the stage of the inflammation. Although excessive thyroid hormones may be released early in the inflammation, transient hypothyroidism may follow before resolution of the inflammation and restoration of euthyroidism. TSH levels are not generally elevated during the course of the thyroiditis and elevated radioactive iodide uptake and serum thyroid antibodies are typically not seen. Although approximately 10% of patients have permanent hypothyroidism, more typically the thyroid disorder resolves spontaneously.

Hashimoto's thyroiditis is a common cause of acquired hypothyroidism. It is an autoimmune disorder characterized by the presence of thyroid antibodies. The antibodies are produced by lymphocytes that become sensitized to thyroidal antigens. Common thyroidal antigens are TPO and TG. In Hashimoto's thyroiditis, the gland becomes inflamed and lymphocytes infiltrate the gland. Structural damage of the gland occurs and TG is released into serum. Hyperthyroidism may be present early in the progression of Hashimoto's thyroiditis and Hashimoto's thyroiditis and Graves' disease can occur simultaneously. However, as the disease progresses and the gland is destroyed, hypothyroidism develops, serum T_4 and T_3 levels fall, and TSH levels rise. The patient usually has a goiter and most typically is either euthyroid or hypothyroid. Radioactive iodine uptake may be low, normal, or high—depending on the nature of the disorder. However, high antibody titers to TPO or TG are typical. Hashimoto's thyroiditis can sometimes be part of a syndrome involving multiple autoimmune endocrine disorders that can include the adrenals, pancreas, parathyroids, and ovaries (Schmidt's syndrome).

SUMMARY

1. The biologically active thyroid hormones are iodothyronines. Whereas T_4 is the predominant hormone secreted by the gland, T_3 is the most potent hormone at the receptor level. Most circulating T_3 is produced peripherally from T_4, and the reaction is catalyzed primarily by D1.

2. Thyroid hormones are major regulators of the body's energy metabolism. They also regulate many aspects

of maturation and development as well as growth. They have neurologic, cardiovascular, musculoskeletal, and reproductive functions.

3. Growth of the thyroid is stimulated by TSH; therefore physiologic changes resulting in increased TSH secretion can produce goiters. The size of the gland is not indicative of the level of function of the gland.

4. Congenital hypothyroidism can produce permanent brain damage if it occurs during the "critical period" that begins in utero and extends until age 2.

5. Common symptoms of hypothyroidism include decreased BMR, cold intolerance, prolonged reflex times, myxedema, and constipation. Common symptoms of hyperthyroidism include increased BMR, heat intolerance, shortened reflex times, diarrhea (or frequent bowel movements), and tremor. The most common form of hyperthyroidism is Graves' disease. It is an autoimmune disease associated with the production of antibodies sensitized to the TSH receptor. Exophthalmos is frequently associated with Graves' disease.

KEY WORDS AND CONCEPTS

- Bruit
- Follicular cells
- Colloid
- Thyroglobulin (TG)
- Iodothyronines
- Thyroxine (T_4)
- Triiodothyronine (T_3)
- Reverse T_3 (rT_3)
- Iodotyrosines
- Monoiodotyrosine (MIT)
- Diiodotyrosine (DIT)
- Iodide
- Iodide trap
- T/S [I^-]
- Thyrotropin, thyroid-stimulating hormone (TSH)
- Radioactive iodide uptake (RAIU)
- Thyroid peroxidase (TPO)
- Organification
- Coupling
- Phagosome (endosome)
- Thyroid deiodinase (D1, D2, D3)
- Extrathyroidal pools

- Wolff-Chaikoff effect
- Goitrogens
- Thioureas (propylthiouracil [PTU])
- Thyroxine-binding globulin (TBG)
- Transthyretin (TTR) (thyroxine-binding prealbumin)
- T_2, T_1, T_0
- Triac
- Tetrac
- T_3-amine
- T_4-amine
- Thyrotropin-releasing hormone (TRH)
- Hypothyroid
- Goiter
- Euthyroid (or hyperthyroid)
- Graves' disease
- Thyroid-responsive element (TSab)
- Sporadic congenital hypothyroidism
- Myxedema madness
- Basal metabolic rate (BMR)
- Endemic cretinism
- Myxedema
- Glycosaminoglycans (GAGs)
- Pretibial myxedema
- Lid retraction
- Exophthalmos
- Subacute thyroiditis
- Hashimoto's thyroiditis

SELF-STUDY PROBLEMS

1. Why is hypercholesterolemia common in hypothyroidism?
2. How does hypothyroidism affect the half-life ($t_{1/2}$) of administered drugs?
3. What effect would a decrease in TBGs binding affinity for thyroid hormones have on thyroid function?
4. Why do serum T_4 levels approximately double in pregnancy? Are pregnant women hyperthyroid?
5. What effect does T_4 administration have on the size of the thyroid and the secretion of T_4 and TSH in a euthyroid person?

BIBLIOGRAPHY

Bahn RS, Heufelder AE: Retroocular fibroblasts: important effector cells in Graves' ophthalmopathy, *Thyroid* 2:89, 1992.

Benvenga S, Lapa D, Trimarchi F: Re-evaluation of the thyroxine-binding to human plasma lipoproteins using three techniques, *J Endocrinol Invest* 24:RC16-RC18, 2001.

Bianco AC, Larsen PR: Intracellular pathways of iodothyronine metabolism. In LE Braverman, Utiger RD, editors: *Werner & Ingbar's the thyroid*, ed 9, Philadelphia, 2005, Lippincott Williams & Wilkins.

Chin WW: Current concepts of thyroid hormone action: progress notes for the clinician, *Thyroid Today* 15(3), 1992.

Delange F: The disorders induced by iodine deficiency, *Thyroid* 4:107, 1994.

Heufelder AE, Dutton CM, Sarkar G, et al: Detection of TSH receptor RNA in cultured fibroblasts from patients with Graves' ophthalmology and pretibial dermopathy, *Thyroid* 3:297, 1993.

Koenig RJ: Thyroid hormone receptor coactivators and corepressors, *Thyroid* 8:703-713, 1998.

Larsen PR, Davies TF, Hay ID: The thyroid gland. In Wilson JD, Foster DW, Kronenberg HM, Larsen PR, et al, editors: *Williams' textbook of endocrinology*, ed 9, Philadelphia, 1998, WB Saunders.

Lazar MA: Thyroid hormone receptors: multiple forms, multiple possibilities, *Endocr Rev* 14:184, 1993.

Ojamaa K, Klemperer JD, Klein I: Acute effects of thyroid hormone on vascular smooth muscle, *Thyroid* 6:505-512, 1996.

Polikar RA, Burger G, Scherrer U, Nicod P: The thyroid and the heart, *Circulation* 87:1435, 1993.

Porterfield SP, Hendrich CE: The role of thyroid hormones in prenatal and neonatal neurological development—current perspectives, *Endocr Rev* 14:94, 1993.

Schreiber G: The evolutionary and integrative role of transthyretoid hormone homeostasis, *J Endocrinol* 175:61-73, 2002.

Schusser GC: The thyroxine-binding proteins, *Thyroid* 10:141-149, 2000.

Weintraub BD: Molecular biology of thyroid disease, *Forum* (Endocrine Fellows Foundation) 13:1, 1992, Pfizer.

Wiersinga WM: Propranolol and thyroid hormone metabolism, *Thyroid* 1:273, 1991.

Yen, PM: Physiological and molecular basis of thyroid hormone action, *Physiol Rev* 81:1097-1142, 2001.

Yen PM: Genomic and nongenomic actions of thyroid hormones. In LE Braverman, Utiger RD, editors: *Werner & Ingbar's the thyroid*, ed 9, Philadelphia, 2005, Lippincott Williams & Wilkins.

Zang J, Lazar MA: The mechanism of action of thyroid hormones, *Annu Rev Physiol* 62:439-466, 2000.

APPENDIX
LABORATORY DATA ON THYROID FUNCTION

Hormone Production Rates

1. T_4 production is approximately 90 mg/day.
2. T_3 production is approximately 30 mg/day.
3. Normal serum T_4 levels are 5 to 12 mg/dl.
4. Normal serum T_3 levels are 115 to 190 ng/dl.
5. Serum rT_3 levels are approximately 40 ng/dl.
6. $t_{1/2}$ of T_4 is 6 to 8 days.
7. $t_{1/2}$ of T_3 is 24 hours.

Tests of Thyroid Function

Serum TSH represents the single best screening test for thyroid function.

Serum T_4 and T_3 are measured by RIA. These tests do not distinguish bound from free hormone.

T_3 Resin Uptake provides an index of TBG levels (or available hormone binding sites). To measure this uptake, a tracer quantity of radioactive T_3 is mixed with serum. The radioactive T_3 should distribute itself between the bound and free forms in accordance with the ratio of bound and free forms for the nonradioactive hormone. A synthetic resin that binds free T_3 is then added. The radioactive T_3 (and cold T_3) that was originally in the free form will now bind to the resin. The resin can be precipitated from the serum and the radioactivity counted. If the levels of free T_3 are high in the original serum, the percentage of resin ^{125}I-T_3 uptake will be high. This could result from low levels of TBG or excessively high levels of free T_3. If serum TBG levels increase and free T_3 is normal, the percentage of free T_3 is low and the relative distribution of the

TABLE 6-2						
Serum Tests for Thyroid Evaluation						
	T_4	T_3	RESIN T_3 UPTAKE	T_4 INDEX	T_3 INDEX	rT_3	TSH
Hyperthyroidism	↑	↑, N	↑	↑, N	↑	↑	↑, ↓, N
Hypothyroidism	↓	↓, N	↓	↓	↓	↓	↑, ↓, N
↑ TBG	↑	↑	↓	N	N	↑	N
↓ TBG	↓	↓	↑	N	N	↓	N

N, normal; TBG, thyroxine-binding globulin; TSH, thyroid-stimulating hormone.

radioactive T_3 between the free and the bound phases decreases. This reduces the free ^{125}I-T_3 available to bind the resin. Hence, the percentage of resin uptake will decrease. Because the resin uptake basically provides an index of serum binding capacity (predominantly TBG), either T_3 or T_4 can be used. However, because the percentage of free T_3 is higher than the percentage of T_4, the results of the resin uptake tend to be slightly more accurate if ^{125}I-T_3 is used rather than ^{125}I-T_4.

Free T_4/T_3 Index

1. Free T_4 index = $[T_4] \times [T_3$ resin uptake$]$
2. Free T_3 index = $[T_3] \times [T_3$ resin uptake$]$
3. These are nondimensional numbers that are an indirect approximation of the true free T_4 or T_3 levels.

Radioactive Iodide Uptake (RAIU)
Increased

1. The RAIU increases in hyperthyroidism (especially at 4 hours and it is rarely normal at 24 hours).
2. The RAIU increases in iodine deficiency.

Decreased

1. Hypothyroidism
2. After exogenous T_4, T_3 administration
3. Subacute thyroiditis

Thyroid Antibodies

Anti-TPO or anti-TG may be elevated in multiple forms of thyroid disease. Very high titers are common for Hashimoto's thyroiditis.

Serum TG

These levels increase in disorders involving destruction of the thyroid, such as thyroid carcinoma and Hashimoto's thyroiditis. Serum TG levels increase when thyroid hormone synthesis and secretion increase.

TRH Challenge to TSH Secretion

A bolus injection of TRH is given and the effects on serum TSH levels are measured. Responses are listed in Table 6-3.

TABLE 6-3		
Responses to Thyrotropin-Releasing Hormone Challenge		
	BASAL MORNING TSH	**RESPONSE TO TRH**
Normal	0.5-4 µU/ml	6-25 µU/ml; peak at 20-30 min
Hyperthyroid	<0.05 µU/ml	No response
Hypothyroidism		
Primary	>4 µU/ml	Increased response
Secondary	Low to normal	No response
Tertiary	Low to normal	Normal or increased response, often delayed (60 min or later)
Nonthyroidal—illness, starvation	Normal to low	Normal to low
Excess glucocorticoids	Low	Decreased response

TRH, thyrotropin-releasing hormone; TSH, thyroid-stimulating hormone.

THE ADRENAL GLAND

OBJECTIVES

1. Discuss the anatomy of the adrenal gland, including the vascular supply and cortical zonation.

2. Discuss the synthesis and regulated release of catecholamines in the chromaffin cell.

3. Explain the action of catecholamines on different adrenergic receptors and the integrated effects of catecholamines during exercise.

4. Outline the differences between the steroidogenic pathways in each zone of the adrenal cortex.

5. Describe the physiologic actions of cortisol, aldosterone, DHEAS, and other adrenal androgens.

6. Describe the regulation of the zona fasciculata and zona reticularis by the pituitary.

7. Describe the regulation of the zona glomerulosa by the renin-angiotensin II-system.

8. Describe the pathophysiology of adrenal hormone excess and underproduction.

In the adult, the adrenal glands emerge as fairly complex endocrine structures (Box 7-1) that produce two structurally distinct classes of hormones: steroids and catecholamines. The catecholamine hormone, **epinephrine,** acts as a rapid responder to stresses such as hypoglycemia and exercise to regulate multiple parameters of physiology, including energy metabolism and cardiac output. Stress is also a major secretogogue of the longer-acting steroid hormone, **cortisol,** which regulates glucose utilization, immune and inflammatory homeostasis, and numerous other processes. The adrenal glands also regulate salt and volume homeostasis through the steroid hormone, **aldosterone.** The adrenal gland secretes large amount of the androgen precursor, **dehydroepiandrosterone**

sulfate (DHEAS), which plays a major role in fetoplacental estrogen synthesis and as a substrate for peripheral androgen synthesis in women.

ANATOMY

The **adrenal glands** are bilateral structures located immediately above the kidneys (*ad,* near; *renal,* kidney) (Figure 7-1A). In humans, they are also referred to as the **suprarenal glands** because they sit on the superior pole of each kidney. The adrenal glands are similar to the pituitary, in that they are derived from both neuronal tissue and epithelial (or epithelial-like) tissue. The outer portion of the adrenal gland, called the **adrenal cortex,** develops from mesodermal cells in the vicinity of the superior pole of the developing kidney. These cells form cords of epithelial endocrine cells. The cells of the cortex develop into

---

The fetal adrenal and its role in the fetoplacental unit will be discussed in Chapter 10.

steroidogenic cells (see Chapter 1), and produce mineralocorticoids, glucocorticoids and adrenal androgens (Figure 7-1C & 7-2).

Soon after the cortex forms, neural crest–derived cells that are associated with the sympathetic ganglia—called **chromaffin cells** because they stain with chromium stains—migrate into the cortical cells and become encapsulated by them. Thus, the chromaffin cells establish the inner portion of the adrenal gland, which is called the **adrenal medulla** (Figure 7-1C). The chromaffin cells of the adrenal medulla have the potential of developing into postganglionic sympathetic neurons. They are innervated by cholinergic preganglionic sympathetic neurons and can synthesize the catecholamine neurotransmitter, **norepinephrine,** from tyrosine. However, the cells of the adrenal medulla are exposed to high local concentrations of cortisol from the cortex. Cortisol inhibits neuronal differentiation of the medullary cells so that they fail to form dendrites and axons. Additionally, cortisol induces the expression of an additional enzyme, **phenylethanolamine-N-methyl transferase (PNMT),** in the catecholamine biosynthetic pathway. This enzyme adds a methyl group to norepinephrine, producing the catecholamine hormone, epinephrine, which is the primary hormonal product of the adrenal medulla (see Figure 7-2).

The high local concentration of cortisol in the medulla is maintained by the vascular configuration within the adrenal gland. The outer connective tissue capsule of the adrenal gland is penetrated by a rich arterial supply coming from three main arterial branches (i.e., the inferior, middle, and superior suprarenal

arteries) (see Figure 7-1A). These give rise to the following two types of blood vessels that carry blood from the cortex to the medulla (see Figure 7-1B):

1. Relatively few medullary arterioles that provide high oxygen and nutrient blood directly to the medullary chromaffin cells;
2. Relatively numerous cortical sinusoids, into which cortical cells secrete steroid hormones (including cortisol).

Both vessel types fuse to give rise to the medullary plexus of vessels that ultimately drain into a single suprarenal vein. Thus, secretions of the adrenal cortex percolate through the chromaffin cells, bathing them in high concentrations of cortisol before leaving the gland and entering the inferior vena cava.

ADRENAL MEDULLA

Together, the two adrenal medullae weigh about 1 gram. As described, the adrenal medulla is similar to a sympathetic ganglion without postganglionic processes. Instead of being secreted near a target organ and acting as neurotransmitters, adrenomedullary catecholamines are secreted into the blood and act as hormones. About 80% of the cells of the adrenal medulla secrete epinephrine and the remaining 20% secrete norepinephrine. Although circulating epinephrine is derived entirely from the adrenal medulla, only about 30% of the circulating norepinephrine comes from the medulla. The remaining 70% is released from postganglionic sympathetic nerve terminals and diffuses into the vascular system. Because the adrenal medulla is not the sole source of catecholamine production, this tissue is not essential for life.

Synthesis of Epinephrine

The enzymatic steps in the synthesis of epinephrine are shown in Figure 7-3. Synthesis begins with the sodium-linked transport of the amino acid, **tyrosine,** into the chromaffin cell cytoplasm (see Figure 7-3), and the subsequent hydroxylation of tyrosine by the rate-limiting enzyme, **tyrosine hydroxylase,** to produce **dihydroxyphenylalanine (DOPA).** DOPA is converted to **dopamine** by the cytoplasmic enzyme, **aromatic amino acid decarboxylase,** and is then

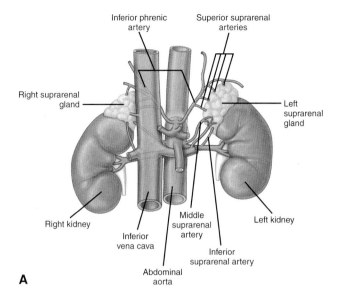

A

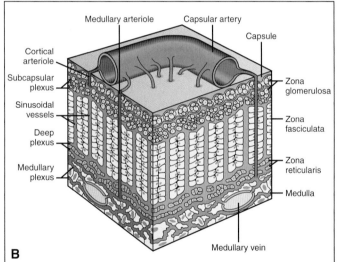

B

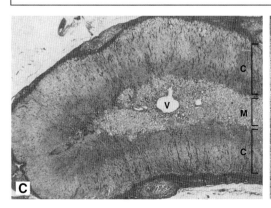

C

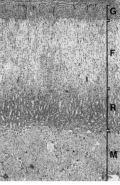

FIGURE 7-1 ■ A, Anatomy of human adrenal glands. Adrenals sit on superior poles of kidneys and thus are also referred to as suprarenal glands. Adrenal glands receive a rich arterial supply from the inferior, middle, and superior suprarenal arteries. In contrast, adrenals are drained by a single suprarenal vein. B, Blood flow through the adrenal gland. Capsular arteries give rise to sinusoidal vessels that carry blood centripetally through the cortex to the medulla. C, Left, Low magnification of adrenal histology (C, cortex; M, medulla; V, central vein.) Right, histological zonation of adrenal gland (G, zona glomerulosa; F, zona fasciculata; R, zona reticularis; M, medulla). (A, From Drake RL, Vogl W, Mitchell AWM: Gray's anatomy for students, Philadelphia, 2005, Elsevier/Churchill Livingstone; B, From Stevens A, Lowe J: Human histology, ed 3, Philadelphia, 2005, Elsevier/Mosby; C, From young B, Lowe JS, Stevens A, Heath JW Wheater's Functional Histology, Philadelphia, 2006, Churchill Livingstone/Elsevier.)

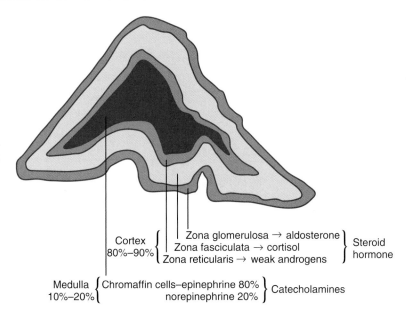

FIGURE 7-2 ■ Zonation and corresponding endocrine function of the adrenal gland.

Cortex 80%–90% {
Zona glomerulosa → aldosterone
Zona fasciculata → cortisol
Zona reticularis → weak androgens
} Steroid hormone

Medulla 10%–20% {
Chromaffin cells–epinephrine 80%
norepinephrine 20%
} Catecholamines

transported into the secretory vesicle (also called the **chromaffin granule**). Within the granule, dopamine is converted to norepinephrine by the enzyme, dopamine-β-hydroxylase. This is an efficient reaction, so essentially all of chromaffin granule dopamine is converted to norepinephrine. In most adrenomedullary cells, essentially all of the norepinephrine diffuses out of the chromaffin granule by facilitated transport and is methylated by the cytoplasmic enzyme, PNMT, to form epinephrine. Epinephrine is then transported back into the granule.

Multiple molecules of epinephrine, and to a lesser extent norepinephrine, are stored in the chromaffin granule complexed with ATP, Ca^{2+}, and proteins called **chromogranins.** These multimolecular complexes are thought to decrease the osmotic burden of storing individual molecules of epinephrine within chromaffin granules. Chromogranins play a role in the biogenesis on secretory vesicles and the organization of components within the vesicles. Chromaffin cells also synthesize several secretory peptides, including adrenomedullin and enkephalins, which can have local, subtle effects on sympathetic input and adrenomedullary response.

Secretion of epinephrine and norepinephrine from the adrenal medulla is regulated primarily by descending sympathetic signals in response to various forms of stress, including exercise, hypoglycemia, and hemorrhagic hypovolemia. The primary autonomic centers that initiate sympathetic responses reside in the hypothalamus and brain stem, and they receive inputs from the cerebral cortex, the limbic system, and other regions of the hypothalamus and brain stem.

The chemical signal for catecholamine secretion from the adrenal medulla is **acetylcholine (ACh)**, which is secreted from **preganglionic sympathetic neurons** and binds to **nicotinic receptors** on chromaffin cells. ACh increases the activity of the rate-limiting enzyme, tyrosine hydroxylase, in chromaffin cells (see Figure 7-3). ACh also increases the activity of dopamine β-hydroxylase and stimulates exocytosis of the chromaffin granules. Synthesis of epinephrine and norepinephrine is closely coupled to secretion so that the levels of intracellular catecholamines do not change significantly—even in the face of changing sympathetic activity. As discussed earlier, cortisol regulates epinephrine production by maintaining adequate expression of the PNMT gene in chromaffin cells (see Figure 7-3).

Mechanism of Action of Catecholamines

Catecholamines act via membrane GPCRs (see Chapter 1). The individual types of **adrenergic receptors** were first classified based on their pharmacology,

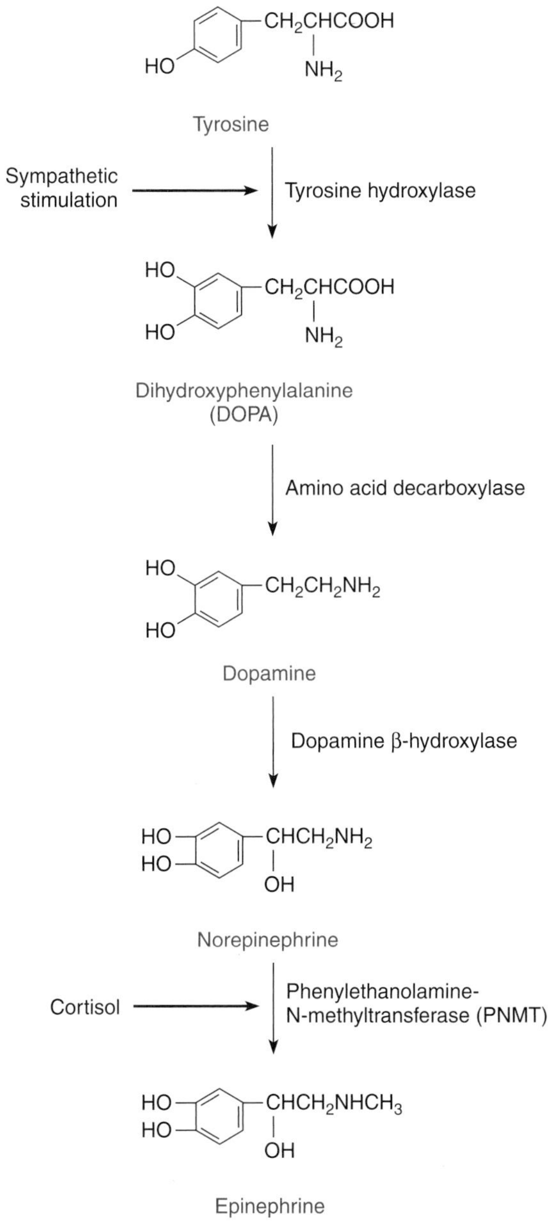

FIGURE 7-3 ■ Steps in the synthesis of catecholamines.

and this classification scheme has been supported by genetics and molecular cloning. Adrenergic receptors are generally classified as **alpha-** and **beta-adrenergic receptors,** with the alphas further divided into α_1 and α_2 **receptors,** and the betas divided into β_1, β_2, and

β_3 receptors (Table 7-1). Each alpha type can be further subdivided into three subtypes (α_{1A}, α_{1B}, α_{1D}, α_{2A}, α_{2B}, α_{2C}). These receptors can be characterized in the following ways according to:

1. The relative potency of endogenous and pharmacologic agonists and antagonists. Epinephrine and norepinephrine are potent agonists for α receptors and the $\beta1$ and $\beta3$ receptors, whereas epinephrine is more potent than norepinephrine for the $\beta2$ receptor. A large number of synthetic selective and nonselective adrenergic agonists and antagonists now exist.
2. Downstream signaling pathways. Table 7-1 shows the primary pathways that are coupled to the different adrenergic receptors. This is an oversimplification because differences in signaling pathways for a given receptor have been linked to duration of agonist exposure and cell type.
3. Location and relative density of receptors. Importantly, different receptor types predominate in different tissues. For example, although both α and β receptors are expressed by islet β cells, the predominant response to a sympathetic discharge is mediated by α_2 receptors.

Physiologic Actions of Adrenomedullary Catecholamines

Because the adrenal medulla is directly innervated by the autonomic nervous system, adrenomedullary responses are very rapid. Because of the involvement of several centers in the CNS, most notably the cerebral cortex, adrenomedullary responses can precede onset of the actual stress (i.e., they can be anticipated). For example, a sprinter at the starting line can experience an adrenomedullary response in anticipation of the starter's gun and of the intense exertion of sprinting. In many cases, the adrenomedullary output, which is primarily epinephrine, is coordinated with sympathetic nervous activity as determined by the release of norepinephrine from postganglionic sympathetic neurons. However, some stimuli (e.g., hypoglycemia) evoke a stronger adrenomedullary response than a sympathetic nervous response, and vice versa.

Many organs and tissues are affected by a sympathoadrenal response. An informative example of the major physiologic roles of catecholamines is the

TABLE 7-1

Catecholamine Receptors

RECEPTOR TYPE	PRIMARY MECHANISM OF ACTION	EXAMPLES OF TISSUE DISTRIBUTION	AGONIST POTENCY
α_1	↑ IP$_3$, DAG	Adrenergic postsynaptic nerve terminals	Epinephrine ≈ norepinephrine
α_2	↓ cAMP	Adrenergic presynaptic terminals (↓ norepinephrine release)	Epinephrine ≈ norepinephrine
β_1	↑ cAMP	Heart	Epinephrine = norepinephrine
β_2	↑ cAMP	Liver	Epinephrine >> norepinephrine
β_3	↑ cAMP	Adipose	Norepinephrine >> epinephrine

cAMP, cyclic adenosine monophosphate; DAG, diacylglycerol; IP$_3$, inositol triphosphate.

sympathoadrenal response to exercise. Exercise is similar to the **"fight or flight" response,** only without the subjective element of fear, and it involves a greater adrenomedullary response (i.e., endocrine role of epinephrine) than a sympathetic nervous response (i.e., neurotransmitter role of norepinephrine). The overall goal of the sympathoadrenal system during exercise is to meet the increased energy demands of skeletal and cardiac muscle while maintaining sufficient oxygen and glucose supply to the brain. The response to exercise includes three of the following major physiologic actions of epinephrine (Figure 7-4):

1. Increased blood flow to the muscles is achieved by the integrated actions of norepinephrine and epinephrine on the heart, veins and lymphatics, and the nonmuscular (e.g., splanchnic) and muscular arteriolar beds. Norepinephrine and epinephrine act on β1 receptors at the heart to increase the rate (chronotropy) and strength (inotropy) of contractions and facilitate ventricular relaxation during diastole (lusitropy). Catecholamines also induce **vasoconstriction through α adrenergic receptors of high capacity vessels (veins and lymphatics),** thereby increasing venous return to the heart. All of these effects increase **cardiac output.** Catecholamines shunt blood away from the GI tract via **vasoconstriction of splanchnic arterioles** (α receptors), and increase blood flow to skeletal muscle by inducing **vasodilation of muscle arteriolar beds** via β2 receptors.
2. Epinephrine promotes **glycogenolysis** in muscle through β2 receptors. Exercising muscle can also

utilize FFAs—and epinephrine and norepinephrine, acting through β2 and β3 receptors, promote **lipolysis** in adipose tissue. The actions just described increase circulating levels of lactate and glycerol, which can be used by the liver as gluconeogenic substrates to increase glucose. Epinephrine does, in fact, increase blood glucose by increasing **hepatic glycogenolysis and gluconeogenesis** through β2 receptors. The promotion of lipolysis in adipose tissue is also coordinated with an epinephrine-induced increase in **hepatic ketogenesis.** Finally, the effects of catecholamines on metabolism are reinforced by the fact that they **stimulate glucagon secretion** (β2 receptors) and **inhibit insulin secretion** (α2 receptors). Efficient production of ATP during normal exercise (i.e., a 1-hour workout) also requires efficient exchange of gases with an adequate supply of oxygen to exercising muscle. Epinephrine promotes this by **relaxation of bronchiolar smooth muscle** through β2 receptors.
3. Catecholamines decrease energy demand by visceral smooth muscle. In general, a sympathoadrenal response **decreases overall motility of the smooth muscle in the GI tract and urinary tract,** thereby conserving energy where it is not needed.

Metabolism of Catecholamines

There are two primary enzymes involved in the degradation of catecholamines: **monoamine oxidase (MAO)** and **catechol-O-methyltransferase (COMT).** Although MAO is the predominant enzyme in neuronal mitochondria, both enzymes are found in many

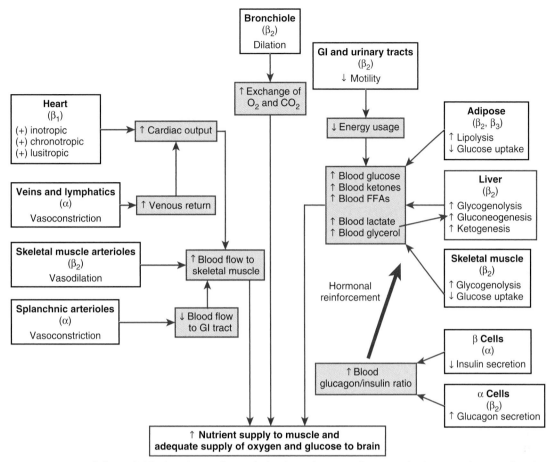

FIGURE 7-4 ■ Some of the individual actions of catecholamines that contribute to the integrated sympathoadrenal response to exercise.

nonneuronal tissues, including liver and kidney. The neurotransmitter norepinephrine is degraded by MAO and COMT after uptake of the compound into the presynaptic terminal. This mechanism is also involved in the catabolism of circulating adrenal catecholamines. However, the predominant fate of adrenal catecholamines is methylation by COMT in nonneuronal tissues such as the liver and kidney. The metabolism of catecholamines is shown in Figure 7-5. Urinary **vanillylmandelic acid (VMA)** and **metanephrine** are sometimes used clinically to assess the level of catecholamine production in a patient. Much of the urinary VMA and metanephrine is derived from neuronal, rather than adrenal, catecholamines.

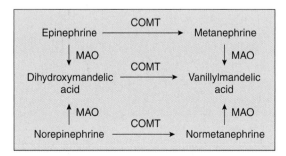

FIGURE 7-5 ■ Degradative metabolism of catecholamines. Monoamine oxidase (MAO) stimulates deamination; catechol-O-methyltransferase (COMT) stimulates methylation.

Pathologic Conditions Involving the Adrenal Medulla

A **pheochromocytoma** is a tumor of the chromaffin tissue that produces excessive quantities of catecholamines. These are commonly adrenal medullary tumors, but they can occur in other chromaffin cells of the autonomic nervous system. Although pheochromocytomas are not common tumors, they are the most common source of hyperadrenal medullary function and are often used as an example to demonstrate the functions of the adrenal medulla. The catecholamine most frequently elevated in pheochromocytoma is norepinephrine. For unknown reasons, the symptoms of excessive catecholamine secretion (Box 7-2) are often sporadic rather than continuous. The symptoms include hypertension, headaches (from hypertension), sweating, anxiety, palpitations, and chest pain. In addition, patients with this disorder may experience orthostatic hypotension (despite the tendency for hypertension). This occurs because hypersecretion of catecholamines can decrease the postsynaptic response to norepinephrine as a result of down-regulation of the receptors. Consequently, the baroreceptor response to the blood shifts that occur on standing is blunted.

ADRENAL CORTEX

The cortex of the adult human adrenal shows distinct zonation with respect to histologic appearance, steroidogenesis, and regulation. The adrenal cortex is made up of three zones: the outer **zona glomerulosa,** the middle **zona fasciculata,** and the inner **zona reticularis** (see Figure 7-2). Each zone expresses a distinct complement of steroidogenic enzymes, resulting in the production of a different steroid hormone as the major endocrine product for each zone as summarized in Figure 7-6. This means that the steroidogenic endocrine cells are characterized by the enzymes they express—as well as their final hormonal product. Associated with the production of a different steroid hormone, each zone has unique aspects concerning its regulation and/or feedback characteristics.

ZONA FASCICULATA

The Zona Fasciculata Makes Cortisol

The largest and most actively steroidogenic zone is the middle zona fasciculata. The zona fasciculata produces the glucocorticoid hormone, **cortisol.** This zone is an actively steroidogenic tissue composed of straight cords of large cells. These cells have a foamy cytoplasm because they are filled with lipid droplets that represent stored cholesterol esters. Although the cells make some cholesterol de novo from acetate, they are very efficient at capturing cholesterol from the blood circulating in the form of low-density lipoprotein and high-density lipoprotein particles. Free cholesterol is then esterified and stored in lipid droplets (Figure 7-7). The stored cholesterol is continually turned back into free cholesterol by a **cholesterol ester hydrolyase,** a process that is increased in response to stimuli of cortisol synthesis (e.g., adrenocorticotropic hormone—see later).

Free cholesterol is modified by five reactions within a steroidogenic pathway to form cortisol. However, cholesterol is stored in the cytoplasm and the first enzyme of the pathway, CYP11A1, is located on the inner mitochondrial membrane (see Figure 7-7). Thus, the rate-limiting reaction in steroidogenesis is the transfer of cholesterol from the outer mitochondrial membrane to the inner mitochondrial membrane. Although several proteins appear to be involved, one protein, called **Steroidogenic Acute Regulatory Protein (StAR Protein),** is indispensable in the process of transporting cholesterol to the inner mitochondrial membrane (see Figure 7-7). In patients with inactivating mutations in StAR protein, cells of the

---

BOX 7-2
COMMON SYMPTOMS ASSOCIATED WITH PHEOCHROMOCYTOMA

- Hypertension
- Headaches
- Sweating
- Anxiety
- Palpitations
- Chest pain
- Orthostatic hypotension

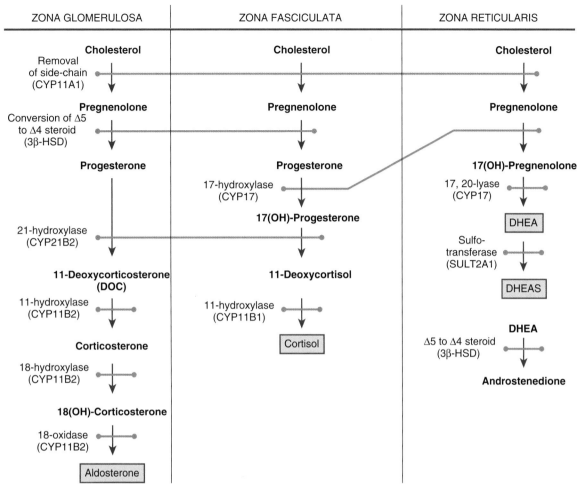

ZONA GLOMERULOSA	ZONA FASCICULATA	ZONA RETICULARIS

FIGURE 7-6 ■ Summary of the steroidogenic pathways for each of the three zones of the adrenal cortex. The major products of each zone are shown in *orange-filled boxes*.

zona fasciculata become excessively laden with lipid ("lipoid") because cholesterol cannot be accessed by CYP11A1 within the mitochondria and utilized for cortisol synthesis.

The pathway by which cortisol is synthesized involves three enzymes that are not specific to the adrenal, and two enzymes that are specifically adrenocortical in their expression. Four of these enzymes belong to the **cytochrome p450 mono-oxidase gene family**, and thus are referred to as **CYPs.** The fifth enzyme is **3β-hydroxysteroid dehydrogenase (3β-HSD).**

The steroidogenic pathway from cholesterol to cortisol is as follows:

Reaction 1. The **side-chain of cholesterol** (carbon 22 to 27) is removed by **CYP11A1** to generate a C21 steroid intermediate, **pregnenolone** (Figure 7-8). Generating a C21 intermediate is a key step because cortisol (as well as aldosterone and progesterone) is a 21-carbon steroid.

Reactions 2a/b and 3a/b. The next two enzymes compete with each other for pregnenolone, so they will be presented as Reactions 2a and 2b. The products of Reactions 2a and 2b are then modified by

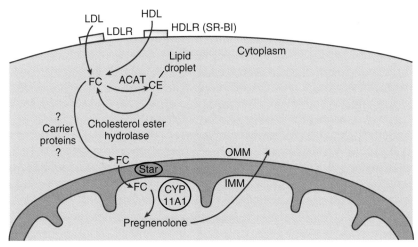

FIGURE 7-7 ■ Events involved in the first reaction in the steroidogenic pathway (conversion of cholesterol to pregnenolone) in zona fasciculata cells. Cholesterol is made de novo from acetate to a limited extent (*not shown*), and a significant amount of cholesterol is imported from low-density lipoprotein particles (LDL) via receptor-mediated endocytosis of the LDL receptor (LDLR) or through transfer of cholesterol from high density lipoproteins (HDL) mediated by the high-density lipoprotein receptor (HDLR), which is also called the scavenger receptor BI (SR-BI). Free cholesterol (FC) is converted to the storage form of cholesterol esters (CEs) by the enzyme, acyl CoA:cholesterol acyltransferase (ACAT). CEs coalesce to form lipid droplets. FC is mobilized for steroidogensis by cholesterol ester hydrolase and transported to the outer mitochondrial membrane by one or more cytoplasmic carrier proteins. FC must then be transported from the outer mitochondrial membrane (OMM) to the inside of the inner mitochondrial membrane (OMM) where CYP11A1 is localized. The critical protein that carries out this transport is steroidogenic acute regulatory (StAR) protein.

the reciprocal enzymes in Reactions 3a and 3b, to generate the final product, **17-hydroxyprogesterone** (Figure 7-9).

Reaction 2a. Pregnenolone is a substrate for the enzyme, **3β-hydroxysteroid dehydrogenase (3β-HSD),** which converts the hydroxyl group on the 3 carbon to a ketone and moves the double bond from the 5-6 ($\Delta5$) position to the 4-5 ($\Delta4$) position. *All active steroid hormones must be converted to $\Delta4$ structures.* This reaction converts **pregnenolone** (also called **P5,** because it is a $\Delta5$ steroid) to **progesterone** (also called **P4,** because it is a $\Delta4$ steroid).

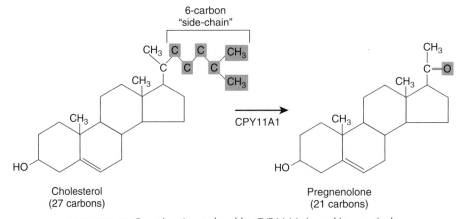

FIGURE 7-8 ■ Reaction 1, catalyzed by CYP11A1, in making cortisol.

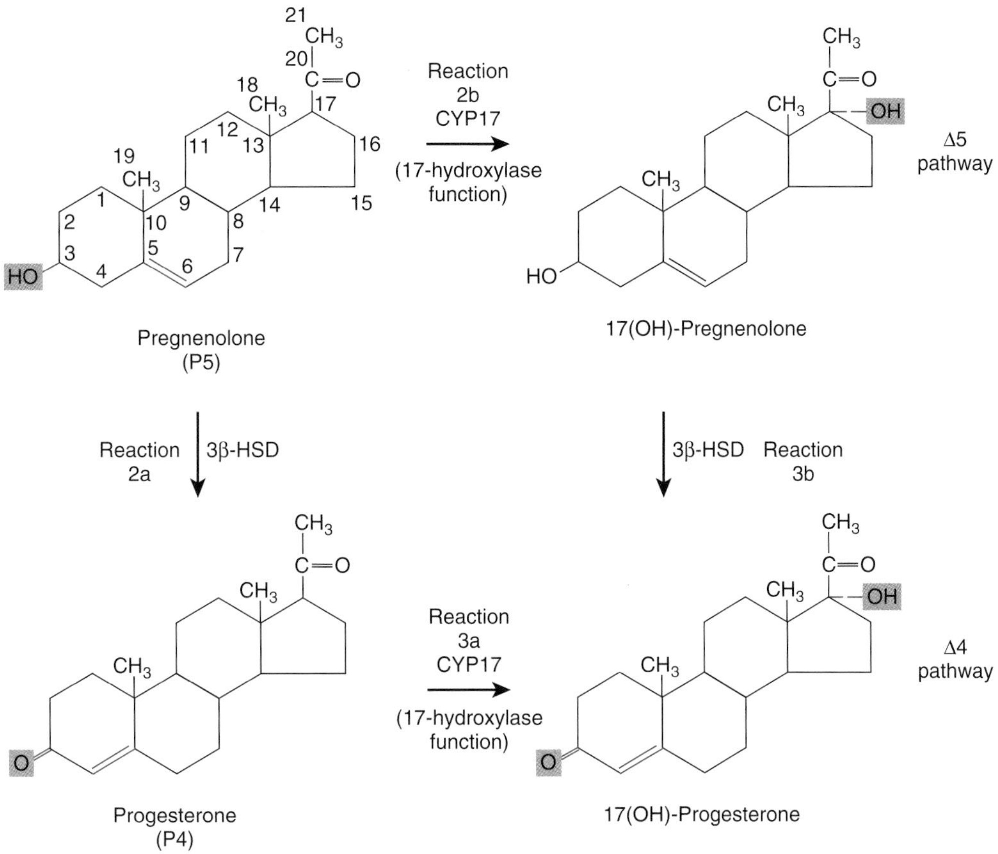

FIGURE 7-9 ■ Reactions 2a/b, and reactions 3a/b, involving CYP17 (17-hydroxylase function) and 3β hydroxysteroid dehydrogenase (3β-HSD), in making cortisol. The Δ5 versus Δ4 pathway is shown.

Reaction 3a. Progesterone is then hydroxylated to **17-hydroxyprogesterone** by **CYP17.** 17-Hydroxylation is an indispensable step for the formation of cortisol (and sex steroids). We will see that the presence or absence of CYP17 plays an important role in defining the nature of steroidogenic tissue.

Reaction 2b. Pregnenolone can also be hydroxylated by CYP17 to **17-hydroypregnenolone** (this is called the Δ5 pathway).

Reaction 3b. 17-Hydroxypregnenolone can then be converted to 17-hydroxyprogesterone by 3ß-HSD (Δ4 pathway).

It should be noted that CYP17 has two separate activities: a **17-hydroxylase function,** and a **17,20-lyase function.** This latter function removes the 20 and 21 carbons, reducing the steroid to a 19-carbon precursor

of active androgens. The zona fasciculata does not express cofactors that promote the 17,20-lyase activity of CYP17, and therefore, does not produce significant amounts of androgen precursors. Instead, 17-hydroxyprogesterone is efficiently funneled into the cortisol-specific pathway, which involves two subsequent hydroxylations by adrenocortical-specific enzymes.

Reactions 4 and 5. 17-Hydroxyprogesterone is hydroxylated on the 21 carbon by **CYP21,** producing **11-deoxycortisol.** 11-Deoxycortisol is then efficiently hydroxylated on the 11 carbon by **CYP11B1,** producing **cortisol** (Figure 7-10). Note that progesterone (the product of reaction 2a) can also enter this pathway of 21- and 11-hydroxylations, producing **deoxycorticosterone (DOC)** and **corticosterone,** respectively (see Figure 7-10). However, CYP17 activity is robust in the

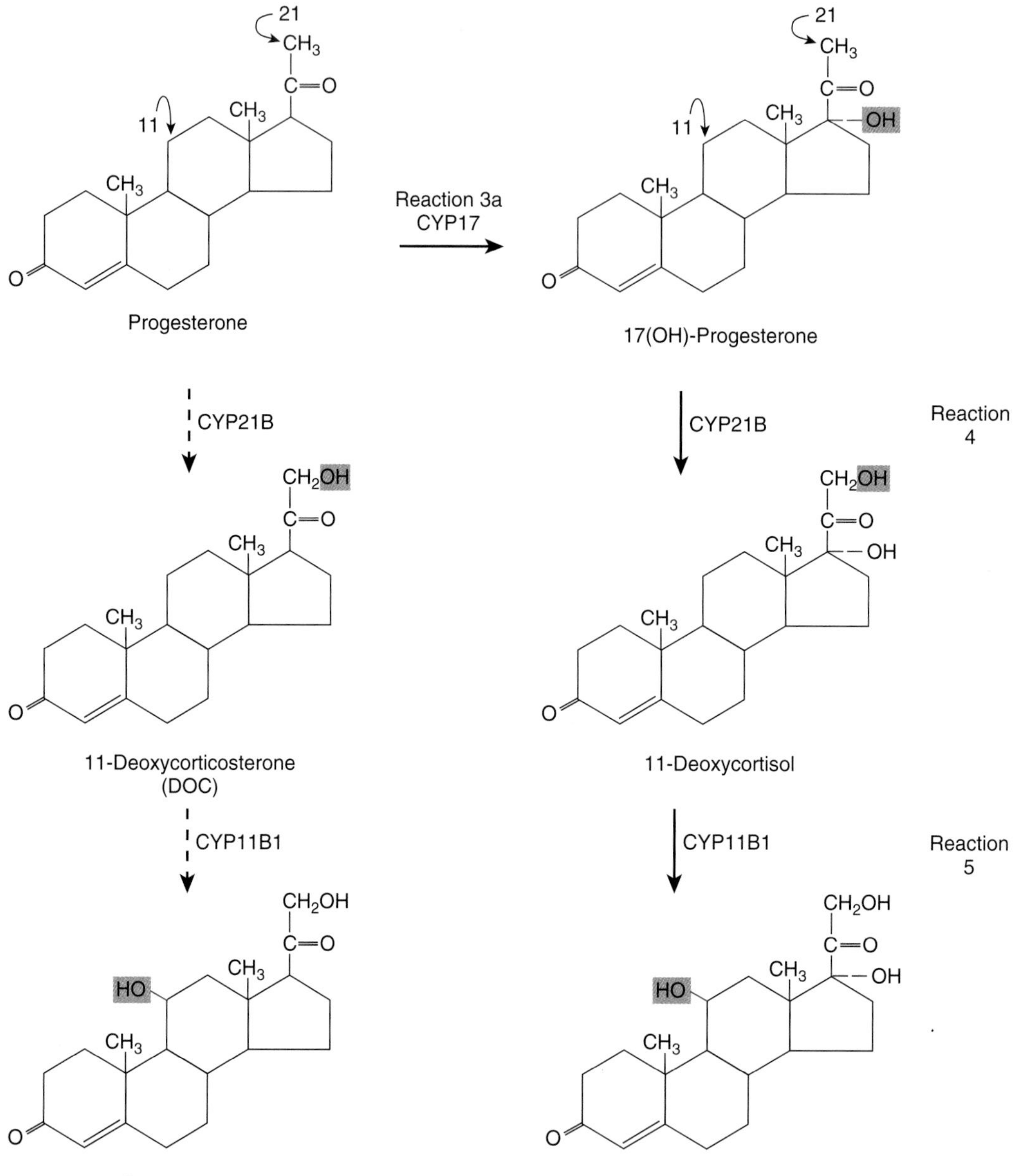

FIGURE 7-10 ■ Reactions 4 and 5, involving CYP21β and CYP11B1, that carry out the last two steps of the synthesis of cortisol. Also shown is the minor pathway leading to the synthesis of corticosterone in the zona fasciculata.

human zona fasciculata, so that DOC and corticosterone are normally minor products.

Transport and Metabolism of Cortisol

Cortisol is transported in blood predominantly bound to proteins. These are primarily **corticosteroid-binding globulin (CBG)** (also called **transcortin**), which binds about 90%, and albumin, which binds 5% to 7 %, of the circulating hormone. The liver is the predominant site of steroid inactivation. It inactivates cortisol and conjugates active and inactive steroids with glucuronide or sulfate so they can be excreted more readily by the kidney (see Chapter 1). The circulating half-life of cortisol is about 70 minutes.

Cortisol is reversibly inactivated by conversion to **cortisone** (see later). This is catalyzed by the enzyme, **11β-hydroxysteroid dehydrogenase type 2 (11β-HSD2)**. The inactivation of cortisol by 11ß-HSD2 is reversible in that another enzyme, **11β-HSD1**, converts cortisone back to cortisol. This occurs in tissues expressing the glucocorticoid receptor (GR), including liver, adipose, and CNS—as well as in skin (which is why cortisone-based creams can be applied to skin to stop inflammation).

Mechanism of Action of Cortisol

Cortisol acts primarily through the **glucocorticoid receptor (GR),** which regulates gene transcription (see Chapter 1). In the absence of hormone, the GR resides in the cytoplasm in a stable complex with several **molecular chaperones,** including heat-shock protein 90 and cyclophilins. Cortisol-GR binding promotes dissociation of the chaperone proteins, followed by:

1. Rapid translocation of the cortisol-GR complex into the nucleus;
2. Dimerization and binding to the **glucocorticoid-response elements (GREs)** near the basal promoters of cortisol-regulated genes;
3. Recruitment of **co-activator proteins** and the assembly of the general transcription factors, leading to increased transcription of the targeted genes.

Physiologic Actions of Cortisol

Cortisol has a broad range of actions on several organ systems (Box 7-3). Several of the actions of cortisol

---

BOX 7-3
BIOLOGIC ACTIONS OF CORTISOL

Metabolic
Hyperglycemic
Glycogenic
Gluconeogenic
Lipolytic
Protein catabolic
Insulin antagonist in muscle and adipose tissue
Inhibits bone formation, stimulates bone resorption
Necessary for vascular response to catecholamines
Anti-inflammatory
Suppresses immune system
Inhibits antidiuretic hormone secretion and action
Stimulates gastric acid secretion
Necessary for integrity and function of gastrointestinal tract
Stimulates red blood cell production
Alters mood and behavior
Permissive for calorigenic, lipolytic effects of catecholamine

---

were put forth as an integrated response to stress by Hans Selye in the 1930s, and cortisol is often characterized as a "stress hormone." In general, cortisol maintains blood glucose, CNS function and cardiovascular function during fasting—and increases blood glucose during stress at the expense of muscle protein. Cortisol protects the body against the self-injurious effects of unbridled inflammatory and immune responses. Cortisol also partitions energy to cope with stress by inhibiting reproductive function. As stated subsequently, cortisol has several other effects on bone, skin, connective tissue, the gastrointestinal tract, and the developing fetus that are independent of its stress-related functions.

Metabolic Actions As the term **glucocorticoid** implies, cortisol is a **steroid** hormone from the adrenal **cortex** that regulates blood **glucose.** Cortisol increases blood glucose by stimulating gluconeogenesis (Figure 7-11). Cortisol enhances the gene expression of the **hepatic gluconeogenic enzymes, phosphoenolpyruvate carboxykinase (PEPCK), fructose-1,6-bisphosphatase,** and **glucose-6-phosphatase.**

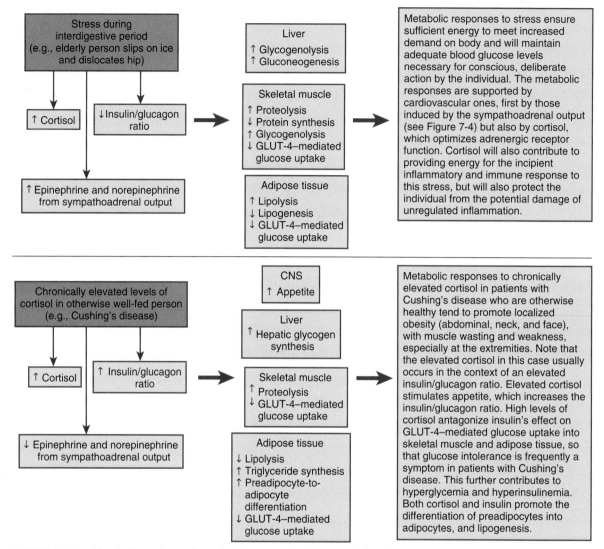

FIGURE 7-11 ■ Metabolic actions of cortisol (integrated with catecholamines and glucagon) in response to stress (*upper panel*), and contrasted to actions of chronically elevated cortisol (integrated with insulin) in an otherwise healthy individual (*lower panel*).

Cortisol also decreases **GLUT-4–mediated glucose uptake** in skeletal muscle and adipose tissue. During the interdigestive period (low insulin/glucagon ratio), cortisol promotes glucose sparing by potentiating the effects of catecholamines on **lipolysis,** thereby making FFAs available as energy sources. Cortisol inhibits protein synthesis and increases **proteolysis,** especially in skeletal muscle, thereby providing a rich source of carbon for hepatic gluconeogenesis.

Figure 7-11 also contrasts the normal role of cortisol in response to a stress and the effects of **chronically elevated cortisol** owing to a pathologic condition. As discussed subsequently, there are important differences in the overall metabolic effects of cortisol between these two states, particularly with respect to lipid metabolism. During stress, cortisol synergizes with catecholamines and glucagon to promote a lipolytic, gluconeogenic, and glycogenolytic metabolic response, while synergizing with catecholamines to promote an appropriate cardiovascular response. During chronically elevated levels of cortisol owing to a pathologic overproduction, cortisol synergizes with insulin in the context of elevated levels of glucose (because of an **increased appetite**) and **hyperinsulinemia** (because of elevated glucose and **glucose intolerance**) to promote **lipogenesis** and **truncal (abdominal, visceral) adiposity.**

Cardiovascular Actions Cortisol reinforces its effects on blood glucose by its positive effects on the cardiovascular system. Cortisol is permissive on the actions of catecholamines and thereby contributes to cardiac output and blood pressure. Cortisol stimulates **erythropoietin** synthesis and, hence, increases red blood cell production. **Anemia** occurs when cortisol is deficient and **polycythemia** occurs when cortisol levels are excessive.

Anti-inflammatory and Immunosuppressive Actions **Inflammation and immune responses** are often part of a response to stress. However, inflammation and immune responses have the potential of doing significant harm, even to the extent of causing death, to the organism they are designed to protect if they are not held in homeostatic balance. As a stress hormone, cortisol plays an important role in maintaining **immune homeostasis**. Cortisol, along with epinephrine and norepinephrine, represses the production of pro-inflammatory cytokines, and stimulate the production of anti-inflammatory cytokines.

The inflammatory response to injury consists of local dilation of capillaries and increased capillary permeability with a resultant local edema and accumulation of white blood cells. These steps are mediated by prostaglandins, thromboxanes, and leukotrienes. Cortisol inhibits **phospholipase A$_2$**, a key enzyme in prostaglandin, leukotriene, and thromboxane synthesis. Cortisol also stabilizes lysosomal membranes, thereby decreasing the release of the proteolytic enzymes that augment local swelling. In response to injury, leukocytes normally migrate to the site of injury and leave the vascular system. These changes are inhibited by cortisol, as is the phagocytic activity of the neutrophils, although bone marrow release of neutrophils is stimulated. Cortisol decreases the number

of circulating eosinophils. The fibroblastic proliferation involved in inflammation is also inhibited. This latter response is important in the formation of barriers to the spread of certain infectious agents. Analogs of glucocorticoid are frequently used pharmacologically because of their anti-inflammatory properties. When cortisol levels are high, many of the body's defense mechanisms against infection are inhibited. For this reason, glucocorticoid therapy is contraindicated as the sole medication for the treatment of infections.

Cortisol inhibits the immune response and, for this reason, glucocorticoid analogs have been used as **immunosuppressants** in organ transplants. High cortisol levels decrease the number of circulating T lymphocytes (particularly helper T lymphocytes) and decrease their ability to migrate to the site of antigenic stimulation. Glucocorticoids promote atrophy of the thymus and other lymphoid tissue. Although corticosteroids inhibit cellularly mediated immunity, antibody production by B lymphocytes does not appear to be impaired.

Action on Reproductive Systems Reproduction exacts a considerable anabolic cost on the organism. In humans, reproductive behavior and function are dampened in response to stress. Cortisol **decreases the function of the reproductive axis at the hypothalamic, pituitary, and gonadal levels.**

Actions on Bone Glucocorticoids increase **bone resorption.** They have multiple actions that alter bone metabolism. Glucocorticoids decrease intestinal calcium absorption and decrease renal calcium reabsorption. Both mechanisms lower serum calcium concentrations. As the serum calcium level drops, the secretion of parathyroid hormone (PTH) increases and PTH mobilizes calcium from bone both by stimulating resorption of bone. In addition to this action, glucocorticoids directly inhibit osteoblast bone-forming functions (see Chapter 4). Although glucocorticoids are useful for treating the inflammation associated with arthritis, excessive use will result in bone loss (osteoporosis).

Actions on Connective Tissue Cortisol **inhibits fibroblast proliferation and collagen formation.**

In the presence of excessive amounts of cortisol, the skin thins and is more readily damaged. The connective tissue support of capillaries is impaired and capillary injury (bruising) is increased.

Actions on Kidney Cortisol **inhibits ADH secretion and action**, so it is an ADH antagonist. In the absence of cortisol, the action of ADH is potentiated, making it difficult to increase the free-water clearance in response to a water load and increasing the likelihood of water intoxication. As discussed earlier, cortisol binds to the mineralocorticoid receptor with high affinity, but this action is normally blocked by the inactivation of cortisol to cortisone by the enzyme 11β-HSD2. However, the mineralocorticoid activity (i.e., Na^+ and H_2O retention, K^+ and H^+ excretion) of cortisol depends on the relative amount of cortisol (or synthetic glucocorticoids) and the activity of 11β-HSD2. Certain agents (such as compounds in black licorice) inhibit 11β-HSD2 and thereby increase the mineralocorticoid activity of cortisol. Cortisol increases the glomerular filtration rate by increasing cardiac output and acting directly on the kidney.

Actions on Muscle Cortisol actions on muscle are complex. When cortisol levels are excessive, **muscle weakness and pain are common symptoms.** The weakness has multiple origins. In part it is a result of the excessive proteolysis that cortisol produces. High cortisol levels can result in hypokalemia (via the mineralocorticoid actions), which can produce muscle weakness because it hyperpolarizes and stabilizes the muscle cell membrane, thereby making stimulation more difficult.

Gastrointestinal Actions Cortisol exerts a **trophic effect on the gastrointestinal (GI) mucosa.** In the absence of cortisol, GI motility decreases, GI mucosa degenerates, and GI acid and enzyme production decrease. Because cortisol stimulates appetite, hypercortisolism is frequently associated with weight gain. The cortisol-mediated stimulation of gastric acid and pepsin secretion increases the risk of ulcer development.

Psychologic Actions The normal range of daily cortisol levels maintains optimal psychological function in humans. **Psychiatric disturbances** are associated with either excessive or deficient levels of corticosteroids. Excessive corticosteroids can initially produce a feeling of well-being but continued excessive exposure eventually leads to emotional lability and depression. Frank psychosis can occur with either excess or deficient hormone. Cortisol has been shown to increase the tendency for insomnia and decrease rapid eye movement (REM) sleep. People who are deficient in corticosteroids tend to be depressed, apathetic, and irritable.

Effects of Cortisol During Fetal Development Cortisol is required for **normal development of the CNS, retina, skin, GI tract, and lungs.** The best-studied system is the lungs, in which cortisol induces differentiation and maturation of type II alveolar cells. These cells produce **surfactant** during late gestation that reduces surface tension in the lungs and thus allows for the onset of breathing at birth.

Regulation of Cortisol Production

Cortisol production by the zona fasciculata is regulated by a standard hypothalamus-pituitary-adrenal axis involving CRH, ACTH, and cortisol (see Chapter 5). The hypothalamus and pituitary stimulate cortisol production and cortisol negatively feeds back on the hypothalamus and pituitary to maintain its set-point.

A subset of the hypophysiotropic parvicellular neurons secrete **corticotropin-releasing hormone (CRH),** which binds to the Gs-coupled **CRH receptor** on **pro-opiomelanocortin (POMC) cells** (also called **corticotropes**) in the pars distalis (see Chapter 5). Both neurogenic (e.g., fear) and systemic (e.g., hypoglycemia, hemorrhage, cytokines) forms of stress stimulate CRH release (Box 7-4). CRH is also under strong

---

BOX 7-4
STIMULI FOR CRH SECRETION

- Diurnal input from suprachiasmatic nucleus
- Proinflammatory cytokines
- Hypoglycemia
- Hemorrhage
- Neurogenic stress (e.g., fear)

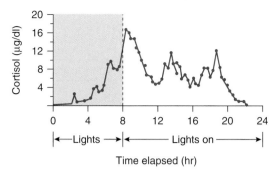

FIGURE 7-12 ■ Pattern of cortisol secretion over 24-hour period in normal subject. *(Redrawn from Weitzman, ED, et al: J Clin Endocrinol Metab 33:14, 1971.)*

diurnal rhythmic regulation emerging from the suprachiasmatic nucleus, so that cortisol levels surge during early predawn and morning hours and then continually decline throughout the day and evening (Figure 7-12). CRH acutely stimulates **adrenocorticotropic hormone (ACTH)** release and chronically increases POMC gene expression and corticotrope hypertrophy and proliferation. Some parvicellular neurons coexpress CRH and **vasopressin** (also called **ADH**). Vasopressin that reaches the anterior pituitary binds to the Gq-coupled vasopressin-3 receptor (V_3 receptor) on corticotropes and potentiates the actions of CRH.

ACTH binds to the **melanocortin-2 receptor (MC2R)** located on cells in the zona fasciculata. The MC2R is coupled primarily to a Gs/cAMP/PKA signaling pathway. The effects of ACTH can be subdivided into three phases:

1. The acute effects of ACTH occur within minutes. Cholesterol is rapidly mobilized from lipid droplets by posttranslational activation of cholesterol ester hydrolase and transported to the outer mitochondrial membrane. ACTH both rapidly increases StAR protein gene expression and activates StAR protein through PKA-dependent phosphorylation. Collectively, these acute actions of ACTH increase pregnenolone levels.
2. The chronic effects of ACTH occur over a period of several hours. These involve increasing the transcription of the genes encoding the steroidogenic

enzymes and their coenzymes. ACTH also increases the expression of the **LDL receptor and scavenger receptor-BI (SR-BI; the HDL receptor).**
3. The trophic actions of ACTH on the zona fasciculata and reticularis occur over a period of weeks and months. This last effect is exemplified by atrophy of the zona fasciculata in patients receiving therapeutic (i.e., supraphysiologic) levels of glucocorticoid analogs for at least 3 weeks. Under these conditions, the exogenous corticosteroids completely repress CRH and ACTH production, resulting in the atrophy of the zona fasciculata and decline in endogenous cortisol production (Figure 7-13). At the end of therapy, such patients need to be slowly weaned from exogenous glucocorticoids to allow the hypothalamus-pituitary-adrenal axis to reestablish itself and for the zona fasciculata to enlarge and produce adequate amounts of cortisol.

Cortisol inhibits both POMC gene expression at the corticotropes and pro-CRH gene expression at the hypothalamus. However, intense stress can override the negative feedback effects of cortisol at the hypothalamus, thereby resetting the set-point at a higher level.

ZONA RETICULARIS

The innermost zone, the zona reticularis, begins to appear after birth at about age 5. **Adrenal androgens,** especially **dehydroepiandrosterone (DHEAS)**—the main product of the zona reticularis, become detectable in the circulation at about 6 years of age. This onset of adrenal androgen production is called **adrenarche,** and contributes to appearance of axillary and pubic hair at about age 8. DHEAS levels continue to increase, peak during the midtwenties, and then progressively decline with age.

The Zona Reticularis Makes Adrenal Androgens

The zona reticularis differs from the zona fasciculata in several important ways with respect to steroidogenic enzyme activity. First, 3β-HSD is expressed at a much lower level in the zona reticularis than in the zona fasciculata, so the Δ5 pathway predominates in the zona reticularis.

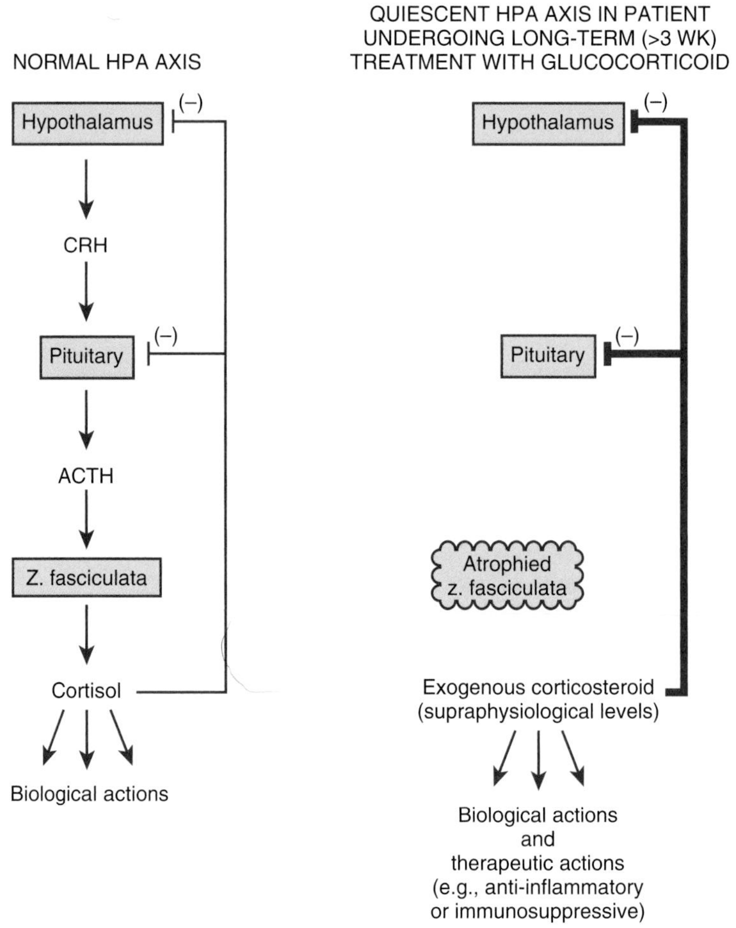

FIGURE 7-13 ■ Comparison of normal hypothalamus-pituitary-adrenal (HPA) axis to quiescent HPA in individual receiving exogenous glucocorticoid therapy. The latter causes the zona fasciculata to atrophy after 3 weeks, requiring a careful withdrawal regimen that allows rebuilding of the adrenal tissue before total cessation of exogenous corticosteroid administration.

Second, the zona reticularis expresses cofactors or conditions that enhance the 17,20-lyase function of CYP17, thereby generating the 19-carbon androgen precursor molecule, dehydroepiandrosterone (DHEA), from 17-hydroxypregnenolone. Additionally, the zona reticularis expresses **DHEA-sulfotransferase (SULT2A1 gene)**, which converts DHEA into DHEAS (Figure 7-14). A limited amount of the Δ4 androgen, **androstenedione,** is also made in the zona reticularis. Small amounts of potent androgens (e.g., testosterone) or 18-carbon estrogens are normally produced by the human adrenal cortex (see Figure 7-6 for summary).

Metabolism and Fate DHEAS and DHEA

DHEAS can be converted back to DHEA by peripheral **sulfatases** and DHEA and androstenedione can be converted to active androgens (testosterone, dihydrotestosterone) peripherally in both sexes. DHEA binds to albumin and other transport globulins with low affinity and so is excreted efficiently by the kidney. The half-life of DHEA is 15 to 30 minutes. In contrast, DHEAS binds to albumin with very high affinity and has a half-life of 7 to 10 hours.

Physiologic Actions of Adrenal Androgens

In men, the contribution of adrenal androgens to active androgens is negligible. However, in women, the adrenal gland contributes to about 50% of circulating active androgens, which are required for axillary and pubic hair growth as well as libido. Under conditions of adrenal androgen excess (adrenal tumor, Cushing's

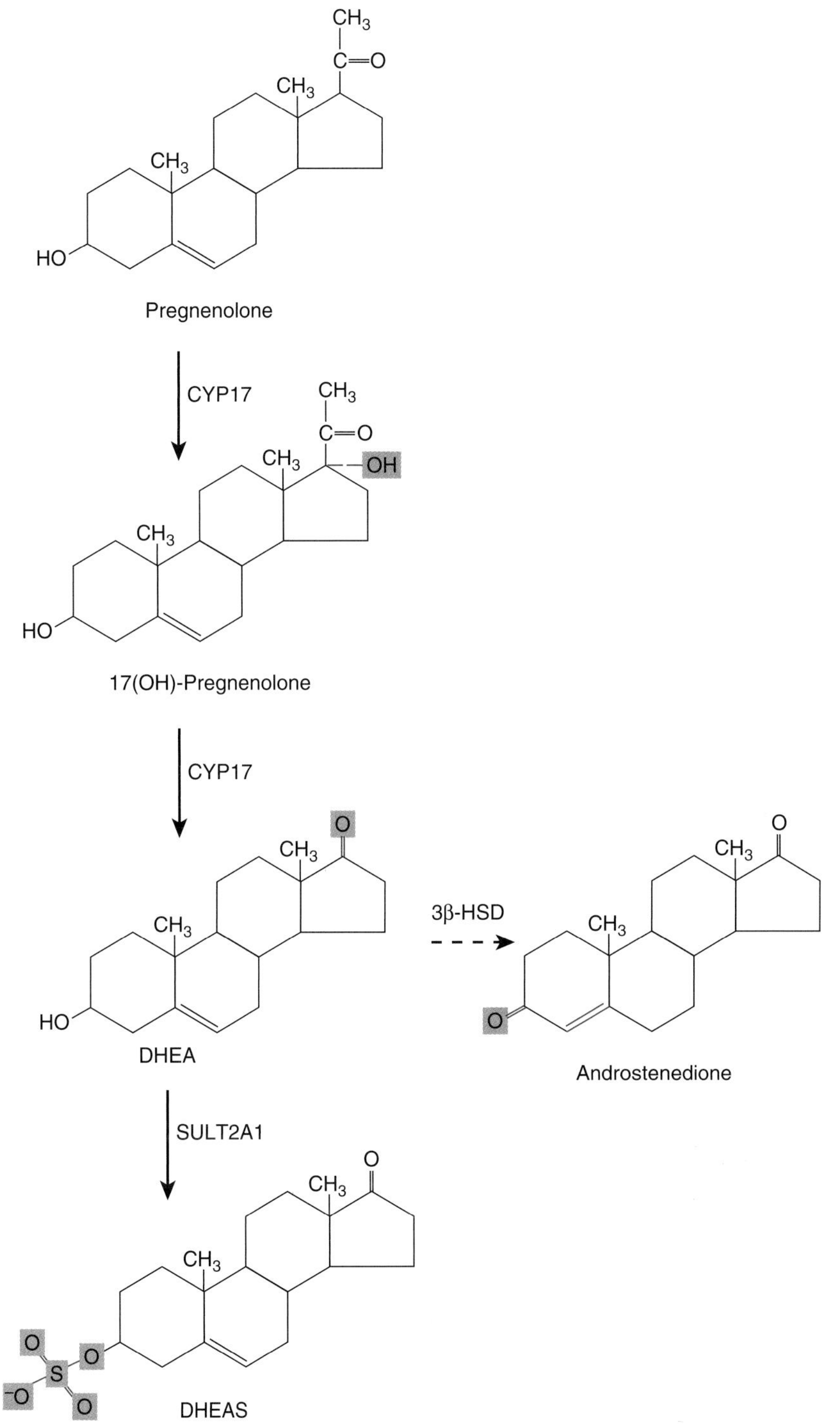

FIGURE 7-14 ■ Steroidogenic pathways in the zona reticularis. The first common reaction in the pathway, conversion of cholesterol to pregnenolone by CYP11A1, is not shown. The expression of 3β-hydroxysteroid dehydrogenase (3β-HSD) is relatively low in the zona reticularis, so that androstenedione is a minor product compared to DHEA and DHEAS. The zona reticularis also makes a small amount of testosterone and estrogens (*not shown*).

syndrome, congenital adrenal hyperplasia—(See p. 191), **masculinization of women** can occur. This involves masculinization of external genitalia (e.g., enlarged clitoris) in utero, and excessive facial and body hair (called **hirsutism**) and acne in adult women. Excessive adrenal androgens also appear to play a role in ovarian dysovulation (i.e., polycystic ovarian syndrome).

Apart from providing androgen precursors, it is not clear what other role(s), if any, the zona reticularis plays in the adult human. DHEAS is the most abundant circulating hormone in young adults. DHEAS increases steadily until it peaks in the midtwenties and then steadily declines thereafter. Thus, there has been considerable interest in the possible role of DHEAS in the aging process. However, the function of this abundant steroid in young adults and the potential impact of its gradual disappearance on aging are still poorly understood. It should be noted that the age-related decline in DHEA and DHEAS has been associated with the popular use of these steroids as dietary supplements, even though there are few (if any) studies to currently support the efficacy or safety of this practice.

Regulation of Zona Reticularis Function

ACTH is clearly a regulator of the zona reticularis. Both DHEA and androstenedione display the same diurnal rhythm as cortisol (DHEAS does not because of its long circulating half-life). The zona reticularis shows the same atrophic changes as the zona fasciculata under conditions of little or no ACTH. However, other factors must regulate adrenal androgen function. Adrenarche occurs in the face of constant ACTH and cortisol levels and the rise and decline of DHEAS is not associated with a similar pattern of ACTH or cortisol production. However, the other factors, whether extra-adrenal or intra-adrenal, remain unknown.

A crucial clinical aspect of the regulation of the zona reticularis is that, although ACTH stimulates production of adrenal androgens, neither adrenal androgens nor their more potent metabolites (e.g., testosterone, dihydrotestosterone, estradiol-17β) negatively feed back on ACTH or CRH. This means that an enzymatic defect associated with the synthesis of cortisol (e.g., CYP21B deficiency) is associated with a dramatic increase in both ACTH (no negative feedback from

cortisol) and in adrenal androgens (due to the elevated ACTH). It is this "loophole" in the hypothalamus-pituitary-adrenal axis that gives rise to congenital adrenal hyperplasia (Figure 7-15) (see later for further of **congenital adrenal hyperplasia**).

ZONA GLOMERULOSA

The thin, outermost zone is called the **zona glomerulosa.** This zone produces the **mineralocorticoid, aldosterone,** which regulates salt and volume homeostasis. The zona glomerulosa is only secondarily influenced by ACTH. Rather, it is regulated primarily by the renin-angiotensin system, extracellular K^+ and atrial natriuretic peptide (ANP).

The Zona Glomerulosa Makes Aldosterone

An important feature in the steroidogenic capacity of the zona glomerulosa is that it does *not* express CYP17.

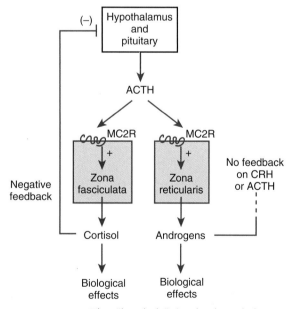

FIGURE 7-15 ■ The "loophole" in the hypothalamus-pituitary-adrenal axis. ACTH stimulates the production of both cortisol and adrenal androgens but only cortisol negatively feeds back on ACTH and CRH. Thus, if cortisol production is blocked (i.e., CYP11B1 deficiency), ACTH levels increase, along with adrenal androgens.

Therefore, zona glomerulosa cells never make cortisol—nor do they make adrenal androgens in any form. Pregnenolone is converted to progesterone and deoxycorticosterone (DOC) by 3β-HSD and CYP21, respectively (Figure 7-16).

A completely unique feature of the zona glomerulosa among the steroidogenic glands is the expression of **CYP11B2.** CYP11B2 lies close to CYP11B1 (i.e., the enzyme that catalyzes the 11-hydroxylation of 11-deoxycortisol in the zona fasciculata to form cortisol—(see Figures 7-6 and 7-10) on the same chromosome in humans but CYP11B2 has a different promoter that is regulated by different signaling pathways. The enzyme itself, called **aldosterone synthase,** catalyzes the last three reactions from DOC to aldosterone within the zona glomerulosa. These reactions are: 11-hydroxylation of DOC to form **corticosterone,** 18-hydroxylation to form **18-hydroxycorticosterone,** and 18-oxidation to form **aldosterone** (see Figure 7-16) (summarized in Figure 7-6).

Transport and Metabolism of Aldosterone

Aldosterone binds to transport proteins (albumin, corticosteroid-binding protein) with low affinity) and therefore has a short biological half-life of about 20 minutes. Almost all of aldosterone is inactivated by the liver in one pass, conjugated to a glucuronide group, and excreted by the kidney.

Mechanism of Aldosterone Action

Aldosterone acts much like cortisol (and other steroid hormones) in that its primary mechanism of action is through binding to a specific intracellular receptor (i.e., **mineralocorticoid receptor [MR]**). After dissociation of chaperone proteins, nuclear translocation, dimerization, and binding to **mineralocorticoid-response element,** the aldosterone-MR complex regulates the expression of specific genes. Cortisol binds equally well to the MR and activates the same genes as does aldosterone. However, as discussed earlier, these cells also express 11β-HSD2, which converts cortisol to the inactive steroid, cortisone (Figure 7-17). Cortisone can be converted back to cortisol by 11β-HSD1, which is expressed in several glucocorticoid-responsive tissues, including the liver and skin.

Physiologic Actions of Aldosterone*

*Actions on Kidney** The primary action of aldosterone is to increase the reabsorption of Na^+, followed by H_2O, by the distal nephron. About 95% of Na^+ reabsorption in the nephron occurs before the distal nephron, independently of aldosterone regulation. However, the amount of Na^+ reabsorbed by the collecting duct can be regulated by a few percent to match changes in dietary Na^+ intake. Na^+ uptake at the collecting duct is accompanied by Cl^- and H_2O. As emphasized in the Mosby Renal Physiology monograph, "a 2% change in the fractional excretion of Na^+ would produce more than a 3 liter change in the volume of the extracellular fluid." **Salt wasting and dehydration** occur in patients with aldosterone insufficiency.

Aldosterone increases Na^+ reabsorption at the distal nephron (the latter portion of the distal convoluted tubule and the cortical collecting duct) primarily by increasing the expression of the α-subunit of the **epithelial Na^+ channel (ENaC).** Aldosterone also increases the stability of ENaC in the apical (luminal) membrane (Figure 7-18). This action of aldosterone is mediated by the **aldosterone-inducible serine/threonine kinase, SGK-1.** SGK-1 gene expression is rapidly and profoundly increased by aldosterone. SGK-1 prevents the ability of a protein, called Nedd 4-2, from targeting ENaC for degradation. The importance of ENaC in the actions of aldosterone is made apparent by forms of aldosterone resistance (**type 1 pseudohypoaldosteronism; PHA1).** PHA1 is characterized by symptoms related to lack of aldosterone (salt-wasting, dehydration, hyperkalemia, with very high levels of renin, angiotensin and aldosterone—[see later for regulation of aldosterone], and hypertension). Some cases of PHA1 are due to inactivating mutations in one of the subunits of the ENaC. In the presence of these mutations, aldosterone cannot efficiently increase Na^+ reabsorption. In contrast to PHA1, **Liddle's syndrome** is characterized by hypertension, hypokalemia, and low renin and aldosterone levels. In these patients, ENaC subunits have mutations that prevent Nedd 4-2 from interacting with them and targeting them for degradation. Therefore, in Liddle's syndrome, the

---

*For more information on this subject, see Koeppen BM, Stanton BA: *Renal physiology,* ed 3, St. Louis, 2001, Mosby Monograph Series.

CH₃
C=O
CH₃

CH₃

HO

Pregnenolone

3β-HSD

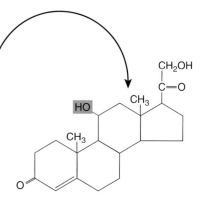

CH₂OH
C=O
CH₃

HO

CH₃

O

Corticosterone

CYP11B2

FIGURE 7-16 ■ Steroidogenic pathways in the zona glomerulosa. The first common reaction in the pathway, conversion of cholesterol to pregnenolone by CYP11A1, is not shown. Note that the last three reactions are catalyzed by CYP11B2.

CH₃
C=O
CH₃

CH₃

O

Progesterone

CYP21B

CH₂OH
C=O
CH₃

HO

CH₃

O

18(OH)-Corticosterone

CYP11B2

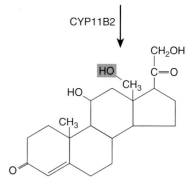

CH₂OH
C=O
CH₃

CH₃

O

11-Deoxycorticosterone
(DOC)

CYP11B2

CH₂OH
C=O
CH
CH₃

HO

CH₃

O

Aldosterone

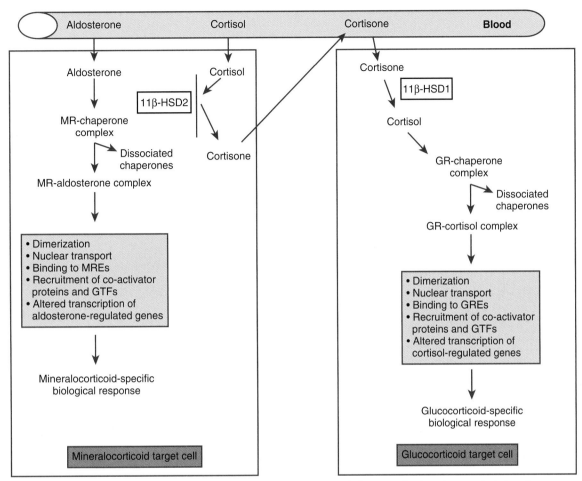

FIGURE 7-17 ■ The mineralocorticoid receptor (MR) is protected from activation by cortisol by the enzyme, 11β-hydroxysteroid dehydrogenase type 2 (11β-HSD2), which converts cortisol to inactive cortisone. Cortisone can be converted back to cortisol in glucocorticoid target cells by the enzyme, 11β-HSD type 1. Cortisol binds to the glucocorticoid receptor (GR) in cortisol target cell.

ENaCs reside in the apical membrane much longer and transport more Na^+ independently of aldosterone.

Aldosterone also promotes Na^+ reabsorption by increasing the activity of the basolateral Na^+/K^+ ATPase in the distal nephron, although the hormone does not acutely increase gene expression of this transporter.

Aldosterone also stimulates K^+ and H^+ secretion. Aldosterone increases gene expression of the **renal outer medullary K^+ (ROMK) channel** and density of this channel in the apical membrane of the distal nephron (see Figure 7-18). The excretion of K^+ is linked to the reabsorption of Na^+, in that the ENaC and the Na^+/K^+-ATPase establish the electrochemical conditions for apical secretion of K^+. In this sense SGK-1 indirectly promotes K^+ secretion. Additionally, SGK-1 increases ROMK channel insertion into the apical membrane and increases its transporting activity. The importance of aldosterone on K^+ and H^+ homeostasis is emphasized by the findings that hyperaldosteronism leads to **hypokalemia and metabolic alkalosis.**

Continuous aldosterone administration will result in **aldosterone escape** in 2 to 3 days. Initially there will be sodium retention and volume expansion, but the

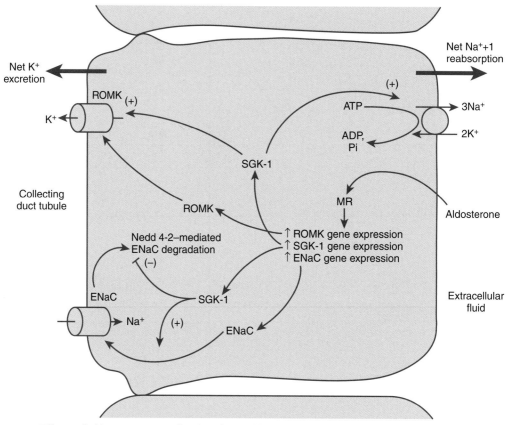

FIGURE 7-18 ■ Effects of aldosterone on collecting duct. Aldosterone increases gene expression of the kinase, SGK-1, the epithelial sodium channel, ENaC, and the renal outer medullary potassium channel, ROMK. SGK-1 kinase activity reinforces aldosterone actions by increaseing ENaC insertion into the membrane and inhibiting Nedd 4-2–dependent degradation of ENaC. SGK-1 also increases the activity of ROMK and the basolateral sodium-potassium ATPase.

volume expansion will not continue indefinitely. As extracellular volume and therefore vascular volume increases, the glomerular filtration rate increases. This increases the rate of sodium delivery to the nephron and therefore the rate of renal sodium excretion, which limits the ability of aldosterone to continue expanding extracellular volume. The increase in vascular volume will stimulate the release of **atrial natriuretic peptide (ANP),** which promotes renal Na⁺ excretion. However, "escape" from the effects of aldosterone on potassium and hydrogen ion secretion does not occur and potassium depletion and metabolic alkalosis can persist.

Actions on Other Epithelia   The colon is an important extrarenal site in terms of aldosterone regulation of salt and water homeostasis. As in the distal nephron, aldosterone increases sodium and water reabsorption and increases K⁺ excretion in the colon. Aldosterone has similar effects on epithelia of salivary glands, sweat glands, and gastric glands.

Actions on Heart Muscle   Clinical studies in humans have revealed a deleterious effect of aldosterone on cardiovascular function independent of its effects on renal sodium and water reabsorption. Aldosterone has a **proinflammatory, profibrotic effect** on the

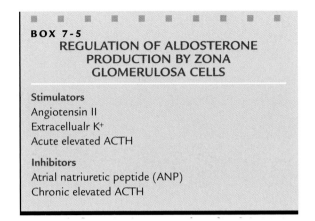

cardiovascular system and causes left ventricular hypertrophy and remodeling. This effect of aldosterone is associated with increased morbidity and mortality in patients with essential hypertension.

Regulation of Aldosterone Secretion

Given that Na^+ reabsorption and water uptake represent major actions of aldosterone, it would make sense that Na^+ levels and volume would feed back on aldosterone production (Box 7-5). This occurs through the **renin-angiotensin-system (RAS)**. In the kidney, the vascular smooth muscle cells of the afferent arteriole adjacent to the glomerulus, called **juxtaglomerular (JG) cells,** are specialized to secrete a proteolytic enzyme called **renin.** Juxtaglomerular cells release renin in response to a decrease in blood pressure in the afferent arteriole—as detected by baroreceptors in the wall of the afferent arteriole. Juxtaglomerular cells also release renin in response to decreased systemic blood pressure—as detected by baroreceptors. Decreased systemic blood pressure leads to activation of sympathetic fibers that directly innervate juxtaglomerular cells via $\beta 1$-adrenergic receptors. In addition to stimulation by decreased blood pressure (i.e., decreased volume), decreased delivery of Na^+ to specialized cells of the ascending loop of Henle, collectively called the **macula densa,** causes these cells to signal to the juxtaglomerular cells to release renin (Figure 7-19).

Once secreted, renin acts on circulating **angiotensinogen (renin substrate)** to produce the decapeptide, **angiotensin I.** Angiotensin I is converted to **angiotensin II** (eight amino acids) by **angiotensin-converting enzyme (ACE)** in the lungs (see Figure 7-19). **Angiotensin II** binds to the Gq-coupled **AT1 receptor**

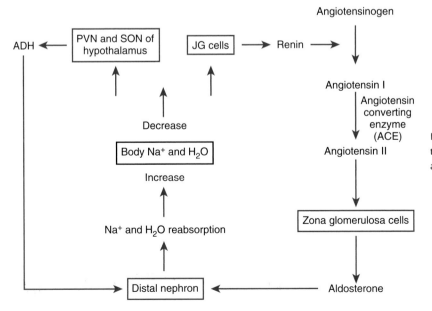

FIGURE 7-19 ■ Control of aldosterone by renin-angiotensinogen-angiotensin system.

on zona glomerulosa cells and most vascular smooth muscle cells. Angiotensin II is a potent stimulus for aldosterone production. Angiotensin II increases StAR and CYP11B2 (aldosterone synthase) expression. As the name suggests, angiotensin II is also a potent vasoconstrictor and plays a direct role in compensation for vascular volume depletion. Rising serum potassium levels depolarize the glomerulosa cell membrane, thereby stimulating voltage-sensitive calcium channels to open. The resultant calcium influx stimulates aldosterone production (Figure 7-19). In contrast to angiotensin II and **extracellular K$^+$**, atrial natriuretic peptide (ANP) acts directly on zona glomerulosa cells to inhibit aldosterone production. Note that ANP also inhibits aldosterone indirectly by inhibiting renin release and plays an important role in the "aldosterone escape response" (see earlier).

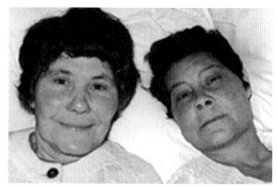

FIGURE 7-20 ■ Woman on right has Addison's disease. Note increased pigmentation relative to her healthy twin sister on left. *(From Hall R, Evered DC: Color atlas of endocrinology, ed 2, London, 1990, Mosby-Wolfe.)*

PATHOLOGIC CONDITIONS INVOLVING THE ADRENAL CORTEX

Adrenocortical Insufficiency

In the absence of cortisol, peripheral resistance drops. Orthostatic hypotension (inability to maintain normal mean arterial pressure when going from lying to standing position) occurs because of decreased baroreceptor-mediated vasoconstriction. **Addison's disease** is primary adrenal insufficiency in which both mineralocorticoids and glucocorticoids are usually deficient. In North America and Europe, the most prevalent cause of Addison's disease is autoimmune destruction of the adrenal cortex. Because of the cortisol deficiency, ACTH secretion increases. Elevated levels of ACTH can compete for the MC1R in melanocytes, causing an increase in skin pigmentation, particularly in skin creases, scars, and gums (Figure 7-20) (see also Chapter 5). The loss of the mineralocorticoids results in contraction of extracellular volume, producing circulatory hypovolemia and therefore a drop in blood pressure. Because the loss of cortisol decreases the vasopressive response to catecholamines, peripheral resistance drops, thereby adding to the tendency toward hypotension. Hypotension predisposes people to circulatory shock. These people are also prone to have hypoglycemia

when stressed or fasting. The hyperglycemic actions of other hormones, such as glucagon, epinephrine, and growth hormone, generally will prevent hypoglycemia at other times. Although volume depletion occurs because of the loss of mineralocorticoids, water intoxication can develop if a water load is given. The loss of cortisol impairs the ability to increase free-water clearance in response to a water load and hence rid the body of the excess water. Patients with this condition will exhibit hyperkalemic acidosis. Because cortisol is important for muscle function, muscle weakness occurs in cortisol deficiency. The loss of cortisol results in anemia, decreased GI motility and secretion, and decreased iron and vitamin B$_{12}$ absorption. The appetite will decrease because of the cortisol deficiency and this decreased appetite, coupled with the GI dysfunction, will predispose these persons to weight loss. These patients often show disturbances in mood and behavior and are more susceptible to depression (Box 7-6).

Adrenocortical Excess

Cushing's Syndrome Adrenocortical hormone excess is termed **Cushing's syndrome.** Pharmacologic use of exogenous corticosteroids is now the most common cause of Cushing's syndrome. The next most prevalent cause is ACTH-secreting tumors. The form of Cushing's syndrome caused by a functional pituitary adenoma

BOX 7-6
MANIFESTATIONS OF PRIMARY ADRENOCORTICAL INSUFFICIENCY

Cortisol deficiency
Gastrointestinal disturbances
Anorexia
Nausea
Vomiting
Diarrhea
Abdominal pain
Weight loss
Mental confusion
Psychosis
Metabolic hypoglycemia
Impaired gluconeogenesis
Increased insulin sensitivity
Cardiovascular/renal disorders
Impaired free-water clearance
Impaired pressor response to catecholamines
Hypotension
Pituitary
Increased adrenocorticotropic hormone secretion
Hyperpigmentation
Aldosterone deficiency
Inability to conserve sodium
Decreased extracellular fluid volume
Decreased blood volume
Weight loss
Decreased cardiac output
Increased renin production
Hypotension
Shock
Impaired renal secretion of potassium and hydrogen
Hyperkalemia
Metabolic acidosis

TABLE 7-2

Clinical Manifestations of Hypercortisolism

SYMPTOM	METABOLIC RESULTS
Weight gain	Centripetal fat distribution, increased appetite
Protein wasting	Thin skin, abdominal striae
Capillary fragility (ecchymoses)	
Muscle wasting, muscle weakness	
Osteoporosis	
Poor wound healing	
Growth retardation	
Carbohydrate intolerance	Impaired glucose use, hyperglycemia
Insulin resistance	
Mineralocorticoid effects of cortisol	Hypertension, hypokalemia
Immunologic suppression	Increased susceptibility to infections
Other manifestations	Hirsutism, oligomenorrhea, polycythemia, personality changes

is called **Cushing's disease.** A fourth cause is primary hypercortisolism resulting from a functional adrenal tumor. If the disorder is primary or if it is a result of corticosteroid treatment, ACTH secretion will be suppressed and increased skin pigmentation will not occur. However, if the hypersecretion of the adrenal is a result of an ACTH-secreting nonpituitary tumor, ACTH levels sometimes become high enough to increase skin pigmentation.

Increased cortisol secretion causes a tendency to gain weight, with a characteristic centripetal fat distribution and a "buffalo hump" (Table 7-2). The face will appear round (fat deposition), and the cheeks may be reddened, in part because of the polycythemia. The limbs will be thin as a result of skeletal muscle wasting (from increased proteolysis), and muscle weakness will be evident (from muscle proteolysis and hypokalemia). Proximal muscle weakness is apparent, so the patient may have difficulty with stair climbing or rising from a sitting position. The abdominal fat accumulation, coupled with atrophy of the abdominal muscles and thinning of the skin, will produce a large, protruding abdomen. Purple abdominal striae are seen as a result of the damage to the skin by the prolonged proteolysis, increased intra-abdominal fat, and loss of abdominal muscle tone (Figure 7-21).

Capillary fragility is seen as a result of damage to the connective tissue supporting the capillaries. Patients are likely to show signs of osteoporosis and poor wound healing. They have metabolic disturbances that include glucose intolerance, hyperglycemia, and insulin resistance. Prolonged hypercortisolism can lead to manifestations of diabetes mellitus. However, the lipolytic effect of cortisol by itself is so minor that if high insulin levels are present, lipogenesis rather than lipolysis, predominates.

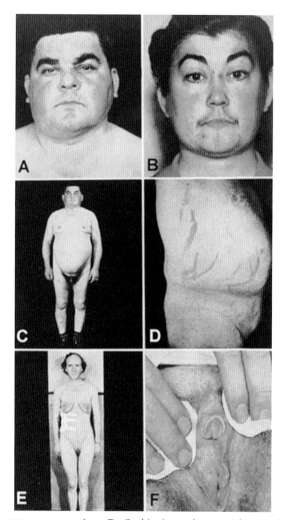

FIGURE 7-21 ■ A to D, Cushing's syndrome with typical moon face, reddish cheeks, truncal obesity, and abdominal striae. E and F, Woman with adrenogenital syndrome. *(From Wilson JD, Foster DW: Williams' textbook of endocrinology, ed 8, Philadelphia, 1992, WB Saunders.)*

effect of catecholamines, whose levels are low in the face of high blood glucose levels.

Insulin probably plays an important role in the increased adipose tissue mass typically seen with hypercortisolism. In fact, cortisol interacts with insulin to promote the differentiation of preadipocytes into adipocytes. For reasons not fully understood, hypercortisolism is associated with a peculiar pattern of fat deposition, which is called centripetal fat distribution because the adipose tissue is concentrated in the trunk, whereas wasting is seen in the arms and legs. Adipose tissue tends to accumulate in the abdomen. Visceral adipose tissue expresses a high level of 11β-HSD1, thereby efficiently converting cortisone to cortisol and increasing differentiation of preadipocytes to adipocytes. However, other mechanisms are likely to contribute. Also, hypercortisolism increases the size of subclavicular fat pads, producing the **buffalo hump** characteristic of this endocrine imbalance (see Table 7-2).

Because there are many hyperglycemic hormones, a cortisol deficiency is not likely to produce hypoglycemia unless food is withheld or the person is stressed. However, cortisol is essential for proper mobilization of proteins for glucose production. Changes in the serum after cortisol administration include increased blood urea nitrogen; decreased serum alanine (because it is used in gluconeogenesis); increased branched-chain amino acids leucine, isoleucine, and valine; increased serum fatty acid levels. The change in branched-chain amino acid levels is indicative of decreased muscle protein synthesis and increased

Excess cortisol increases total body fat. This increase in body fat results from two factors: (1) cortisol stimulates appetite (a CNS effect), so the obesity is a result of increased caloric consumption; and (2) cortisol increases the blood glucose level, which increases insulin secretion. Insulin is a strong lipogenic hormone, whereas cortisol is a weak lipolytic hormone. Cortisol acts primarily as a permissive agent on the

TABLE 7-3		
Relative Potencies of Corticosteroids Compared with Cortisol		
	GLUCOCORTICOID ACTIVITY	MINERALOCOR-TICOID ACTIVITY
Cortisol	1.0	1.0
Corticosterone	0.3	15
Aldosterone	0.3	3000
Deoxycorticosterone	0.2	100
Cortisone	0.7	1.0
Prednisolone	4	0.8
Dexamethasone	25	About 0

proteolysis, whereas the increase in fatty acids reflects adipose tissue lipolysis. Because of the suppression of the immune system caused by the glucocorticoids, patients are more susceptible to infection. Mineralocorticoid activities of the glucocorticoids and the possible elevation of aldosterone secretion produce salt retention and subsequent water retention, resulting in hypertension. Excessive androgen secretion in women can produce hirsutism, male pattern baldness, and clitoral enlargement (adrenogenital syndrome).

Conn's Syndrome Primary hyperaldosteronism is called **Conn's syndrome**. It frequently occurs as a result of aldosterone-secreting tumors. Excessive mineralocorticoid secretion results in potassium depletion, sodium retention, muscle weakness, hypertension, hypokalemic alkalosis, and polyuria. Although extracellular fluid volume increases, edema is not common because of hypervolemia-induced ANP release that results in natriuresis.

Congenital Adrenal Hyperplasia Any enzyme blockage that decreases cortisol synthesis will increase ACTH secretion and produce adrenal hyperplasia. The most common form of congenital adrenal hyperplasia occurs as a result of a deficiency of the enzyme **21-hydroxylase (CYP21)**. These individuals cannot produce normal quantities of cortisol, **deoxycortisol,**

DOC, corticosterone, or aldosterone. Because of impaired cortisol production and resultant elevated ACTH levels, steroidogenesis is stimulated, thereby increasing the synthesis of those products formed before the blockage. Because this includes the adrenal androgens, a female fetus will be masculinized. Because they are unable to produce the mineralocorticoids, aldosterone, DOC, and corticosterone, patients with this disorder have difficulty retaining salt and maintaining extracellular volume. Consequently, they are likely to be hypotensive. If the blockage is at the next step, **11β-hydroxylase (CYP11B1),** DOC will be formed and the levels of DOC will accumulate. Because DOC has significant mineralocorticoid activity and the levels become high, these individuals tend to retain salt and water and become hypertensive. The elevated androgen levels can cause masculinization of a female fetus. If there is a deficiency of 17α-hydroxylase, neither cortisol nor sex hormones are produced. The inability to produce normal androgen levels during fetal development can result in a female phenotype for both males and females. A complete deficiency of **3β-hydroxysteroid dehydrogenase (3β-HSD)** is fatal. An incomplete deficiency results in the inability to produce adequate quantities of mineralocorticoids, glucocorticoids, and strong androgens or estrogens. The adrenal produces large quantities of the weak androgen DHEA. This can result in some masculinization of a female fetus and incomplete masculinization of a male fetus.

SUMMARY

1. The adrenal gland is composed of a cortex, which is of mesodermal origin, and a medulla, which is of neuroectodermal origin. The cortex produces steroid hormones and the medulla produces catecholamines.

2. Rate-limiting enzymes in medullary catecholamine synthesis are tyrosine hydroxylase and β-dopamine hydroxylase, which are induced by sympathetic stimulation, and phenylethanolamine *N*-methyltransferase, which is induced by cortisol.

3. Catecholamines increase serum glucose and fatty acid levels. They stimulate gluconeogenesis,

glycogenolysis, and lipolysis. Catecholamines increase cardiac output but have selective effects on blood flow to different organs.

4. A pheochromocytoma is a tumor of chromaffin tissue that produces excessive quantities of catecholamines. Symptoms of pheochromocytoma are often sporadic and include hypertension, headaches, sweating, anxiety, palpitations, chest pain, and orthostatic hypotension.

5. The adrenal cortex displays clear structural and functional zonation: the zona glomerulosa produces the mineralocorticoid, aldosterone; the zona fasciculata produces the glucocorticoid, cortisol; and

the zona reticularis produces the weak androgens, DHEA and DHEAS.

6. Cortisol acts by binding to the glucocorticoid receptor. During stress, cortisol increases blood glucose by increasing gluconeogenic gene expression in the liver and breaking down muscle protein to supply gluconeogenic precursors. Cortisol also decreases glucose uptake by muscle and adipose tissue and has permissive actions on glucagon and catecholamines. Cortisol has multiple effects on other tissue. From a pharmacologic point of view, the immunosuppressive/anti-inflammatory effect is the most important.

7. Cortisol is regulated by the CRH-ACTH-cortisol axis. Cortisol negatively feeds back at both the hypothalamus on CRH-producing neurons and on the pituitary corticotropes. CRH is regulated by several forms of stress, including proinflammatory cytokines, hypoglycemia, neurogenic stress, and hemorrhage, and by diurnal inputs.

8. Adrenal androgens, DHEA, DHEAS, and androstenedione, are androgen precursors. They can be converted to active androgens peripherally and provide about 50% of circulating androgens in women. In adult men, the role of adrenal androgens, if any, remain obscure. In women, adrenal androgens promote pubic and axillary hair growth and libido. Excessive adrenal androgens in women can lead to various degrees of virilization and ovarian dysfunction.

9. The zona glomerulosa of the adrenal cortex is the site of aldosterone production. Aldosterone is the strongest naturally occurring mineralocorticoid in humans. Aldosterone promotes Na$^+$ and water uptake by the distal nephron, while promoting renal K$^+$ and H$^+$ excretion. Aldosterone promotes Na$^+$ and water uptake in the colon and salivary glands. Aldosterone has a proinflammatory, profibrotic effect on the cardiovascular system, and causes left ventricular hypertrophy and remodeling.

10. Major actions of angiotensin II on the adrenal cortex are increased growth and vascularity of the zona glomerulosa, increased StAR and CYP11B2 enzyme activity, and increased aldosterone synthesis.

11. Major stimuli for aldosterone production are a rise in angiotensin II and a rise in serum potassium concentration. The major inhibitory signal is ANP.

12. Addison's disease is adrenocortical insufficiency. Common symptoms include hypotension, hyperpigmentation, muscle weakness, anorexia, hypoglycemia, and hyperkalemic acidosis.

13. Cushing's syndrome results from hypercortisolemia. If the basis of the disorder is increased pituitary adrenocorticotropin secretion, the disorder is called *Cushing's disease.* Common symptoms of Cushing's syndrome include centripetal fat distribution, muscle wasting, proximal muscle weakness, thin skin with abdominal striae, capillary fragility, insulin resistance, and polycythemia.

14. Congenital adrenal hyperplasia results from a congenital enzyme deficiency that blocks production of cortisol. The enzyme blockage results in elevated ACTH secretion, which stimulates adrenal cortical growth and secretion of precursors produced before the block. A 21-hydroxylase (CYP21B) deficiency is the most common form.

KEY WORDS AND CONCEPTS

- Epinephrine
- Cortisol
- Aldosterone
- Dehydroepiandrosterone sulfate (DHEAS)
- Adrenal glands
- Suprarenal glands
- Adrenal cortex
- Chromaffin cells
- Adrenal medulla
- Norepinephrine
- Phenylethanolamine-*N*-methyl transferase (PNMT)
- Tyrosine
- Tyrosine hydroxylase
- Dihydroxyphenylalanine (DOPA)
- Dopamine
- Aromatic amino acid decarboxylase
- Chromaffin granule
- Chromogranins
- Acetylcholine (ACh)

- Preganglionic sympathetic neurons
- Alpha- and beta-adrenergic receptors
- Fight or flight response
- Cardiac output
- Glycolysis
- Lipolysis
- Hepatic glycogenolysis and gluconeogenesis
- Hepatic ketogenesis
- Monoamine oxidase (MAO)
- Catechol-O-methyltransferase (COMT)
- Vanillylmandelic acid (VMA)
- Metanephrine
- Pheochromocytoma
- Zona glomerulosa
- Zona fasciculata
- Zona reticularis
- Cholesterol ester hydroxylase
- Steroidogenic Acute Regulatory Protein (StAR Protein)
- Cytochrome p450 mono-oxidase gene family (CYPs)
- side-chain of cholesterol
- CYP11A1
- progesterone (P4)
- 17-hydroxyprogesterone
- 3β-hydroxysteroid dehydrogenase (3β-HSD)
- pregnenolone (P5)
- Δ5 pathway
- Δ4 pathway
- 17-Hydroxylase function
- 17,20-Lyase function
- CYP21
- 11-deoxycortisol
- CYP11B1
- Deoxycorticosterone (DOC)
- Corticosterone
- Corticosteroid-binding globulin (CBG; transcortin)
- Cortisone
- 11β-Hydroxysteroid dehydrogenase type 2 (11β- HSD2)
- 11β-HSD1
- Glucocorticoid receptor (GR)
- Molecular chaperones
- Glucocorticoid-response elements (GREs)
- Co-activator proteins
- Glucocorticoid
- Hepatic gluconeogenic enzymes
- GLUT-4–mediated glucose uptake
- Lipolysis
- Proteolysis
- Increased appetite
- Hyperinsulinemia
- Glucose intolerance
- Lipogenesis
- Truncal (abdominal, visceral) adiposity
- Anti-inflammatory and immunosuppressive actions
- Erythropoietin
- Anemia
- Inflammation and immune responses
- Immune homeostasis
- Phospholipase A$_2$
- Anti-inflammatory properties
- Immunosuppressants
- Bone resorption
- Hypothalamus-pituitary-adrenal axis
- Corticotropin-releasing hormone (CRH)
- CRH receptor
- Pro-opiomelanocortin (POMC) cells (corticotropes)
- Adrenocorticotropic hormone (ACTH)
- Vasopressin (ADH)
- Melanocortin-2 receptor (MC2R)
- LDL receptor
- Scavenger receptor-BI (SR-BI; the HDL receptor)
- Adrenal androgens
- Adrenarche
- DHEA-sulfotransferase (SULT2A1 gene)
- Androstenedione
- Sulfatases
- Masculinization of women
- Hirsutism
- Congenital adrenal hyperplasia
- Mineralocorticoid
- CYP11B2
- Aldosterone synthase
- Corticosterone
- 18-Hydroxycorticosterone
- Aldosterone
- Mineralocorticoid receptor (MR)
- Mineralocorticoid-response element
- Salt wasting and dehydration

- Epithelial Na$^+$ channel (ENaC)
- Aldosterone-inducible serine/threonine kinase, SGK-1
- Type 1 pseudohypoaldosteronism; PHA1
- Liddle's syndrome
- Renal outer medullary K$^+$ (ROMK) channel
- Hypokalemia and metabolic alkalosis
- Aldosterone escape
- Atrial natriuretic peptide (ANP)
- Proinflammatory, profibrotic effect (of aldosterone)
- Renin-angiotensin-system (RAS)
- Juxtaglomerular cells
- Renin
- Macula densa
- Angiotensinogen (renin substrate)
- Angiotensin I
- Angiotensin II
- Angiotensin-converting enzyme (ACE)
- AT1 receptor
- Extracellular K$^+$
- Adrenocortical insufficiency

- Addison's disease
- Cushing's syndrome
- Cushing's disease
- Buffalo hump
- Adrenogenital syndrome
- Conn's syndrome
- 21-Hydroxylase (CYP21)
- Deoxycortisol
- 11β-Hydroxylase (CYP11B1)
- 3β-Hydroxylase dehydrogenase (3β-HSD)

SELF-STUDY PROBLEMS

1. Describe how norepinephrine in the cytoplasm is converted to epinephrine in the chromaffin granule.
2. How does epinephrine influence metabolic pathways in the liver? adipose tissue?
3. Explain how catecholamines can cause vasoconstriction in some blood vessels, while causing vasodilation in others.
4. Complete the following chart:

	3β-HSD	CYP17 (17-HYDROXYLASE FUNCTION)	CYP17 (17,20-LYASE FUNCTION)	CYP21B	CYP11B1	CYP11B2
Zona glomerulosa	(+)			(+)		
Zona fasciculata		(+)	(−)		(+)	
Zona reticularis						(−)

5. Why may the adrenal cortex atrophy when synthetic glucocorticoids are administered?
6. Why may masculinization of women (adrenogenital syndrome) occur in patients with Cushing's disease?
7. Explain the interaction of ENaC and SGK-1 in the actions of aldosterone.
8. Explain the differences between the cause of orthostatic hypotension in patients with orthostatic hypotension associated with pheochromocytoma and orthostatic hypotension associated with Addison's disease.

9. Why are the consequences of a secondary pituitary ACTH insufficiency generally less severe than those of a primary adrenal insufficiency?

BIBLIOGRAPHY

Bassett MH, White PC, Rainey WE: The regulation of aldosterone synthase expression, *Mol Cell Endocrinol* 217:67-74, 2004.

Connell JM, Davies E: The new biology of aldosterone, *J Endocrinol* 186:1-20, 2005.

Dluhy RG, Lawrence JE, Williams GH: Endocrine hypertension. In Larsen PR, Kronenberg HM, Melmed S, Polonsky K, editors: *Williams' textbook of endocrinology*, ed 10, Philadelphia, 2003, Saunders, pp 552-585.

Feldman DS, Carnes CA, Abraham WT, Bristow MR: Mechanisms of disease: beta-adrenergic receptors—alterations in signal transduction and pharmacogenomics in heart failure, *Nat Clin Pract Cardiovasc Med* 2:475-483, 2005.

Stewart PM: The adrenal cortex. In Larsen PR, Kronenberg HM, Melmed S, Polonsky K, editors: *Williams' textbook of endocrinology*, ed 10, Philadelphia, 2003, Saunders.

Vallon V, Lang F: New insights into the role of serum- and glucocorticoid-inducible kinase SGK1 in the regulation of renal function and blood pressure, *Curr Opin Nephrol Hypertens* 14:59-66, 2005.

Zhou J, Cidlowski JA: The human glucocorticoid receptor: One gene, multiple proteins and diverse responses, *Steroids* 70:407-417, 2005.

THE MALE REPRODUCTIVE SYSTEM

O B J E C T I V E S

1. Describe the organization of the male gonad, the testis, and the process of spermatogenesis, and discuss how this process is supported by Sertoli cells.

2. Describe the steroidogenic pathway of Leydig cells that produces testosterone, the peripheral conversion of testosterone to estradiol-17β or dihydrotestosterone (DHT), and the actions of these steroids in men.

3. Discuss the regulation of testicular function by the hypothalamic-pituitary-testicular axis.

4. Describe the role of the proximal male reproductive tract, especially the epididymis, in the further development of sperm.

5. Discuss the more distal segments of the male reproductive tract, including the accessory sex glands, in the context of emission and ejaculation.

6. Describe the neurovascular events in the penis that are involved in erection.

7. Describe the development of the male tract and the events of puberty.

8. Discuss the following pathologic conditions of the male reproductive system: Klinefelter syndrome, androgen insensitivity that is coupled to testicular feminization and male pseudohermaphroditism, 5α-reductase type 2 deficiency, and Kallmann syndrome.

Humans reproduce sexually. After a period of reproductive quiescence during childhood, the reproductive system undergoes maturation, with development of secondary sexual characteristics and heightened interest in sex in both the male and the female. Men produce haploid gametes, called sperm, essentially in a continuous manner, whereas the female gamete, called the egg (or ovum), is produced in a discontinuous manner at a rate of about 1 egg per month. Clinically unassisted fertilization in humans involves internal insemination of the female tract by the male, followed by a 9-month gestational period that is supported by hemochorial placentation.

The two most basic components of the reproductive system are the **gonads** and the **reproductive tract**. The gonads (**testes** in men, **ovaries** in women)

perform an **endocrine function**, which, like the thyroid and adrenal glands, are regulated within a **hypothalamus-pituitary-gonadal axis**. However, the gonads are distinct from other endocrine glands, in that they also perform an exocrine (**gametogenic**) function. The reproductive tract serves to transport gametes and, in women, allows for fertilization, implantation, and gestation. *Normal gametogenesis in the gonads, as well as the development and physiology of the male and female reproductive tracts, is absolutely dependent on the endocrine function of the gonads.*

In men, the reproductive system has evolved for **continuous, lifelong gametogenesis**, coupled to occasional **internal insemination** with a **high density of sperm** (greater than 60×10^6/ml in 3 to 5 ml of semen). This means that in adult men the basic roles of

197

gonadal hormones are (1) support of gametogenesis (**spermatogenesis**), (2) maintenance of the male reproductive tract and production of semen, and (3) maintenance of secondary sex characteristics and libido. There is no overall cyclicity of this activity in men.

HISTOPHYSIOLOGY OF THE TESTIS

A major difference between the testes and the ovaries is that the testes reside outside of the abdominal cavity in the **scrotum**. This location maintains the testicular temperature at about 35° C, which is crucial for sperm development. Failure of the testes to descend through the inguinal canal into the scrotum during development results in infertility. The human **testis** is covered by a connective tissue capsule and is divided into about 300 **lobules** by fibrous septa. Within each lobule are two to four loops of **seminiferous tubules**. Each loop empties into an anastomosing network of tubules called the **rete testis**. The rete testis is continuous with small ducts, the **efferent ductules** that lead the sperm out of the testis into the head of the **epididymis** on the superior pole of the testis (Figure 8-1). Once in the epididymis, the sperm pass from the **head**, to the **body**, to the **tail** of the epididymis and then to the **vas (ductus) deferens**. **Spermatozoa** are stored in the tail of the epididymis and the vas deferens for several months as viable sperm.

The presence of the seminiferous tubules in the lobules of the testis creates two compartments within each lobule: an intratubular compartment, which is composed of the **seminiferous epithelium** of the seminiferous tubule; and a peritubular compartment, which is composed of neurovascular elements, connective tissue cells, immune cells, and the interstitial **cells of Leydig,** whose main function is to produce **testosterone** (see p. 204).

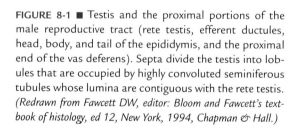

FIGURE 8-1 ■ Testis and the proximal portions of the male reproductive tract (rete testis, efferent ductules, head, body, and tail of the epididymis, and the proximal end of the vas deferens). Septa divide the testis into lobules that are occupied by highly convoluted seminiferous tubules whose lumina are contiguous with the rete testis. *(Redrawn from Fawcett DW, editor: Bloom and Fawcett's textbook of histology, ed 12, New York, 1994, Chapman & Hall.)*

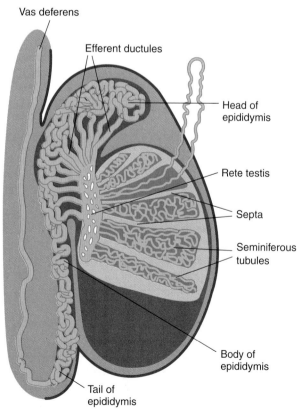

Vas deferens

Efferent ductules

Head of epididymis

Rete testis

Septa

Seminiferous tubules

Body of epididymis

Tail of epididymis

The Intratubular Compartment

The seminiferous tubule is lined by a complex **seminiferous epithelium** composed of two cell types: (1) **sperm cells** in various stages of **spermatogenesis** and (2) the **Sertoli cell,** which is a nurse cell in intimate contact with all sperm cells and which regulates many aspects of spermatogenesis (Figure 8-2).

Developing Sperm Cells Spermatogenesis involves the processes of **mitosis** and **meiosis** (Figure 8-3). Stem cells, called **spermatogonia,** reside at the basal level of the seminiferous epithelium. Spermatogonia divide mitotically to generate daughter spermatogonia (**spermatocytogenesis**). One or more remain within the stem cell population, firmly adhered to the basal lamina. A majority of these daughter spermatogonia, however, commit to meiotic division, which will result in haploid spermatozoa on completion. Of note, these divisions are accompanied by **incomplete cytokinesis,** so that all daughter cells remain interconnected by a cytoplasmic bridge. This configuration probably contributes to the synchrony of development of a clonal population of sperm cells.

Spermatogonia migrate apically away from the basal lamina as they enter the first meiotic prophase. At this time, they are called **primary spermatocytes**. During first meiotic prophase, the hallmark processes of sexual reproduction involving chromosomal reduplication, synapsis, crossing-over, and homologous recombination take place. Completion of the first meiotic division gives rise to **secondary spermatocytes**, which quickly (within 20 minutes) complete the second meiotic division. The initial products of meiosis are haploid **spermatids**, which reside apically within the seminiferous epithelium, close to the lumen of the seminiferous tubule. Spermatids are small, round cells with a nucleus and cytoplasm of unremarkable appearance. Spermatids undergo a remarkable metamorphosis called **spermiogenesis** (Figure 8-4). As the spermatid matures into a **spermatozoon,** the size of the nucleus decreases and a prominent tail is formed. The tail, which contains microtubular structures similar to those of a flagellum, serves to propel sperm. The chromatin material in the sperm nucleus condenses, and most of the cytoplasm is lost. The acrosome is a membrane-enclosed structure on the head of the sperm that acts as a lysosome and contains proteolytic enzymes that are important for penetration of the ovum. These enzymes remain inactive until the acrosomal reaction occurs (see Chapter 10).

Spermatozoa are found at the luminal surface of the seminiferous tubule. Release of sperm, or **spermiation**, requires the action of Sertoli cells. The products of spermiogenesis are the streamlined spermatozoa. The process of spermatogenesis takes about 72 days. A cohort of adjacent spermatogonia enters the process every 16 days, so that the process is staggered at one point along a seminiferous tubule. Also, the process is staggered along the length of a seminiferous tubule—not all spermatogonia enter the process of spermatogenesis at the same time along the entire length of the tubule, or in synchrony with every other tubule (there are about 500 seminiferous tubules per testis) (see later). Because the seminiferous tubules within one testis total about 400 meters in length, spermatozoa are continually being generated at many sites within the testis at any given time.

The Sertoli Cell (Box 8-1) The **Sertoli cell** represents the true epithelial cell of the seminiferous epithelium and extends from the basal lamina to the lumen. Sertoli cells surround sperm cells, providing structural support within the epithelium, and form adherens-type junctions and gap junctions with all stages of sperm cells (Figure 8-5). Through the formation and breakdown of these junctions, Sertoli cells guide sperm cells toward the lumen as they advance to later stages in spermatogenesis. Accordingly, major secretory products of Sertoli cells are proteases and protease inhibitors. Spermiation requires the final breakdown of Sertoli-sperm cell junctions.

Another important structural feature of Sertoli cells is the formation of tight junctions between adjacent Sertoli cells (see Figure 8-5). These **Sertoli-Sertoli cell occluding junctions** divide the seminiferous epithelium into a **basal compartment**, containing the spermatogonia and early-stage primary spermatocytes, and an **adluminal compartment**, containing later-stage primary spermatocytes and all subsequent stages of sperm cells. As early primary spermatocytes move apically from the basal compartment to the adluminal one, the tight junctions need to be disassembled and reassembled. These tight junctions form

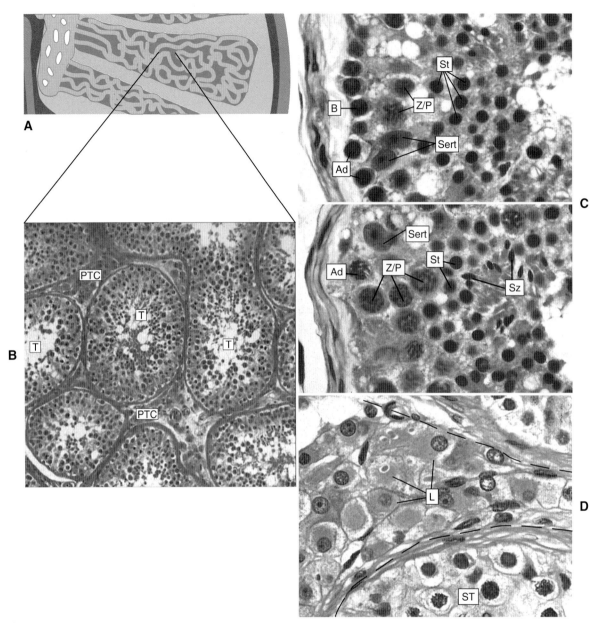

FIGURE 8-2 ■ **A,** Low-magnification drawing showing testicular lobule containing coils of seminiferous tubules. **B,** Higher-magnification histologic organization of a section from the testicular lobule (as drawn in **A**), showing several seminiferous tubules (T) (*shaded*), which collectively make up the intratubular compartment, and the peritubular compartment (PTC). **C,** Higher-magnification histologic organization of two seminiferous tubules (*upper and lower panels*), showing Sertoli cells (Sert), spermatogonia (Ad and B), primary spermatocytes (Z/P), spermatids (St), and spermatozoa (Sz). L, lumen of tubule. Notice that the collection of sperm cells differ in the two adjacent tubules, as a result of differences in their stage of spermatogenesis. **D,** Higher-magnification histologic organization of the peritubular compartment (between *dashed lines*) showing a cluster of Leydig cells (L). (**A** *from Porterfield: Endocrine physiology ed 2 St. Louis, 2001, Mosby.* **B-D** *From Stevens A, Lowe J: Human histology, ed 3, Philadelphia, 2005, Mosby.*)

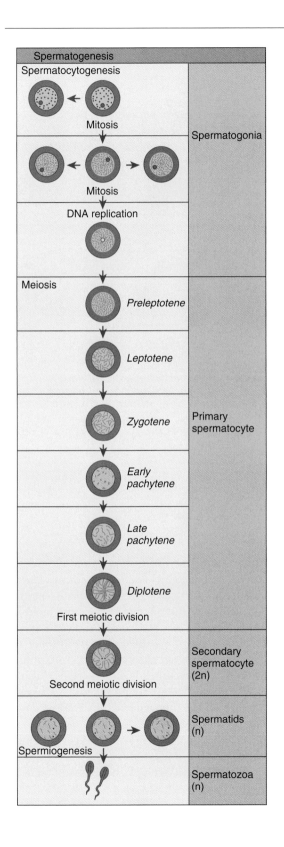

Spermatogenesis

BOX 8-1
FUNCTIONS OF SERTOLI CELLS

Supportive ("Nursing")
- Maintaining, breaking, and re-forming multiple junctions with developing sperm
- Maintaining blood-testis barrier
- Phagocytosis
- Transfer of nutrients and other substances from blood to developing sperm cells
- Expression of paracrine factors and receptors for sperm-derived paracrine factors

Exocrine
- Production of fluid to move immobile sperm out of testis toward epididymis
- Production of androgen-binding protein (ABP)
- Determination of release of spermatozoa (spermiation) from seminiferous tubule

Endocrine
- Expression of androgen receptor (AR) and follicle-stimulating hormone (FSH) receptor
- Production of müllerian-inhibiting substance (MIS)—also called anti-müllerian hormone (AMH)
- Aromatization of testosterone to estradiol-17β (this has local effect—not strictly endocrine)

the physical basis for the **blood-testis barrier**, which creates a specialized, immunologically safe microenvironment for developing sperm. By blocking paracellular diffusion, the tight junctions restrict movement of substances between the blood and the developing germ cells through a trans-Sertoli cell transport

FIGURE 8-3 ■ Major stages of spermatogenesis. Spermatogonia undergo mitosis (spermatocytogenesis) to produce both a reservoir of spermatogonia and maturing spermatogonia that differentiate into primary spermatocytes. These spermatocytes remain joined by cytoplasmic bridges (not shown). Primary spermatocytes undergo the complex process of the first meiotic division to become secondary spermatocytes, and then a rapid second meiotic division (reduction-division) to become haploid spermatids. Spermatids mature into spermatozoa by the process of spermiogenesis.

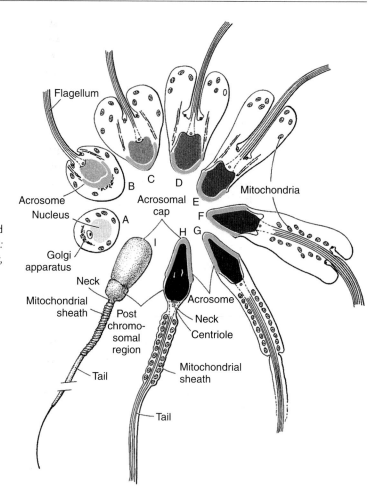

FIGURE 8-4 ■ Spermatocyte (A), spermatid (B–F), and spermatozoon (G–I). *(From Carlson B: Human embryology and developmental biology, St. Louis, 1994, Mosby.)*

pathway and in this manner allow the Sertoli cell to control nutrient availability to germ cells. Accordingly, Sertoli cells also have the responsibility for providing nutrients to this environment, such as transferrin, iron, and lactate. For example, spermatogonia and released spermatozoa utilize glucose and glycolysis for energy. However, sperm undergoing meiosis cannot efficiently utilize glucose as an energy source. Sertoli cells acquire glucose by the GLUT-1 transporter, metabolize it to lactate, and transfer it to developing sperm, which express a sperm-specific lactate transporter. This process is dependent on hormonal stimulation (FSH and testosterone) but also appears to be optimized by local sperm cell–generated paracrine factors.

Thus, healthy Sertoli cell function is essential for sperm cell viability and development. In this respect, it should be noted that spermatogenesis is absolutely dependent on testosterone produced by peritubular Leydig cells (see later), yet it is the Sertoli cells that express the **androgen receptor**, *not* the developing sperm cells. Similarly, the pituitary hormone follicle-stimulating hormone (FSH) also is required for maximal sperm production, and again, it is the Sertoli cell that expresses the **FSH receptor**, not the developing sperm. Thus, these hormones support spermatogenesis indirectly through stimulation of Sertoli cell function.

Sertoli cells have multiple additional functions. Sertoli cells express the enzyme CYP19 (also called

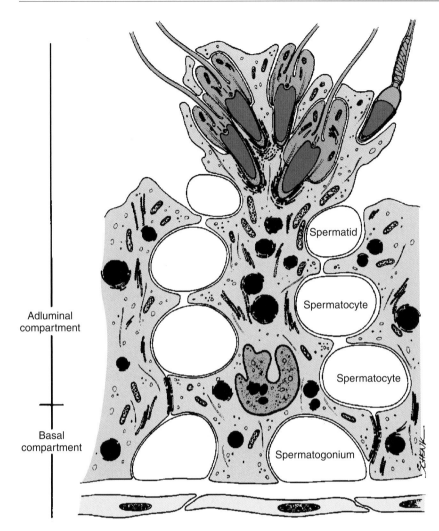

Adluminal compartment

Basal compartment

Spermatid

Spermatocyte

Spermatocyte

Spermatogonium

FIGURE 8-5 ■ Diagram of the Sertoli cell showing the relationship between Sertoli cell cytoplasm and developing spermatocytes. *(From Griffin JE, Wilson JD: Disorders of the testis and the male reproductive tract. In Larsen PR, Kronenberg HM, Melmed S, Polonsky KS, editors: Williams' textbook of endocrinology, ed 10, Philadelphia, 2003, Saunders.)*

aromatase), which converts Leydig cell–derived testosterone to the potent estrogen, estradiol-17β (see later). This local production of estrogen may enhance spermatogenesis in humans. Sertoli cells also produce **androgen-binding protein (ABP).** ABP is encoded by the same gene as for **sex hormone–binding globulin (SHBG)** (see later) but has different carbohydrate groups and is specifically expressed intratesticularly. ABP maintains a high androgen level within the adluminal compartment, the lumina of the seminiferous tubules, and the proximal part of the male reproductive tract. Sertoli cells also produce a large amount of fluid. This fluid provides an appropriate bathing

medium for the sperm and assists in moving the immotile spermatozoa from the seminiferous tubule into the epididymis. Sertoli cells perform an important phagocytic function. This involves engulfing **residual bodies,** which represent cytoplasm that is shed by spermatozoa during spermiogenesis.

Finally, the Sertoli cell has an important endocrine role. During development, Sertoli cells produce **antimüllerian hormone (AMH),** also called **müllerianinhibiting substance (MIS),** which induces regression of the embryonic müllerian duct that is programmed to give rise to the female reproductive tract (see later). The Sertoli cells also produce the hormone **inhibin.**

Inhibin is a heterodimer protein hormone related to the transforming growth factor-β (TGF-β) family. FSH stimulates inhibin production, which then exerts negative feedback on gonadotropes to inhibit FSH production. Thus, inhibin keeps FSH levels within a specific range (p. 207).

The Peritubular Compartment

The peritubular compartment contains the primary endocrine cell of the testis, the **Leydig cell** (see Figure 8-2). This compartment also contains common cell types of loose connective tissue, and an extremely rich peritubular capillary network that must provide nutrients to the seminiferous tubules (by way of Sertoli cells) while conveying testoterone away from the testes to the peripheral circulation.

The Leydig Cell   Leydig cells are steroidogenic stromal cells. These cells synthesize cholesterol de novo, as well as acquiring it through **low-density lipoprotein receptors (LDL receptors)** and **high-density lipoprotein receptors (HDL receptors)** (the HDL receptor also is called **scavenger receptor-BI [SR-BI]**), and store cholesterol as cholesterol esters, as described for adrenocortical cells (see Chapter 7). Free cholesterol is generated by a **cholesterol ester hydrolase**, and transferred to the outer mitochondrial membrane, and then to the inner mitochondrial membrane in a **steroidogenic acute regulatory protein (StAR)**-dependent manner. As in all steroidogenic cells, cholesterol is converted to pregnenolone by **CYP11A1**. Pregnenolone is then processed to progesterone, 17α-hydroxyprogesterone, and androstenedione by 3β-hydroxysteroid dehydrogenase (**3β-HSD**) and **CYP17** (Figure 8-6). Recall from Chapter 7 that CYP17 is a bifunctional enzyme, with a **17-hydroxylase activity** and a **17, 20-lyase activity**. CYP17 displays a robust level of both activities in the Leydig cell. In this respect, the Leydig cell is similar to the zona reticularis cell, except that it expresses a higher level of 3β-HSD, so that the **Δ4 pathway** is ultimately favored. Another major difference is that the Leydig cell expresses a Leydig cell–specific isoform of **17β-hydroxysteroid dehydrogenase (17β-HSD type 3)**, which converts **androstenedione** to **testosterone** (see Figure 8-6).

Mutation of this specific gene in men results in a form of **male pseudohermaphroditism** (see later).

FATES AND ACTIONS OF ANDROGENS

Intratesticular Androgen

The testosterone produced by Leydig cells has several fates and multiple actions (Box 8-2 and Table 8-1). Because of the proximity of Leydig cells to the seminiferous tubules, significant amounts of testosterone diffuse into the seminiferous tubules and become concentrated within the adluminal compartment by androgen-binding protein (ABP) (see Figure 8-6). Testosterone levels within the seminiferous tubules that are greater than 100 times more concentrated than circulating testosterone levels are absolutely required for normal spermatogenesis. As noted, Sertoli cells express the enzyme **CYP19 (aromatase)**, which converts a small amount of testosterone into the highly potent estrogen **estradiol-17β**. Human sperm cells express at least one isoform of the **estrogen receptor (ER)**, and there is some evidence from aromatase-deficient men that this locally produced estrogen optimizes spermatogenesis in humans.

Peripheral Conversion to Estrogen

In several tissues (especially adipose tissue), testosterone is converted to estrogen (see Figure 8-6). Studies in men with aromatase deficiency have shown that inability to produce estrogen results in tall stature, owing to lack of epiphyseal closure in long bones, and accompanying osteoporosis. Thus, peripheral estrogen plays an important role in bone maturation and biology in men. These studies also implicated estrogen in promoting insulin sensitivity, improving lipoprotein profiles (i.e., increasing HDL, decreasing triglycerides and LDL), and exerting negative feedback on pituitary gonadotropins.

Peripheral Conversion to DHT

Testosterone can also be converted into a potent, **nonaromatizable androgen, 5α-dihydrotestosterone (DHT),** by the enzyme **5α-reductase** (see Figure 8-6). There are two isoforms of 5α-reductase, type 1

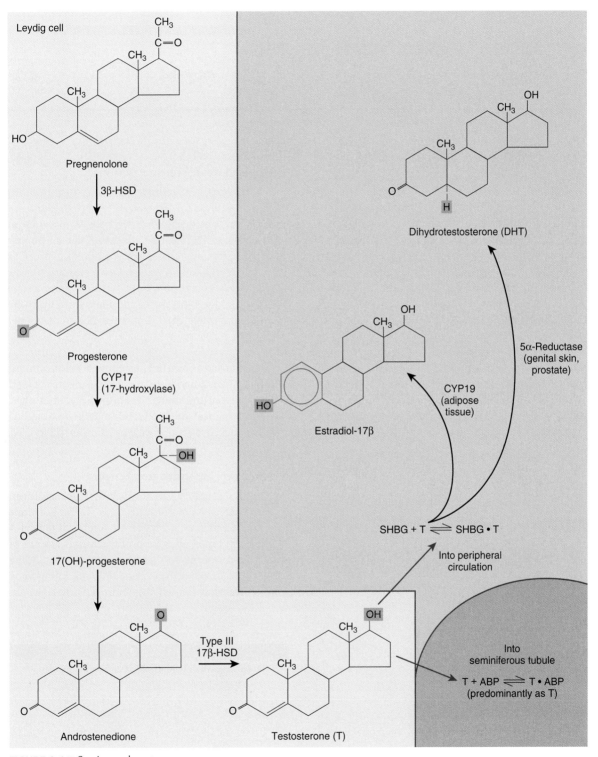

FIGURE 8-6 ■ See Legend next page.

FIGURE 8-6, Cont'd ■ Steroidogenic pathway in Leydig cells leading to testosterone production (conversion of cholesterol to pregnenolone is not shown). Testosterone (T) diffuses both into the neighboring seminiferous tubules and into the peritubular capillary network to be carried into the peripheral circulation. In the lumina of seminiferous tubules, T is concentrated by binding to androgen-binding protein (ABP). T is carried in the peripheral circulation by sex hormone–binding globulin (SHBG) and albumin. The Leydig cell makes limited amounts of DHT and estradiol-17β, but considerably more of these two steroids are made by peripheral conversion.

and type 2. Major sites of 5α-reductase 2 expression are the male urogenital tract, genital skin, hair follicles, and liver. 5α-reductase 2 generates DHT, which is required for masculinization of the external genitalia in utero, and in many of the changes associated with puberty, including growth and activity of the prostate gland (see later), growth of the penis, darkening and folding of the scrotum, growth of pubic and axillary hair, facial and body hair, and increased muscle mass. Onset of 5α-reductase 1 expression occurs at puberty. This isozyme is expressed primarily in the skin and contributes to sebaceous gland activity and acne associated with puberty. Because DHT has strong growth-promoting (i.e., trophic) effects on its target organs, the development of **selective 5α-reductase 2 inhibitors** has benefited the treatment of prostatic hypertrophy and prostatic cancer.

BOX 8-2
ACTIONS OF ANDROGENS

■ Regulation of differentiation of male internal and external genitalia in fetus
■ Stimulation of growth, development, and function of male internal and external genitalia
■ Stimulation of sexual hair development
■ Stimulation of sebaceous gland secretion
■ Stimulation of erythropoietin synthesis
■ Control of protein anabolic effects
■ Stimulation of bone growth and closure of epiphyses
■ Initiation and maintenance of spermatogenesis
■ Stimulation of androgen-binding protein synthesis (synergizes with follicle-stimulating hormone [FSH])
■ Maintenance of secretions of sex glands
■ Regulation of behavioral effects, including libido

Peripheral Testosterone Actions

Individuals with 5α-reductase 2–deficiency are born with ambiguous or feminized external genitalia, thereby demonstrating the need for conversion of testosterone to DHT for an effect on some androgen-responsive tissues. However, testosterone can act as itself in several cell types. As mentioned previously, testosterone regulates Sertoli cell function. Testosterone induces the development of the male tract from the mesonephric duct in the absence of 5α-reductase. Testosterone has several metabolic effects, including increasing very-low-density lipoprotein (VLDL) and LDL while decreasing HDL, promoting the deposition of abdominal adipose tissue, increasing red blood cell production, promoting bone growth and health, and having a protein anabolic effect on muscle. Testosterone is sufficient to maintain erectile function and libido.

Mechanism of Androgen Action

Testosterone and DHT act through the same androgen receptor (AR). As described for other steroid hormone receptors (see Chapter 1), the AR resides in the cytoplasm bound to chaperone proteins in the absence of ligand. Testosterone-AR binding or DHT-AR binding causes dissociation of chaperone proteins, followed by nuclear translocation of the androgen-AR complex,

TABLE 8-1	
Approximate Hormone Production Rates in Adult Man	
Testosterone	5 mg/day
Estradiol	10-15 µg/day
Dihydrotestosterone	50-100 µg/day
17α-Hydroxyprogesterone	1-2 mg/day

dimerization, binding to an **androgen-response element (ARE)**, and recruitment of co-activator proteins and general transcription factors to the vicinity of a specific gene's promoter. It remains unclear how testosterone and DHT differ in their ability to activate the AR in the context of different cell types.

Transport and Metabolism of Androgens

As testosterone enters the peripheral circulation, it quickly reaches equilibrium with serum proteins. About 60% of circulating testosterone is bound to sex hormone–binding globulin (SHBG), 38% is bound to albumin, and about 2% remains as "free" hormone. Testosterone and its metabolites are excreted primarily in the urine (Figure 8-7). Approximately 50% of excreted androgens are found as **urinary 17-ketosteroids**, with most of the remainder being conjugated androgens or diol or triol derivatives. Only about 30% of the 17-ketosteroids in urine are from the testis; the rest are produced from adrenal androgens. Androgens are conjugated with glucuronate or sulfate in the liver, and these **conjugated steroids** are excreted in the urine.

Theoretically, androgens can be administered orally. However, because the absorption of many naturally occurring androgens is minimal and their half-lives are relatively short, synthetic analogs that are more readily absorbed in the gastrointestinal tract and that have longer half-lives generally are used for oral treatment.

HYPOTHALAMUS-PITUITARY-TESTIS AXIS

The testis is regulated by an endocrine axis involving parvicellular hypothalamic **gonadotropin-releasing hormone (GnRH)-secreting neurons** and **pituitary gonadotropes** that produce both **luteinizing hormone (LH)** and **follicle-stimulating hormone (FSH)** (Figure 8-8). Recall from Chapter 5 that LH and FSH are **pituitary glycoprotein hormones**. They are heterodimers, composed of a common α subunit—the α-glycoprotein subunit (α-GSU)—and a specific β subunit (either LH-β or FSH-β).

Regulation of Leydig Cell Function

The Leydig cell expresses the **LH receptor**. LH acts on Leydig cells much like ACTH does on zona fasciculata cells (see Chapter 7). The LH receptor is coupled to a Gs–cyclic adenosine monophosphate cAMP-PKA signaling pathway (see Chapter 1). Rapid effects include hydrolysis of cholesterol esters and new expression of StAR. Less acute effects include an increase in steroidogenic enzyme gene expression, and in the expression of the LDL receptor and SR-BI (the HDL receptor). Over the long term, LH promotes Leydig cell growth and proliferation.

Testosterone has a negative feedback effect on LH production by the pituitary gonadotrope as testosterone, DHT, and estradiol-17β. All three steroid hormones inhibit the expression of LH-β and the GnRH receptor. These steroids also inhibit the release of GnRH by the hypothalamic neurons.

Regulation of Sertoli Cell Function

Although testosterone, DHT, and estrogen exert negative feedback on both LH and FSH, they selectively inhibit LH more effectively than FSH. From a historical standpoint, this finding raised the possibility that a Sertoli cell–derived factor might feed back on FSH production. The Sertoli cell is stimulated by both testosterone and FSH. The **FSH receptor** also is coupled primarily to a Gs-cAMP-PKA pathway. In addition to stimulating the synthesis of proteins involved in the "nurse cell" aspect of Sertoli cell function (e.g., ABP), FSH stimulates the synthesis of the dimeric

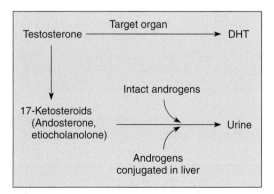

FIGURE 8-7 ■ Metabolism of androgens. DHT, dihydrotestosterone.

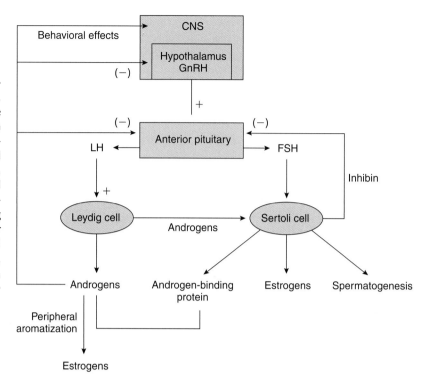

FIGURE 8-8 ■ Summary of regulation of testicular function. Gonadotropin-releasing hormone (GnRH) stimulates secretion of anterior pituitary hormones—luteinizing hormone (LH) and follicle-stimulating hormone (FSH). These hormones act on Leydig and Sertoli cells to stimulate production of hormones, androgen-binding protein, and sperm. Testicular androgens and inhibin can control production of LH and FSH. CNS, central nervous system; DHT, dihydrotestosterone; T, testosterone.

protein **inhibin**. Inhibin has a common α subunit, coupled with either a β_A subunit, called **inhibin A,** or a β_B subunit, called **inhibin B**. Inhibin B is induced by FSH and exerts negative feedback on the gonadotrope to selectively inhibit FSH production.

There exists an important "loophole" in the male reproductive axis, which is based on the fact the intratesticular levels of testosterone need to be greater than 100-fold higher than circulating levels of the hormone in order to maintain normal rates of spermatogenesis, but it is the circulating levels of testosterone that provide the negative feedback to the pituitary and hypothalamus. This means that exogenous administration of testosterone can raise circulating levels sufficient to inhibit LH but not sufficient to concentrate in the testis at the required concentration for normal spermatogenesis. The decreased LH levels, however, will diminish intratesticular production of testosterone by Leydig cells, which will result in reduced levels of spermatogenesis (Figure 8-9). This "loophole" is currently being investigated as a possible strategy for developing a **male oral contraceptive**. It also is the basis for sterility in some cases of steroid abuse in men.

THE MALE REPRODUCTIVE TRACT

Once spermatozoa emerge from the efferent ductules, they leave the gonad and enter the male reproductive tract (Figure 8-10). The segments of the tract are as follows: the **epididymis (head, body,** and **tail),** the **vas deferens,** the **ejaculatory duct,** the prostatic urethra, the membranous urethra and the penile urethra. Unlike in the female tract, there is a **contiguous lumen** from the seminiferous tubule to the end of the male tract (i.e., the tip of the penile urethra), and the male tract connects to the **distal urinary tract** (i.e., **male urethra**). In addition to conveying sperm, the primary functions of the male reproductive tract are as follows:

1. Sperm spend about a month in the epididymis, where they undergo further maturation. The epithelium of the epididymis is actively secretory and adds numerous proteins and glycolipids to the seminal fluid. Spermatozoa that enter the head of the epididymis are weakly motile but are strongly unidirectionally motile by the time they exit the tail.

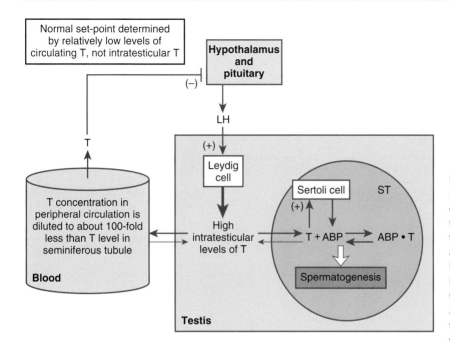

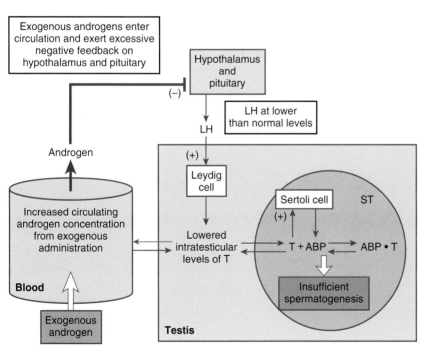

FIGURE 8-9 ■ The difference in intratesticular testosterone versus circulating testosterone concentrations, and its importance in the hypothalamus-pituitary-testis axis. **Upper panel,** The feedback loop in the normal adult man. **Lower panel,** Administration of testosterone (or an androgenic analog) increases circulating testosterone (androgen) levels, which in turn increases the negative feedback on LH release. Decreased LH levels diminish Leydig cell activity and intratesticular production of androgen. Lowered intratesticular testosterone levels result in reduced sperm production and can cause infertility. Note that the inhibin feedback loop has been omitted from this diagram. ABP, androgen-binding protein; LH, luteinizing hormone; ST, seminiferous tubule; T, testosterone.

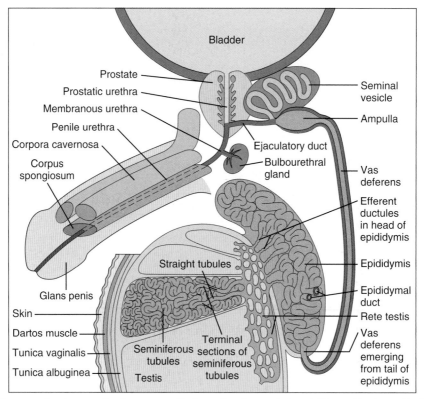

FIGURE 8-10 ■ Diagram of male reproductive system. *(Redrawn from Stevens A, Lowe J: Human histology, ed 3, Philadelphia, 2005, Mosby.)*

Spermatozoa also undergo the process of **decapacitation**, which involves the addition of molecules to their membranes order to prevent spermatozoa from undergoing the acrosomal reaction before contact with an egg (see Chapter 10). Sperm become capacitated by the female reproductive tract within the oviduct (see Chapter 9). The function of the epididymis is dependent on luminal testosterone-ABP complexes that come from the seminiferous tubules, and on testosterone from the blood. Of note, the epididymal epithelium is extremely tight, so that a **blood-epididymis barrier** exists.

2. Sperm are stored in the tail of the epididymis and vas deferens. Sperm can be stored for several months without loss of viability. The primary function of the vas deferens, besides providing a storage site, is to propel sperm during sexual intercourse into the male urethra. The vas deferens has a very thick muscularis that is richly innervated by sympathetic nerves. Normally in response to repeated tactile stimulation of the penis during coitus, the muscularis of the vas deferens receives bursts of sympathetic stimulation, causing peristaltic contractions. The emptying of the contents of the vas deferens into the prostatic urethra is called **emission**. Emission immediately precedes **ejaculation**, which is the propulsion of semen out of the male urethra.

3. During emission, contraction of the vas deferens coincides with contraction of the muscular coats of the two accessory sex glands, the **seminal vesicles** (right and left) and the **prostate gland** (which surrounds the prostatic urethra). At this point, sperm become mixed with all the components of **semen**. The seminal vesicles secrete approximately 60% of

the volume. These glands are the primary source **fructose,** a critical nutrient for sperm. Seminal vesicles also secrete **semenogelins,** which induce coagulation of semen immediately after ejaculation. The alkaline secretions of the prostate, which make up about 30% of the volume, are high in **citrate**, **zinc**, **spermine**, and **acid phosphatase. Prostate-specific antigen (PSA)** is a serine protease that liquefies coagulated semen after a few minutes. PSA can be detected in the blood under conditions of prostatic infection, benign prostatic hypertrophy and prostatic carcinoma, and is currently used as one indicator of prostatic health. The predominant buffers in semen are phosphate and bicarbonate. A third accessory gland, the **bulbourethral glands** (also called Cowper's glands), empty into the penile urethra in response to sexual excitement prior to emission and ejaculation. This secretion is high in mucus, which lubricates, cleanses and buffers the urethra. Average sperm counts are reported to be from 60 to 100 million/ml semen. Men with sperm counts below 20 million/ml, less than 50% motile sperm, or less than 60% normally conformed sperm usually are infertile.

4. As noted, emission and ejaculation occur during coitus in response to a reflex arc that involves sensory stimulation from the penis (via the pudendal nerve) followed by sympathetic motor stimulation to the smooth muscle of the male tract and somatic motor stimulation to the musculature associated with the base of the penis. However, in order for sexual intercourse to occur in the first place, the male partner has to achieve and maintain an **erection** of the **penis**. The penis has evolved as an intromittent organ designed to separate the walls of the vagina, pass through the potential space of the vaginal lumen and deposit semen at the deep end of the vaginal lumen near the cervix. This process of **internal insemination** can be performed only if the penis is stiffened from the process of erection.

Erection is a neurovascular event. The penis is composed of three erectile bodies: two **corpora cavernosa** and one **corpus spongiosum**. The penile urethra runs through the corpus spongiosum. These three bodies are composed of **erectile tissue**—an anastomosing network of potential **cavernous vascular spaces** lined with continuous endothelia within a loose connective tissue support. During the **flaccid state**, blood flow to the cavernous spaces is minimal. This is due to vasoconstriction of vasculature that shunts blood flow away from the cavernous spaces. In response to sexual arousal, parasympathetic nerves innervating the vascular smooth muscle of the arterial supply to the cavernous spaces release nitric oxide (NO). NO activates guanylyl cyclase, increasing cyclic guanosine monophosphate (cGMP), which decreases intracellular Ca^{2+} and causes muscular relaxation. The vasodilation allows blood to flow into the spaces, causing engorgement and erection. The engorged tissue also presses on veins in the penis, reducing venous drainage.

Inability to achieve or maintain an erection is termed **erectile dysfunction (ED)** and is a basis for infertility. Multiple factors can lead to ED, including insufficient androgen production, neurovascular damage (e.g., from diabetes mellitus, spinal cord injury), structural damage to the penis, perineum or pelvis, psychogenic factors (e.g., depression, performance anxiety), prescribed medications, and recreational drugs, including alcohol and tobacco. A major development in the treatment of some forms of erectile dysfunction is availability of **selective cGMP phosphodiesterase inhibitors**, which assist in the maintenance of an erection.

DEVELOPMENT OF THE MALE REPRODUCTIVE SYSTEM

The genetic sex of a fetus depends on the nature of the sex chromosomes contributed by the egg and the sperm. Normally there are 46 chromosomes, consisting of 22 sets of **autosomes** and a set of sex chromosomes. The **sex chromosomes** are called X and Y chromosomes; XX is the normal pattern for the female, and XY is the normal pattern for the male. The short arm of the Y chromosome contains the gene regulating the differentiation of the primitive gonad into a testis.

Before 6 weeks of gestation, the fetus contains indifferent gonads that have formed from the gonadal ridge. By the beginning of the sixth week of development, the genital ridges have been invaded by migratory germ cells from the yolk sac. At this stage, the gonads have the potential of becoming either ovaries or testes. By 6 weeks of gestation, the gonads contain germ cells, stromal cells that will become either Leydig cells or theca cells (see Chapter 9), and supporting cells that will become either Sertoli cells or granulosa cells (see Chapter 9). Located on the short arm of the Y chromosome is the testis-determining gene referred to as *SRY* (**sex-determining region Y**). *SRY* encodes the testicular-determining factor that allows for the development of the testis. The *SRY* gene product inhibits the action of another transcription factor, DAX-1, in stromal and supporting cells, but not germ cells. DAX-1 promotes the later development of ovarian tissue, unless blocked by SRY. If SRY is present, the undifferentiated somatic cells of the gonad can respond to another transcription factor, SOX-9, and develop into Sertoli cells (Figure 8-11). Leydig cells appear later (week 8) and start producing the androgens necessary for male reproductive tract

development (see later). Further development leads to the structural and vascular characteristics of a testis. Sertoli cells surround primordial germ cells, which now become the spermatogonia. Sertoli cells remain unresponsive to androgens in the fetus, and essentially no meiosis occurs in the testis until puberty. The testis develops between 6 and 8 weeks of gestation.

Although genes regulate the development of the ovaries and testes, hormones mediate phenotypic gender expression. The fetus originally develops with multipotential internal and external genitalia (Figure 8-12). Internally there are two **mesonephric** (also called **wolffian**) **ducts,** which have the potential for becoming male internal genitalia, and two **paramesonephric** (also called **müllerian**) **ducts,** which have the potential for becoming female internal genitalia. Whether male or female internal genitalia develop depends on the presence or absence of two

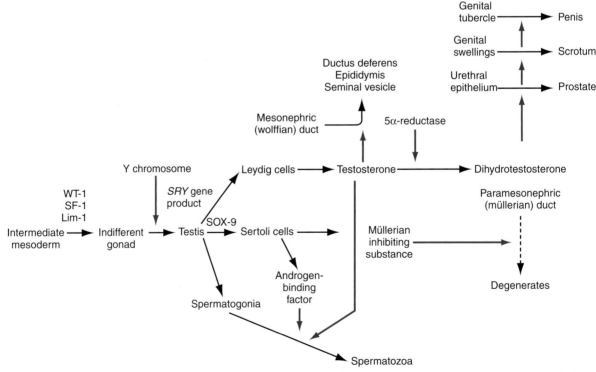

FIGURE 8-11 ■ Differentiation of the male phenotype. (*Redrawn from Carlson BM: Human embryology and developmental biology, updated ed, Philadelphia, 2004, Mosby.*)

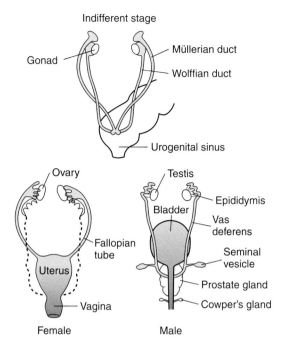

FIGURE 8-12 ■ Differentiation of internal genitalia and primordial ducts. *(Redrawn from George FW, Wilson JD: Embryology of the genital tract. In Walsh PC, et al, editors: Campbell's urology, ed 6, Philadelphia, 1992, WB Saunders.)*

hormones produced by the fetal testis—**testosterone** and **müllerian-inhibiting substance (MIS)** (Box 8-3).

Testosterone is produced by the Leydig cells of the testis, and MIS is produced by the Sertoli cells of the seminiferous tubules. By 8 weeks of gestation, the fetal testis is actively producing testosterone. Because the fetal pituitary is not yet secreting luteinizing hormone (LH),

testosterone production is regulated by **placental human chorionic gonadotropin (hCG),** which resembles LH structurally. Testosterone acts in a paracrine manner to unilaterally stimulate growth and development of the mesonephric ducts into the epididymis, vas deferens, seminal vesicles, and ejaculatory ducts (Figure 8-13). The Sertoli cells of the fetal testis produce the peptide hormone MIS, which stimulates regression of the müllerian ducts. In the absence of MIS, the müllerian ducts are retained and become female internal genitalia—fallopian tubes, uterus, cervix, and upper one third of the vagina (see Chapter 9). In the absence of testosterone, the mesonephric ducts regress. This effect is local; if a testis is absent on one side, the müllerian duct will be retained on that side. If high testosterone levels are present in a female fetus because of a congenital adrenal disorder, or because of a maternal endocrine disorder, both sets of ducts can be retained. Dihydrotestosterone (DHT) is not involved in the masculinization of these internal genitalia because the enzyme 5α-reductase is not expressed in these tissues at the time of differentiation of the mesonephric duct.

Development of the external genitalia also is hormonally regulated, and differentiation occurs between 9 and 12 weeks of gestation (Box 8-4). Androgens, particularly DHT, are responsible for transforming the multipotential fetal external genitalia (genital tubercle, genital fold, genital swelling, and urogenital sinus) into the male prostate, penis, penile urethra, and scrotum (Figure 8-14 and Table 8-2). These tissues remain ones in which DHT is produced and where DHT serves as the most potent androgen.

In the absence of androgen exposure, the external genitalia develop into the labia, clitoris, and lower two thirds of the vagina. If **5α-reductase,** the enzyme required to convert testosterone to DHT, is deficient, the appearance of the external genitalia may be ambiguous, so that the affected infant can be mistaken for a genetic female.

The ovary is quiescent during gestation. Ovarian secretions are not involved in fetal differentiation of the female reproductive system. In the absence of either ovary or testis, female internal and external genitalia develop.

■ ■ ■ ■ ■ ■ ■ ■ ■ ■

BOX 8-3
REGULATION OF DEVELOPMENT OF INTERNAL GENITALIA

The wolffian ducts, *when stimulated with testosterone,* become the epididymis, vas deferens, seminal vesicles, and ejaculatory ducts.

The müllerian ducts, *in the absence of Sertoli cell müllerian-inhibiting substance,* become the fallopian tubes, uterus, cervix, and upper one third of the vagina.

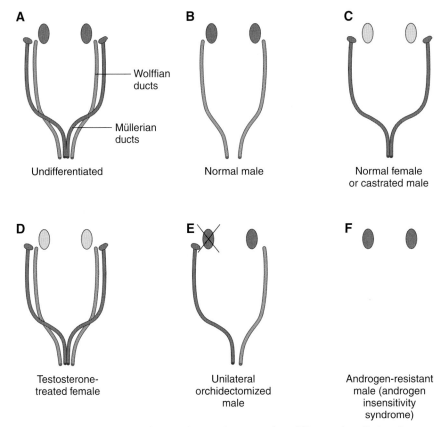

FIGURE 8-13 ■ Regulation of development of internal genitalia. **A,** Both wolffian and müllerian ducts are originally present in both male and female fetuses (undifferentiated). **B,** If functional testes are present, wolffian ducts develop and müllerian ducts regress. **C,** If no testes are present, müllerian ducts develop and wolffian ducts are lost. **D,** If a female fetus is exposed to testosterone, both ductile systems can remain. **E,** If a testis is removed unilaterally (orchidectomized), the müllerian duct will develop and the wolffian duct will regress on one side. **F,** A male with functional testes but androgen insensitivity will show regression of both ductile systems.

Puberty and Senescence

The reproductive axis is driven by GnRH-secreting neurons in the mediobasal hypothalamus. These "GnRH neurons" display activity during gestation and in the neonate, but soon after there is a long period of quiescence of the reproductive axis in humans. This period lasts from infancy through childhood, and ends during early teenage years. The reappearance of activity within the reproductive system is called **puberty** and induces dramatic phenotypic and behavioral changes (Figure 8-15).

The period of reproductive quiescence during childhood is due to an inhibition of GnRH neurons by

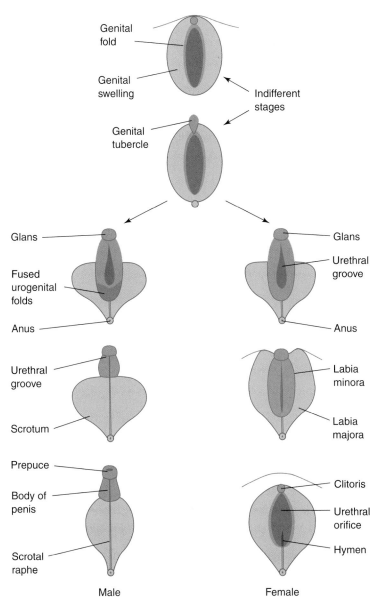

FIGURE 8-14 ■ Regulation of development of external genitalia. In the presence of DHT between 9 and 12 weeks of gestation, male external genitalia develop from the genital tubercle, genital fold, genital swelling, and urogenital sinus. In the absence of DHT, female external genitalia develop.

TABLE 8-2
Time Frame for Fetal Development of Male Reproductive System

6 to 8 weeks gestation	Differentiation of testes
8 weeks gestation	Retention of wolffian ducts
	Regression of müllerian ducts
9 to 12 weeks gestation	Development of male-type external genitalia

the central nervous system (CNS), and to an exquisite sensitivity of the negative feedback of steroids on the hypothalamus and pituitary (i.e., a low "set-point," or **gonadostat**). Puberty is associated with a removal of the CNS inhibition on the GnRH neurons, and the resetting of the gonadostat to a higher level (i.e., less sensitive feedback). Immediately before puberty, during the peripubertal period, intermittent sleep-associated

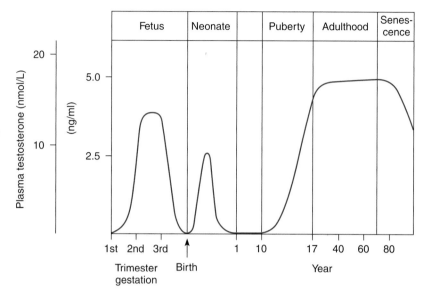

FIGURE 8-15 ■ Plasma testosterone levels during life span of normal male.

surges in GnRH begin to occur (Figure 8-16). Gonadotrope sensitivity to GnRH increases, resulting in an increase in LH secretion. At puberty, the frequency and amplitude of the GnRH pulses increase. This change increases LH and FSH secretion throughout the day and ultimately testicular androgen production.

An important hallmark of puberty in males is an increase in testicular volume (Figure 8-17). Before puberty, there are a few partially differentiated Leydig cells. During puberty, Leydig cells differentiate from mesenchymal peritubular cells and divide to form the typical clusters seen in the adult testis. Within the seminiferous tubules, spermatogenesis is initiated at puberty, and as testosterone and FSH levels increase, the rate of spermatogenesis reaches adult levels. Sertoli cells divide and become more active at puberty,

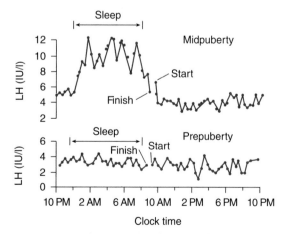

FIGURE 8-16 ■ Sleep-associated rises in luteinizing hormone (LH) secretion in the pubertal male. *(Redrawn from Wilson GD, Foster DW, editors: Williams' textbook of endocrinology, ed 8, Philadelphia, 1992, WB Saunders.)*

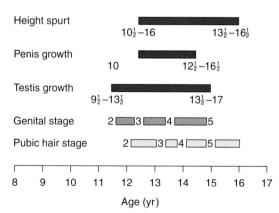

FIGURE 8-17 ■ Normal sequence of changes of male puberty. Numbers 2 to 5 refer to Tanner stages (see Table 8-3). *(Data from Marshall WA, Tanner JM: Arch Dis Child 45:13, 1970.)*

STAGE	GENITALS	PUBIC HAIR
TABLE 8-3		
Tanner Pubertal Stages in Male		
1	Preadolescent	Preadolescent—no pubic hair
2	Scrotum and testes enlarge, change in scrotal skin texture	Sparse, long, downy pubic hair, chiefly at base of penis
3	Growth of penis in length and further growth of testes and scrotum	Hair darker and coarser
4	Growth of penis in length and breadth, darkening of scrotal skin	Adult-type hair, but area covered is less than that in adult
5	Adult-sized genitalia	Adult hair texture and quantity; hair is distributed in diamond-shaped escutcheon with hair extending up linea alba

Data from Marshall WA, Tanner JM: *Arch Dis Child* 45:13, 1970.

forming the occluding junctions and performing other hormonally dependent functions.

Puberty is associated with numerous primary and secondary sexual changes, including growth and onset of function of the prostate and seminal vesicles; increased growth of the penis; increased muscle mass; thickening of vocal cords; appearance of pubic, facial, and body hair; and development of libido (see Figure 8-17) (Table 8-3). Many of these changes are dependent on the conversion of testosterone to DHT. The pubertal growth spurt in males requires several hormones, including growth hormone, insulin-like growth factor-1, testosterone, and estrogen.

There is no distinct **andropause** in men. As men age, however, gonadal sensitivity to LH decreases and androgen production drops (see Figure 8-15). As this occurs, serum LH and FSH levels rise. Although sperm production typically begins to decline after age 50 years, many men can maintain reproductive function and spermatogenesis throughout life. Figure 8-15 shows how plasma testosterone levels change throughout the life span.

Disorders Involving the Male Reproductive System

Klinefelter Syndrome Men with an extra X chromosome have the genetic disorder called **Klinefelter syndrome (seminiferous tubular dysgenesis)**. Although there are multiple permutations of the disorder, the most common form results in a 47,XXY karyotype. Affected persons are phenotypically male because of

the presence of the Y chromosome, but they typically have small testes and decreased germ cells (Figure 8-18). The testosterone levels are low to normal, and estradiol and gonadotropin levels are high. An elevated estradiol-to-testosterone ratio can lead to moderate feminization, including the potential for limited

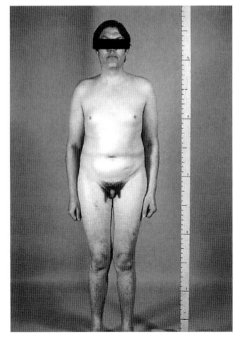

FIGURE 8-18 ■ Klinefelter syndrome in a young man. Limited gynecomastia is present, and body shape is somewhat feminine. (*From Besser GM, Thorner MO: Clinical endocrinology ed 2, London, 1994, Mosby-Wolfe.*)

gynecomastia (inappropriate development of breasts). Patients with this disorder do not have normal spermatogenesis, and FSH levels are high because of abnormal Sertoli cell function.

Androgen Insensitivity Syndrome **Androgen insensitivity syndrome (AIS)** results from a hereditary defect of the X chromosome gene controlling androgen receptor (AR) expression. Because the defect can range from partial to complete inability of the AR to respond to androgens, the degree of feminization of AIS is variable. Because the karyotype is 46,XY, the gonad develops into the testis, which produces testosterone and MIS in utero. The mesonephric (wolffian) duct does not develop into male structures, however, because androgen action is deficient, and MIS causes the müllerian duct to regress. Consequently, there are no functional internal genitalia.

The external genitalia typically develop as female, and the phenotype is female (Figure 8-19). In severe AIS, the affected person has labia, a clitoris, and a short vagina. Pubic and axillary hair is absent or sparse because the development of sexual hair is androgen dependent. Menstruation does not occur (see Chapter 9), and serum androgen levels are high or normal. When androgen production rises at puberty, estradiol production increases, both from the testes and from peripheral aromatization of androgens. LH levels remain elevated throughout adulthood, because testosterone and DHT cannot exert negative feedback on the pituitary and hypothalamus because of a defective AR. The increase leads to dividing, hypertrophic Leydig cells that produce enhanced amounts of androstenedione, testosterone, and estradiol-17β. The androgens are peripherally converted to estrogens, which feminize the individual in a manner unopposed by androgenic actions. This phenotype that is derived from hyperstimulated Leydig cells secreting steroids that are converted into estrogens and lead to feminization is called **testicular feminization**. The overall condition generally is referred to as **male pseudohermaphroditism**. The designator *male* is appropriate because the genotype of the affected person is XY. The term *pseudohermaphroditism* refers to the presence of an incomplete mix of external genitalia, which are feminine in this case, and internal genitalia, which is a male gonad in this case. Note that the testes typically remain in

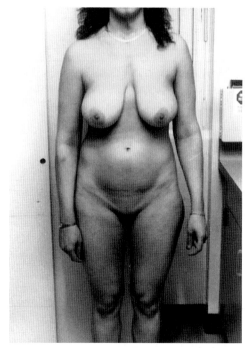

FIGURE 8-19 ■ A 46,XY patient with complete androgen insensitivity and female phenotype. Full breast development and female body form (e.g., widened pelvis) constitute evidence of testicular feminization. *(From Quigley CA, et al: Endocr Rev 16:271, 1995.)*

the abdomen, because androgens are required for testicular descent. Because of gonadotropic hyperstimulation, the gonads represent a probable site for cancerous growth and are surgically removed as a precaution.

5α-Reductase 2 Deficiency A **5α-reductase 2–deficiency** results in decreased DHT formation. Affected persons typically have normal internal genitalia but incompletely masculinized external genitalia (i.e., **ambiguous genitalia**). They often are mistaken for females at birth. The testosterone production is normal, and at puberty, when testosterone production occurs, some masculinization of the external genitalia may occur. As discussed previously, 5α-reductase 1 activity appears at puberty, which may generate enough DHT to induce the pubertal changes.

Kallmann Syndrome **Kallmann syndrome** is primary isolated gonadotropin deficiency. This genetic disorder is often associated with anosmia, or the loss of smell. It is due to the inability of GnRH neurons to properly migrate to the mediobasal hypothalamus from the nasal placode (see Chapter 5). People affected with this disorder have undescended testes (cryptorchism). Although there is normal embryonic development of the mesonephric (wolffian) duct–derived structures, penis development is deficient and microphallus results. These effects probably result from the fact that early fetal development of the internal genitalia is controlled by testicular androgens that are regulated by placental hCG (see Chapter 10), rather than fetal LH. The inability of the fetus to secrete normal quantities of LH has an impact on testicular function later in development, when androgens regulate growth of the external genitalia. The severity of the impairment of LH secretion is variable, as is the severity of the reproductive problems associated with the disorder.

SUMMARY

1. The human reproductive system is composed of a pair of gonads (testes or ovaries) and a reproductive tract. The gonads have two major functions: to produce hormones (endocrine function) and to produce gametes (exocrine function). The gametogenic function of the gonads and the physiology of the reproductive tract are critically dependent on the endocrine function of the gonads.

2. Seminiferous tubules (the intratubular compartment) contain Sertoli cells and developing sperm. Sertoli cells have a "nursing" function, providing the proper microenvironment for sperm development. Sertoli cells also have an important exocrine function, producing fluid and androgen-binding protein. In addition, Sertoli cells have an endocrine function, producing müllerian-inhibiting substance (i.e., anti-müllerian hormone) and inhibin. Sertoli cells express the androgen receptor and the FSH receptor.

3. Spermatogenesis involves mitosis and meiosis. The final product is haploid spermatozoa. Normal spermatogenesis is dependent on FSH and high intratesticular levels of testosterone. However, sperm cells do *not* express the androgen receptor or the FSH receptor and are completely dependent on Sertoli cells for their development.

4. Leydig cells reside in the peritubular compartment. Leydig cells express the LH receptor and produce testosterone, as well as small amounts of DHT and estradiol-17β.

5. Testosterone can be converted peripherally to DHT (e.g., in the prostate gland) or estradiol-17β (e.g., in adipose tissue). Testosterone and DHT regulate secondary sex characteristics and are required for the normal development, growth, and function of the male reproductive tract. Estrogen is required for normal bone growth and epiphyseal plate closure in men, and for modulation of lipoprotein profile (lowered VLDL and LDL, increased HDL).

6. The endocrine function is regulated within a hypothalamus-pituitary-testis axis. GnRH is produced by hypothalamic neurons and stimulates LH and FSH production by pituitary gonadotropes. Circulating levels of testosterone, and to some extent DHT and estradiol-17β, exert a negative feedback at both the pituitary and the hypothalamus.

7. The male reproductive tract includes the epididymis, the vas deferens, the ejaculatory duct, and the male urethra. The male tract also includes accessory sex glands, the seminal vesicles, and the prostate gland. The secretions of these glands produce most of the volume of semen. Semen serves to provide bulk to sperm, maintain an alkaline environment for sperm, provide nutrients to sperm, prevent sperm capacitation, and inhibit sperm motility in the male reproductive tract. Emission and ejaculation are achieved through primarily sympathetic stimulation of the muscularis of the male tract and somatic stimulation of pelvic muscles.

8. The male tract also includes a copulatory organ, the penis. Erection of the penis is required for internal insemination of the female tract. Erection of the penis is a neurovascular process, involving parasympathetic stimulation of erectile tissue arterioles leading to vasodilation and engorgement of

the cavernous spaces. Multiple factors can lead to erectile dysfunction.

9. Development of the gonad is genetically determined. The presence of a Y chromosome allows for the expression of the *SRY* gene, which induces somatic cells to develop into Sertoli cells at week 6. Leydig cells develop by week 8. If the *SRY* gene is not expressed, the gonad will develop later into an ovary.

10. Development of the fetal reproductive system is hormonally regulated. The original fetal reproductive system is multipotential and contains both müllerian and wolffian ducts. If testes are present and produce müllerian-inhibiting substance (MIS) at approximately 8 weeks of gestation, the müllerian ducts regress. If testosterone is produced, the wolffian ducts develop into the epididymis, vas deferens, seminal vesicles, and ejaculatory ducts. If neither MIS nor testosterone is present, the wolffian ducts regress and the müllerian ducts develop into the fallopian tubes, uterus, cervix, and upper one third of the vagina.

11. At approximately 9 to 12 weeks of gestation, the external genitalia develop. If dihydrotestosterone (DHT) is present, a penis and scrotum develop. DHT also regulates the development of the prostate. If DHT is absent, labia, clitoris, and lower two thirds of the vagina develop.

12. At puberty, the gonadostat is "reset" so that the sensitivity to negative feedback inhibition of testosterone on GnRH and LH secretion decreases. Also, a CNS-derived inhibition of the GnRH neurons diminishes. LH and FSH secretion rises, which stimulates testicular growth and testosterone production. Sertoli cells divide and mature, and spermatogenesis begins. Spermatogonia do not enter meiosis until puberty.

13. Klinefelter syndrome (gonadal dysgenesis) results when men have an extra X chromosome.

14. Androgen insensitivity syndrome results from a hereditary defect in the gene controlling androgen receptor expression. As a result of diminished feedback, LH levels are elevated, as are testosterone levels. More testis-derived testosterone is converted to estrogens, resulting in a female phenotype (enhanced breast development, female pelvis). This process is called testicular feminization. The overall condition (high estrogen levels in the absence of androgen effects) gives rise to male pseudohermaphroditism.

15. Deficiency of 5α-reductase can result in ambiguous genitalia at birth.

16. Kallmann syndrome is an example of tertiary hypogonadism, due to the inability of GnRH neuronal precursors to migrate from the nasal placode to the mediobasal hypothalamus during development. This genetic disorder is associated with loss of the sense of smell and cryptorchism.

KEY WORDS AND CONCEPTS

- Gonad
- Reproductive tract
- Testes
- Ovaries
- Endocrine function
- Hypothalamus-pituitary-gonadal axis
- Gametogenic
- Continuous, lifelong gametogenesis
- Internal insemination
- High density of sperm
- Spermatogenesis
- Scrotum
- Lobules
- Seminiferous tubules
- Rete testis
- Efferent ductules
- Epididymis—head, body, and tail
- Vas (ductus) deferens
- Spermatozoa
- Seminiferous epithelium
- Interstitial cells of Leydig
- Testosterone
- Spermatogenesis
- Sertoli cell
- Mitosis
- Meiosis
- Spermatogonia
- Spermatocytogenesis
- Incomplete cytokinesis
- Primary spermatocytes
- Secondary spermatocytes
- Spermatids
- Spermiogenesis

- Spermatozoon
- Spermiation
- Sertoli-Sertoli cell occluding junctions
- Basal compartment
- Adluminal compartment
- Blood-testis barrier
- Androgen receptor
- FSH receptor
- Androgen-binding protein (ABP)
- Sex hormone–binding globulin (SHBG)
- Residual bodies
- Anti-müllerian hormone (AMH)
- Müllerian-inhibiting substance (MIS)
- Inhibin
- Leydig cell
- Low-density lipoprotein receptors (LDL receptors)
- High-density lipoprotein receptors (HDL receptors)
- Scavenger receptor-BI (SR-BI)
- Cholesterol ester hydrolase
- Steroidogenic acute regulatory protein (StAR)
- CYP11A1
- 3β-HSD
- CYP17
- 17-hydroxylase activity
- 17,20-lyase activity
- Δ4 pathway
- 17β-hydroxysteroid dehydrogenase (17β-HSD type 3)
- Androstenedione
- Male pseudohermaphroditism
- CYP19 (aromatase)
- Estradiol-17β
- Estrogen receptor (ER)
- Non-aromatizable androgen
- 5α-dihydrotestosterone (DHT)
- 5α-reductase
- Selective 5α-reductase 2 inhibitors
- Androgen-response element (ARE)
- Urinary 17-ketosteroids
- Conjugated steroids
- Gonadotropin-releasing hormone (GnRH) neurons
- Pituitary gonadotropes
- Luteinizing hormone (LH)
- Follicle-stimulating hormone (FSH)
- Pituitary glycoprotein hormones
- LH receptor
- Inhibin A
- Inhibin B
- Male oral contraceptive
- Ejaculatory duct
- Contiguous lumen
- Distal urinary tract
- Male urethra
- Decapacitation
- Blood-epididymis barrier
- Emission
- Ejaculation
- Seminal vesicles
- Prostate gland
- Semen
- Fructose
- Semenogelins
- Citrate
- Zinc
- Spermine
- Acid phosphatase
- Prostate-specific antigen (PSA)
- Bulbourethral glands
- Erection
- Penis
- Corpora cavernosa
- Corpus spongiosum
- Erectile tissue
- Cavernous vascular spaces
- Flaccid state
- Erectile dysfunction (ED)
- Selective cGMP phosphodiesterase inhibitors
- Autosomes
- Sex chromosomes
- SRY (sex-determining region Y)
- Mesonephric (wolffian) ducts
- Paramesonephric (müllerian) ducts
- Placental human chorionic gonadotropin (hCG)
- Puberty
- Gonadostat
- Andropause
- Klinefelter syndrome
- Seminiferous tubular dysgenesis
- Gynecomastia

- Androgen insensitivity syndrome (AIS)
- Testicular feminization
- 5α-reductase 2–deficiency
- Ambiguous genitalia
- Kallmann syndrome

SELF-STUDY PROBLEMS

1. What is the relationship of Sertoli cells to the basal and adluminal compartments of the seminiferous tubules?

2. Explain how the loss of 17β-hydroxysteroid dehydrogenase (type 3) would affect the following: spermatogenesis, external genitalia, breast development.

3. Why does a congenital 5α-reductase deficiency have the potential to result in a pseudohermaphroditic condition when internal genitalia are male and external genitalia appear female?

4. How does abuse of androgens cause low sperm count?

5. Name one event that occurs in developing sperm cells during the following: spermatocytogenesis, spermiogenesis, passage through the epididymis, emission.

BIBLIOGRAPHY

Bhasin S, Berman J, Berman L, Hellstrom WJG: Sexual dysfunction in men and women. In Larsen PR, Kronenberg HM, Melmed S, Polonsky K, editors: *Williams textbook of endocrinology*, ed 10, Philadelphia, 2003, Saunders, pp 771-793.

Dehm, SM, Tindall, DJ: Regulation of androgen receptor signaling in prostate cancer, *Expert Rev Anticancer Ther* 5:63-74, 2005.

Ebling FJ: The neuroendocrine timing of puberty, *Reproduction* 129:675-683, 2005.

Griffin JE, Wilson JD: Disorders of the testes and male reproductive tract. In Larsen PR, Kronenberg HM, Melmed S, Polonsky K, editors: *Williams textbook of endocrinology*, ed 10, Philadelphia, 2003, Saunders, pp 709-769.

Mruk DD, Cheng CY: Sertoli-Sertoli and Sertoli-germ cell interactions and their significance in germ cell movement in the seminiferous epithelium during spermatogenesis, *Endocr Rev* 25:747-806, 2004.

Poletti A, Negri-Cesi P, Martini L: Reflections on the diseases linked to mutations of the androgen receptor, *Endocrine* 28:243-262, 2005.

Rochira V, Balestrieri A, Madeo B et al: Congenital estrogen deficiency in men: a new syndrome with different phenotypes; clinical and therapeutic implications in men, *Mol Cell Endocrinol* 193:19-28, 2002.

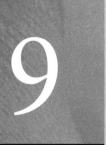

9 THE FEMALE REPRODUCTIVE SYSTEM

OBJECTIVES

1. Describe the anatomy and histology of the ovary and the development of the ovarian follicle.

2. Describe the steroidogenic pathways in the ovarian follicle and the functions of the ovarian steroids, estradiol-17β and progesterone.

3. Discuss the hypothalamus-pituitary-ovarian axis in the context of the monthly menstrual cycle.

4. Discuss the changes in the physiology of the female reproductive tract throughout the menstrual cycle.

5. Describe the anatomy and function of the female external genitalia during the female sexual response.

6. Discuss pathophysiologic conditions of the female reproductive system, including Turner syndrome and polycystic ovarian syndrome.

The physiology of pregnancy and the development and functions of the placenta and mammary glands are discussed in Chapter 10.

The female reproductive system is composed of the gonads, called ovaries, and the female reproductive tract. Like the male gonads, the ovaries perform an **endocrine function** and a **gametogenic function.** The endocrine function is regulated within a hypothalamic-pituitary-ovarian axis, and ovarian hormones are absolutely necessary for the health and normal function of the female tract. The female reproductive system differs from the male system in several important general aspects, including the following (Box 9-1):

1. Anatomically, the ovaries reside within the abdominal cavity, but are not contiguous with the reproductive tract. From a clinical standpoint, this means that cells (e.g., embryo, ovarian cancer, endometrial tissue) can gain access to the abdominal cavity.

2. Whereas the gametogenic function of the ovary is continuous, the release of gametes (as **secondary** oocytes, referred to as **eggs**) through the process of **ovulation** is cyclic. In humans, the ovary ovulates about one egg per month as part of the monthly **human menstrual cycle.** Unlike in the male, meiotic division of female gametes has starts and stops, and meiotic maturation from an **oogonium** to a mature, haploid **ovum** may take decades. There is also a finite number of gametes within the ovary at birth, which becomes depleted by about the fifth decade of life, at the time of **menopause.** From a clinical standpoint, this means that women are more fertile and produce healthier gametes earlier in life. It also means that there is an increasingly large population of postmenopausal women in the Western world who are at risk for various conditions that arise after ovarian function ceases

3. The first half of the ovarian cycle is called the **follicular phase.** The **ovarian follicle** refers to a primary oocyte surrounded by somatic, endocrine

---

BOX 9-1

MAJOR DIFFERENCES BETWEEN MALE AND FEMALE REPRODUCTIVE SYSTEMS

Male Reproductive System	Female Reproductive System
Gonads (testes) reside outside of abdominal cavity, in scrotum	Gonads (ovaries) reside within abdominal cavity
Gonad is contiguous with reproductive tract	Gonad is not contiguous with reproductive tract
Release of gametes (sperm) from gonads is continuous	Release of gamete (egg) from gonads occurs once per month
Gametic reserve is replenished throughout life	Gametic reserve is finite and exhausted by menopause
Testosterone exerts negative feedback on secretion of pituitary LH and FSH	Estrogen exerts both negative and positive feedback on secretion of pituitary LH and FSH
Male tract serves only male gamete transport and maturation	Female tract serves male and female gamete transport and maturation, fertilization, placentation, gestation, and delivery
Activity of male tract does not show rhythm	Activity of female tract is based on the monthly menstrual cycle, or on the length of a pregnancy (normally about 9 months)
Testosterone is always the primary gonadal steroid	Estrogen is the primary gonadal steroid in the first half of the monthly cycle, and progesterone in the second half
The male reproductive system does not prepare for newborn	The female reproductive system prepares for newborn with breast development and milk production and is involved in breast feeding of the newborn

---

cells (see later). Ovulation is induced by a **midcycle gonadotropin** (primarily luteinizing hormone [LH]) **surge**. Follicular cells that remain in the ovary after ovulation develop into the **corpus luteum**, and the second half of the ovarian cycle is called the **luteal phase**. During the follicular phase, a dominant follicle is selected and grows to a large preovulatory follicle. Unlike the testis, which secretes testosterone fairly constantly, the ovary produces the female sex steroids estradiol-17β and progesterone in a cyclic manner during the menstrual cycle. Normally, only the dominant follicle performs a significant steroidogenic function. The dominant follicle secretes increasing amounts of estrogen during the follicular phase. The corpus luteum secretes large amounts of progesterone along with estrogen.

4. The ovary functions in the context of a **hypothalamic-pituitary-ovarian axis**. At low levels, estrogen exerts negative feedback on LH and follicle-stimulating hormone (FSH) production. Progesterone also inhibits LH and FSH secretion, and inhibin (also produced by the follicle and corpus luteum) selectively inhibits FSH secretion. However, unlike the male axis, the female axis also displays a switch from **negative feedback by low levels of estrogen** to **positive feedback by high levels of estrogen** maintained for several days. It is this positive feedback that induces the midcycle LH surge, which in turn induces ovulation. This remarkable interplay among the ovary, pituitary, and hypothalamus drives the human menstrual cycle (see later). However, this elegant multicomponent, time-dependent process can be perturbed by numerous factors, leading to **infertility** and endocrine imbalances.

5. Unlike the male tract, the **female reproductive tract** undergoes cyclic changes in response to the changing levels of ovarian steroids. The most obvious change occurs in the lining of the uterus, called the **uterine endometrium**. Estrogen production during the follicular phase of the ovary drives the **proliferative phase** of the uterus, during which

time the endometrium grows in thickness. Progesterone production during the luteal phase of the ovary drives the **secretory phase** of the uterus, during which time the uterus prepares for an implanting embryo. If fertilization and implantation do not occur, the corpus luteum undergoes programmed cell death (apoptosis) by day 28 of the cycle. The withdrawal of ovarian progesterone causes the collapse of the endometrium and its subsequent loss through the process of **menstruation**, which occurs during the first few days at the beginning of the next cycle (i.e., early follicular phase of the ovary). Unlike the male tract, the female reproductive tract must support **fertilization, implantation, placentation**, and **parturition**. This means that the physiology of women has to adapt to both monthly and longer-term gestational and postgestational changes. From a clinical standpoint, numerous complications can arise from the demands of this ever-changing physiology.

6. Neonatal and infant nutrition is provided naturally by the female. This requires the development and function of the **mammary glands**, which can be considered accessory glands to the female reproductive system.

ANATOMY AND HISTOLOGY OF THE OVARY

The ovary is located within a fold of peritoneum called the **broad ligament**, usually close to the lateral wall of the pelvic cavity (Figure 9-1). The ovary extends into the peritoneal cavity, so that ovulated eggs briefly reside within the peritoneal cavity before they are captured by the oviducts. Nerves and blood vessels enter and exit the ovary at both its lateral and medial poles.

The ovary can be roughly divided into an outer cortex and an inner medulla (Figure 9-2). The neurovascular elements run into the medulla of the ovary. The cortex of the ovary is composed of a densely cellular stroma. Within this stroma reside the **ovarian follicles**, which contain a primary oocyte surrounded by follicle cells (see later). The cortex is covered by a connective tissue capsule, called the tunica albuginea, and a layer of simple epithelium, called **ovarian surface epithelial cells**. There are no ducts emerging from the ovary to convey its gametes to the reproductive tract. Thus, the process of ovulation involves an inflammatory event that erodes the wall of the ovary. After ovulation, the ovarian surface epithelial cells rapidly divide to repair the wall. It is this highly mitogenic population of cells, the ovarian surface epithelial

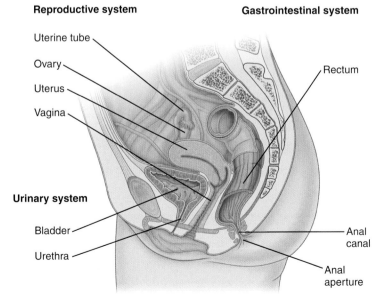

Reproductive system

Uterine tube
Ovary
Uterus
Vagina

Gastrointestinal system

Rectum

Urinary system

Bladder
Urethra

Anal canal

Anal aperture

FIGURE 9-1 ■ Anatomy of the female pelvis—midsagittal section. *(From Drake RL, Vogl W, Mitchell AWM: Gray's anatomy for students, Philadelphia, 2005, Churchill Livingstone.)*

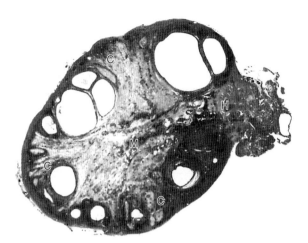

FIGURE 9-2 ■ Histologic features of the ovary. Micrograph of the ovary shows the hilum (H), medulla (M), and cortex (C). Follicular formation and maturation occur in the cortex and are responsible for the cystic spaces seen here. *(From Stevens A, Lowe J: Human histology, ed 3, Philadelphia, 2005, Elsevier/Mosby.)*

cells, which give rise to more than 80% of cases of **ovarian cancer**.

GROWTH, DEVELOPMENT, AND FUNCTION OF THE OVARIAN FOLLICLE

The ovarian follicle is the functional unit of the ovary, performing both gametogenic and endocrine functions. A histologic section of the ovary from a premenopausal cycling woman contains follicular structures at many different points of their development. The life history of a follicle can be divided into the following stages:

1. Resting primordial follicle
2. Growing preantral (primary and secondary) follicle
3. Growing antral (tertiary) follicle
4. Dominant (preovulatory, graafian) follicle
5. Dominant follicle within the periovulatory period
6. Corpus luteum (of menstruation or of pregnancy)
7. Atretic follicles

In this section, follicular biology is discussed in terms of (1) the growth and structure of the follicle, (2) the state of the gamete, and (3) the endocrine function of the follicle cells.

Resting Primordial Follicle

Growth and Structure Resting primordial follicles represent the earliest and simplest follicular structure in the ovary. Primordial follicles appear during midgestation through the interaction of gametes and somatic cells. Primordial germ cells that have migrated to the gonad continue to divide mitotically as oogonia until the fifth month of gestation in humans. At this point, the approximately 7 million oogonia enter the process of meiosis, thereby becoming **primary oocytes**.

During this time, the primary oocytes become surrounded by a simple epithelium of somatic **follicle cells**, thereby creating primordial follicles (Figure 9-3).

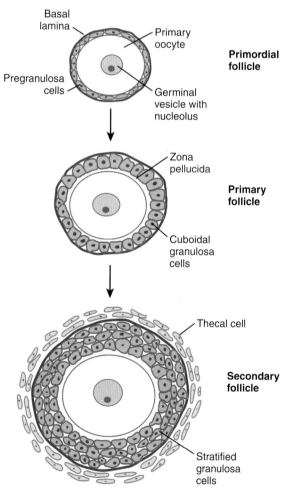

FIGURE 9-3 ■ Early follicular development from a primordial follicle to a secondary, preantral follicle.

The follicle cells (also called **pregranulosa cells**) establish **gap junctions** with each other and the oocyte. The follicle cells themselves represent a true avascular epithelium, surrounded by a basal lamina. As in Sertoli cell–sperm interactions, the granulosa cells remain intimately attached to the oocyte throughout its development. Granulosa cells provide nutrients such as amino acids, nucleic acids, and pyruvate to support oocyte maturation.

Primordial follicles represent the **ovarian reserve** of follicles (Figure 9-4). This is reduced from a starting number of about 7 million to less than 300,000 follicles at reproductive maturity. Of these, a woman will ovulate about 450 between menarche (first menstrual cycle) and menopause (cessation of menstrual cycles). At menopause, less than 1000 primordial follicles are left in the ovary. Primordial follicles are lost primarily from death due to **follicular atresia** (see later). A small subset of primordial follicles, however, will enter follicular growth in waves. Because the ovarian follicular reserve represents a fixed, finite number, the rate at which resting primordial follicles die or begin to develop will determine the reproductive life span of a woman. The determination of the age at menopause has a strong genetic component but also is influenced by environmental factors. For example, cigarette smoking significantly depletes the ovarian reserve. An overly rapid rate of atresia or development also will deplete the reserve, giving rise to **premature ovarian failure**.

Pituitary gonadotropins are likely to maintain a normal ovarian reserve by promoting the general health of the ovary. However, the rate at which resting primordial follicles entering the growth process appears to be independent of pituitary gonadotropins. There is evidence in mice that follicle cells stimulate oocyte growth through the release of the peptide kit ligand, which binds to its tyrosine kinase receptor, **c-Kit**, on the oocyte membrane. Reciprocal regulation of granulosa cell growth by the oocyte also probably occurs, and transforming growth factor-β (TGF-β)–related factors, such as **growth differentiation factor-9 (GDF-9)** and **bone morphogenetic protein-15 (BMP-15)**, play a role in this. Additional evidence indicates that factors from growing follicles provide restraint on the development of too many primordial follicles. One such factor appears to be **anti-müllerian hormone (AMH)**. AMH-knockout mice deplete their ovarian reserve more rapidly than do wild-type mice, as a result of a high rate of follicular development. In summary, whether a resting follicle enters the early growth phase is dependent primarily on intraovarian paracrine factors that are produced by both the follicle cells and oocytes.

The Gamete As mentioned previously, the gamete in primordial follicles is derived from oogonia that have entered the first meiotic division and are now called primary oocytes. These primary oocytes progress through most of prophase of the first meiotic division (termed prophase I) over a 2-week period and then arrest in the **diplotene** stage. This stage is characterized by decondensation of chromatin, which supports transcription needed for oocyte maturation. Meiotic arrest at this stage, which may last for up to 50 years, appears to be due to "maturational incompetence," or the lack of necessary cell cycle proteins to support the completion of meiosis. The nucleus of the oocyte, called the **germinal vesicle**, remains intact at this stage.

Endocrine Function Although primordial follicles release paracrine factors such as Kit ligand, they do not produce ovarian hormones.

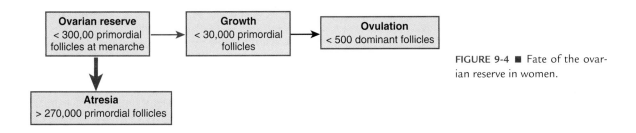

FIGURE 9-4 ■ Fate of the ovarian reserve in women.

Growing Preantral Follicles

Growth and Structure The first stage of follicular growth is **preantral**, which refers to development that occurs *before* the formation of a fluid-filled **antral cavity**. One of the first visible signs of follicle growth is the appearance of cuboidal granulosa cells. At this point, the follicle is referred to as a **primary follicle** (see Figure 9-3). As granulosa cells proliferate, they form a multilayered (i.e., stratified) epithelium around the oocyte. At this stage, the follicle is referred to as a **secondary follicle** (see Figure 9-3).

Once a secondary follicle acquires three to six layers of granulosa cells, it secretes paracrine factors that induce nearby stromal cells to differentiate into epithelioid **thecal cells**. Thecal cells form a flattened layer of cells around the follicle. Once a thecal layer forms, the follicle is referred to as a **mature preantral follicle** (see Figure 9-3). In humans, it takes several months for a primary follicle to reach the mature preantral stage.

Follicular development is associated with an inward movement of the follicle from the outer cortex to the inner cortex, closer to the vasculature of the ovarian medulla. Follicles release angiogenic factors that induce the development of one or two arterioles, which generate a vascular wreath around the follicle.

The Gamete During the preantral stage, the oocyte begins to grow and produce cellular and secreted proteins. The oocyte initiates secretion of extracellular matrix glycoproteins, called **ZP1**, **ZP2**, and **ZP3**, that form the **zona pellucida** (see Figure 9-3). The zona pellucida ultimately increases to a thickness of 13 µm in humans and provides a species-specific binding site for sperm during fertilization (see Chapter 10). Of importance, granulosa cells and the oocyte project cellular extensions through the zona pellucida and maintain gap junctional contacts. The oocyte also continues to secrete paracrine factors (probably members of the TGF-β family) that regulate follicle cell growth and differentiation.

Endocrine Function The granulosa cells express the **FSH receptor** during this period but are dependent primarily on factors from the oocyte to grow. They do not produce ovarian hormones at this early stage of follicular development.

The newly acquired thecal cells are analogous to testicular Leydig cells (see Chapter 8), in that they reside outside of the epithelial "nurse cells," express the **LH receptor**, and produce **androgens**. The main difference between Leydig cells and thecal cells is that thecal cells do not express high levels of a 17β-hydroxysteroid dehydrogenase (17β-HSD). Thus, the major product of the thecal cells is **androstenedione**, as opposed to testosterone. Androstenedione production at this stage is minimal.

Growing Antral Follicles

Growth and Structure Mature preantral follicles develop into **early antral follicles** (Figure 9-5) over a period of about 25 days, growing from a diameter of approximately 0.1 to 0.2 mm. Once the granulosa epithelium increases to six or seven layers, fluid-filled spaces appear between cells and coalesce into the **antrum**. Over a period of about 45 days, this wave of small antral follicles will continue to grow to large, recruitable antral follicles that are 2 to 5 mm in diameter. This period of growth is characterized by about a 100-fold increase in granulosa cells (from about 10,000 to 1,000,000 cells). It also is characterized by swelling of the antral cavity, which increasingly divides the granulosa cells into two discrete populations (Figures 9-5 and 9-6):

- The **mural granulosa cells** (also called **stratum granulosum**) are those that form the outer wall of the follicle. The basal layer is adhered to the basal lamina, and in close proximity to the outerlying thecal layers. Mural granulosa cells become highly steroidogenic, and remain in the ovary after ovulation to differentiate into the corpus luteum.
- The **cumulus cells** are the inner cells that surround the oocyte (they are also referred to as the **cumulus oophorus**). The innermost layer (relative to the oocyte) of cumulus cells maintain gap and adhesion junctions with the oocyte. Cumulus cells are released with the oocyte (collectively referred to as the **cumulus-oocyte complex**) during the process of ovulation. Cumulus cells are crucial for the ability of the fimbriated end of the oviduct to "capture" and move the oocyte by a ciliary transport mechanism along the length of the oviduct to the site of fertilization.

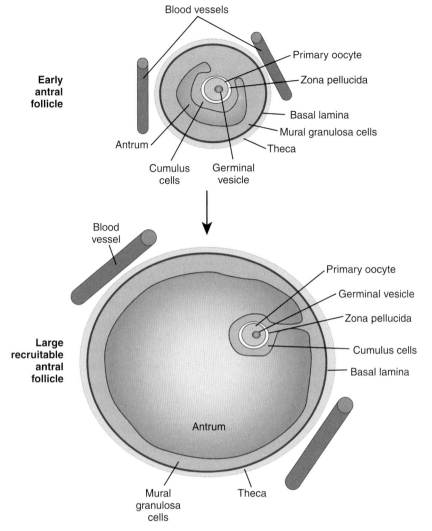

Early antral follicles are dependent on pituitary FSH for normal growth. Large antral follicles become highly dependent on pituitary FSH for their growth and sustained viability. As discussed later (under "Dominant Follicle"), 2- to 5-mm follicles are **recruited** to enter a rapid growth phase by a transient increase in FSH that occurs toward the end of a previous menstrual cycle.

The Gamete The oocyte grows rapidly in the early stages of antral follicles—growth then slows in larger follicles. During the antral stage, the oocyte synthesizes sufficient amounts of cell cycle components so that it becomes competent to complete meiosis I at ovulation (note that the human egg arrests after ovulation at a second point, metaphase II, until it is fertilized by sperm). Thus, in early primary and secondary follicles, the oocyte fails to complete meiosis I because of a dearth of specific meiosis-associated proteins (i.e., they are incompetent to complete meiosis I). Larger antral follicles, however, gain **meiotic competence** but still maintain **meiotic arrest** until the midcycle LH surge. Meiotic arrest is achieved by the maintenance of elevated cyclic adenosine monophosphate (cAMP)

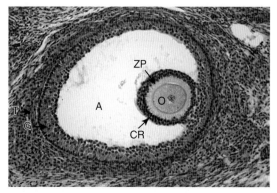

FIGURE 9-6 ■ Histologic features of ovarian graafian follicle. Ovum (O) is surrounded by zona pellucida (ZP). As a result of shrinkage artifacts, the zona pellucida appears larger than normal. Corona radiata (CR) is indicated, as is large antrum (A). G, glomerulosa cell; T, thecal cells.

levels in the mature oocyte. The oocyte expresses a constitutively active (i.e., active without a ligand) G protein–coupled receptor, called **GPR3**, that maintains high cAMP levels (Figure 9-7).

Endocrine Function Thecal cells of large antral follicles produce significant amounts of androstenedione and testosterone. Androgens are converted to estradiol-17β by the granulosa cells (see later). At this stage, however, FSH stimulates proliferation of granulosa cells and induces the expression of CYP19 (aromatase) required for estrogen synthesis. Additionally, the

mural granulosa cells of the large antral follicles produce increasing amounts of **inhibin B** during the early follicular phase. Low levels of estrogen and inhibin exert a negative feedback effect on FSH secretion, thereby contributing to the selection of the follicle with the most FSH-responsive cells.

Dominant Follicle

Growth and Structure At the end of a previous menstrual cycle, a crop of large (2- to 5-mm) antral follicles (see Figure 9-4) are **recruited** to begin rapid, gonadotropin-dependent development. The total number of recruited follicles in both ovaries can be as high as 20 in a younger woman (less than 33 years of age), but rapidly declines at older ages. The number of recruited follicles is reduced to the **ovulatory quota** (which is *one* in humans) by the process of **selection**. As FSH levels decline, the rapidly growing follicles progressively undergo atresia, until one follicle is left. Generally, the largest follicle with the most FSH receptors of the recruited crop becomes the **dominant follicle**. Selection occurs during the early follicular phase. By midcycle, the dominant follicle becomes a large **preovulatory follicle** that is 20 mm in diameter and contains about 50 million granulosa cells by the midcycle gonadotropin surge.

The Gamete The oocyte is competent to complete meiosis I but remains arrested in the dominant follicle. Growth of the oocyte continues, but at a slower

FIGURE 9-7 ■ Phases of oocyte development.

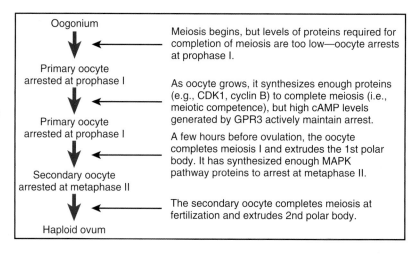

Oogonium	Meiosis begins, but levels of proteins required for completion of meiosis are too low—oocyte arrests at prophase I.
Primary oocyte arrested at prophase I	As oocyte grows, it synthesizes enough proteins (e.g., CDK1, cyclin B) to complete meiosis (i.e., meiotic competence), but high cAMP levels generated by GPR3 actively maintain arrest.
Primary oocyte arrested at prophase I	A few hours before ovulation, the oocyte completes meiosis I and extrudes the 1st polar body. It has synthesized enough MAPK pathway proteins to arrest at metaphase II.
Secondary oocyte arrested at metaphase II	The secondary oocyte completes meiosis at fertilization and extrudes 2nd polar body.
Haploid ovum	

rate—the human oocyte reaches a diameter of about 140 μm by ovulation. The stalk by which cumulus cells are attached to the mural granulosa cells becomes increasingly attenuated.

Endocrine Function   The newly selected follicle emerges for the first time during its development as a significant steroidogenic "gland." Ovarian steroidogenesis requires both theca and granulosa cells (Figures 9-8 and 9-9). As discussed earlier, thecal cells express **LH receptors** and produce androgens. Basal levels of LH stimulate the expression of steroidogenic enzymes, as well as the **LDL receptor** and the **HDL receptor** (**SR-B1**), in the theca. Thecal cells show robust expression of **CYP11A1 (side-chain cleavage enzyme)**, 3β-**hydroxysteroid dehydrogenase** (3β-**HSD**), and **CYP17**, with both 17-hydroxylase activity and 17,20-lyase activity. Androgens (primarily **androstenedione** but also some **testosterone**) released from the theca can diffuse into the mural granulosa cells, or can enter the vasculature surrounding the follicle.

The mural granulosa cells of the selected follicle have a high number of **FSH receptors**, and are very sensitive to FSH signaling. FSH strongly up-regulates **CYP19** (**aromatase**) gene expression and activity. CYP19 converts androstenedione to the weak estrogen, **estrone**, and converts testosterone to the potent estrogen, **estradiol-17β**. Granulosa cells express activating isoforms of **17β-hydroxysteroid dehydrogenase** (**17β-HSD**), which ultimately drives steroidogenesis toward the production of estradiol-17β. FSH also induces the expression of inhibin B during the follicular phase.

Of importance, FSH also induces the expression of LH receptors in the mural granulosa cells during the second half of the follicular phase. Thus, mural granulosa cells become responsive to both gonadotropins, allowing these cells to maintain high levels of CYP19 in the face of declining FSH levels. Acquisition of LH receptors also ensures that mural granulosa cells will respond to the LH surge (see later).

The Dominant Follicle During the Periovulatory Period

The **periovulatory period** can be defined as the time from the onset of the LH surge to the expulsion of the cumulus-oocyte complex out of the ovary (i.e., ovulation). This process lasts for 32 to 36 hours in women.

Starting at the same time, and superimposed on the process of ovulation, is a change in the steroidogenic function of the theca and mural granulosa cells. This process is called **luteinization** and culminates in the formation of a **corpus luteum** that is capable of producing large amounts of **progesterone**, along with estrogen, within a few days after ovulation. Thus, the LH surge induces the onset of complex processes during the periovulatory period that (1) completes the gametogenic function of the ovary for a given month and (2) switches the endocrine function to one that prepares the female reproductive tract for implantation and gestation.

Growth and Structure   The LH surge induces dramatic structural changes in the dominant follicle that involve its rupture, ovulation of the cumulus-oocyte complex and the biogenesis of a new structure called the corpus luteum from the remaining thecal cells and mural granulosa cells. Major structural changes occur during this transition (Figure 9-10):

1. Before ovulation, the large preovulatory follicle presses against the ovarian surface, generating a poorly vascularized bulge of the ovarian wall called the **stigma**. The LH surge induces the release of inflammatory cytokines and hydrolytic enzymes from the theca and granulosa cells. These secreted components lead to the breakdown the follicle wall, tunica albuginea and surface epithelium in the vicinity of the stigma. At the end of this process, the antral cavity becomes continuous with the peritoneal cavity.

2. The attachment of the cumulus cells to the mural granulosa cells degenerates, so that the cumulus-oocyte complex becomes free-floating within the antral cavity. Cumulus cells also respond to the LH surge by secreting hyaluronic acid and other extracellular matrix components. These enlarge the entire cumulus oocyte complex, a process called **cumulus expansion**. This enlarged cumulus-oocyte complex is more easily captured and transported by the oviduct. The expanded cumulus also makes the cumulus-oocyte complex easier for spermatozoa to find. Sperm express a **membrane hyaluronidase** that allows them to penetrate the expanded cumulus (see Chapter 10). The cumulus-oocyte complex is released through the ruptured

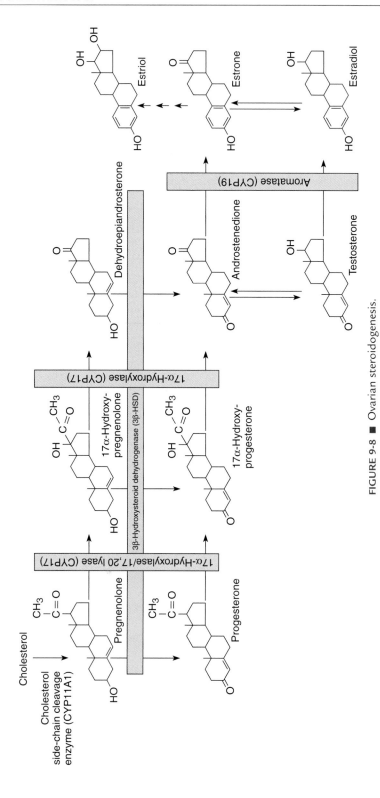

FIGURE 9-8 ■ Ovarian steroidogenesis.

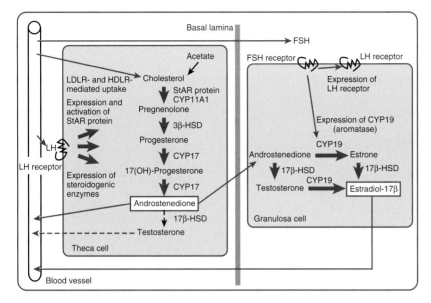

FIGURE 9-9 ■ Two-cell model of ovarian steroidogenesis. FSH, follicle-stimulating hormone; HDLR, high-density lipoprotein receptor; 3β-HSD, 3β-hydroxysteroid dehydrogenase; 17β-HSD, 17β-hydroxysteroid dehydrogenase; LDLR, low-density lipoprotein receptor; LH, luteinizing hormone; StAR protein, steroidogenic acute regulatory protein.

stigma in a slow, gentle process, indicating that the follicular fluid in the antrum is not under increased pressure. The specific forces that lead to expulsion of the cumulus-oocyte complex are unknown.

3. The basal lamina of the mural granulosa cells is broken down, so that blood vessels and outerlying theca can push into the granulosa cells. Granulosa cells secrete **angiogenic factors**, such as vascular endothelial growth factor (VEGF), angiopoietin 2, and basic fibroblast growth factor (bFGF), which significantly increase the blood supply to the new corpus luteum.

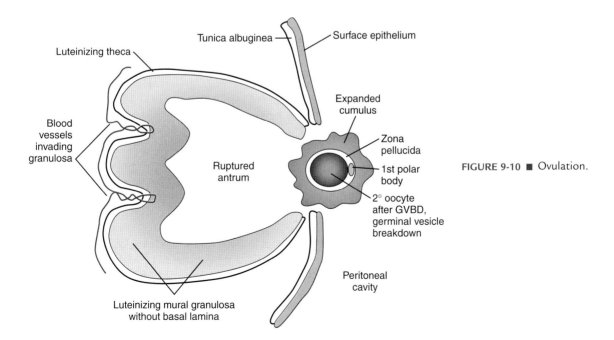

FIGURE 9-10 ■ Ovulation.

The Gamete Before ovulation, the primary oocyte is competent to complete meiosis, but is arrested in prophase I as a result of high cAMP levels (see Figure 9-7). The LH surge induces the oocyte to progress to metaphase II. The oocyte subsequently arrests at metaphase II until fertilization. LH receptors are only present on the mural granulosa cells. The LH surge induces the mural granulosa cells to release **epidermal growth factor (EGF)-related paracrine factors** (e.g., amphiregulin, epiregulin) that bind to their receptors on the cumulus cells. It is not clear how this signal to the cumulus cells is transduced into a signal to the oocyte. Release from arrest presumably involves a decrease in cAMP, although it is unknown at present whether there is a downregulation of its synthesis (i.e., a decrease in GPR3 activity) or an enhancement of cAMP degradation (i.e., an increase in phosphodiesterase activity). In any case, the decrease in cAMP and **Protein Kinase A (PKA)** activity leads indirectly to activation of a complex called **maturation-promoting factor (MPF)**. MPF is composed of a **cyclin-dependent kinase**, called **CDK1**, and **cyclin B**, which activates CDK1. Cyclin B synthesis is elevated during the periovulatory period, thereby increasing CDK1 activity. CDK1 activity is further enhanced by dephosphorylation, which is an indirect result of decreased PKA activity. The fully active MPF drives nuclear events that complete meiosis I with the extrusion of the first polar body. The secondary oocyte then arrests in **metaphase II**. This is achieved by an increase in an activity called **cytostatic factor (CSF)**. It is now known that CFS is composed of the kinase **c-Mos**, its target **mitogen-activated kinase kinase (MAPKK)**, also called **MEK 1** (Chapter 1), and **MAPK**. Thus, elevation of the MAPK signaling pathway is required for arrest at metaphase II, and fertilization leads to the rapid degradation of MAPK. It should be emphasized that our understanding of normal oocyte maturation has had a major impact on the ability to treat infertile couples through the process of **in vitro fertilization (IVF)**. Normal oocyte biology dictates the type of hormonal treatment, the timing of egg retrieval, and the meiotic stage of eggs used for fertilization (see later).

Endocrine Function Both theca and mural granulosa express LH receptors at the time of the LH surge. The LH surge induces differentiation of the granulosa cells—a process that will continue for several days after ovulation. During the periovulatory period, the LH surge induces the following shifts in the steroidogenic activity of the mural granulosa cells (Figure 9-11):

1. It transiently inhibits CYP19 expression and, consequently, estrogen production. The rapid decline in estrogen helps to turn off the positive feedback on LH secretion.
2. By inducing the breakdown of the basal lamina, the LH surge causes the direct vascularization of the granulosa cells. This makes LDL and HDL cholesterol accessible to these cells for steroidogenesis. The LH surge also increases the expression of the LDL receptor and HDL receptor (SR-BI) in granulosa cells.
3. The LH surge increases the expression of **StAR protein**, CYP11A1 (side-chain cleavage enzyme), and 3β-HSD. Because CYP17 activity, especially the 17,20-lyase function, is largely absent in granulosa cells, these cells begin to secrete progesterone, and progesterone levels will gradually increase over the next week.

The Corpus Luteum

Growth and Structure After ovulation, the remnant of the antral cavity fills with blood from damaged blood vessels in the vicinity of the stigma. This gives rise to a **corpus hemorrhagicum**. Within a few days, red blood cells and debris are removed by macrophages, and fibroblasts fill in the antral cavity with a hyaline-like extracellular matrix. In the mature **corpus luteum** (Figure 9-12), the granulosa cells, now called **granulosa lutein cells**, enlarge and become filled with lipid (cholesterol esters). The enlarged granulosa lutein cells collapse into and partially fill in the old antral cavity. Proliferation of these cells is very limited. The theca, along with blood vessels, mast cells, macrophages, leukocytes and other resident connective tissue cells, infiltrate the granulosa layer at multiple sites.

The human corpus luteum is programmed to live for 14 ± 2 days (**corpus luteum of menstruation**), unless "rescued" by the LH-like hormone **human chorionic gonadotropin (hCG)** that originates from an implanting embryo. If rescued, the **corpus luteum of pregnancy** will remain viable for as long as the pregnancy (usually about 9 months). The mechanism

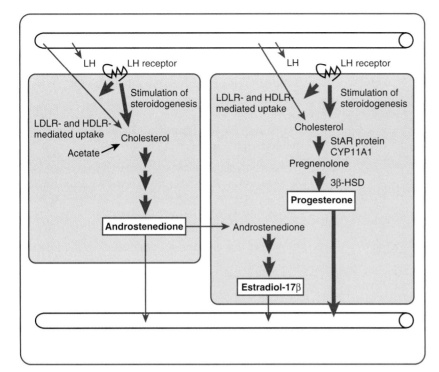

FIGURE 9-11 ■ Two-cell model of ovarian steroidogenesis during the luteal phase. HDLR, high-density lipoprotein receptor; 3β-HSD, 3β-hydroxysteroid dehydrogenase; LDLR, low-density lipoprotein receptor; LH, luteinizing hormone; StAR protein, steroidogenic acute regulatory protein.

by which the corpus luteum of menstruation regresses in 14 days is not fully understood. Regression appears to involve the release of the **prostaglandin PGF2α** from both the granulosa lutein cells and the uterus, in response to declining levels of progesterone during the second week of the luteal phase. Several paracrine factors (endothelin, monocyte chemotactic protein-1) from immune and vascular cells probably play a role in the demise and removal of granulosa lutein cells. The corpus luteum ultimately is turned into a scar-like body called the **corpus albicans**, which sinks into the medulla of the ovary and is slowly absorbed.

The Gamete The LH surge induces two parallel events, ovulation and luteinization. If ovulation occurs normally, the corpus luteum is devoid of a gamete.

Endocrine Function Progesterone production by the corpus luteum (see Figure 9-11) increases steadily from the onset of the LH surge and peaks during midluteal phase. The main purpose of this timing is to transform the uterine lining into an adhesive and supportive structure for implantation and early pregnancy. As discussed in Chapter 10, the midluteal

phase is synchronized with early embryogenesis, so that the uterus is optimally primed when a blastocyst tumbles into the uterus around day 22 of the menstrual cycle. Estrogen production transiently decreases in response to the LH surge but then rebounds and also peaks at midluteal phase.

Luteal hormonal output is absolutely dependent on basal LH levels (see Figure 9-11). In fact, progesterone output is closely correlated with the pulsatile pattern of LH release in women. Both FSH and LH are reduced to basal levels during the luteal phase by the negative feedback from progesterone and estrogen. Also, granulosa lutein cells secrete **inhibin A**, which selectively represses FSH secretion. The elevated estrogen levels at midluteal phase may be responsible for the decrease in the sensitivity of the corpus luteum to LH, so that progesterone and estrogen levels decline during the second half of the luteal phase unless an increase in circulating LH-like activity (i.e., in the form of hCG) compensates for the decreased sensitivity to LH.

The corpus luteum must generate large amounts of progesterone for an adequate number of days that are sufficient to support implantation and early pregnancy.

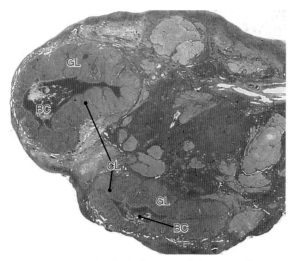

FIGURE 9-12 ■ Histologic features of the corpus luteum. Micrograph of an ovary containing two corpora lutea (CL). These arise from the co-ovulation of two dominant follicles, creating the potential for nonidentical twins. Each corpus luteum shows a central blood clot (BC) (at this stage, it would be more accurate to refer to each of them as a corpus hemorrhagicum) surrounded by a thick layer of lipid-rich granulosa lutein cells (GL). *(From Stevens A, Lowe J: Human histology, ed 3, Philadelphia, 2005, Elsevier/ Mosby.)*

Thus, the duration of the life of the corpus luteum is very regular, and a shortened luteal phase typically leads to infertility. The quality of the corpus luteum is largely dependent on the size and health of the dominant follicle from which is developed, which in turn was dependent on normal hypothalamic and pituitary stimulation during the follicular phase. Numerous factors that perturb hypothalamic and pituitary output during the follicular phase, including heavy exercise, starvation, high prolactin levels, abnormal thyroid function, and so on, can lead to **luteal phase deficiency (LPD)** and **infertility**.

The corpus luteum of other mammalian species also produces an insulin-like hormone called **relaxin**. The human corpus luteum produces very low levels of relaxin, however, and the physiologic role of circulating relaxin in humans has not been established.

Follicular Atresia

Follicular atresia refers to the demise of an ovarian follicle. During atresia, the granulosa cells and oocytes undergo **apoptosis**. The thecal cells typically persist and repopulate the cellular stroma of the ovary. The thecal cells retain LH receptors and the ability to produce androgens and collectively are referred to as the **interstitial gland** of the ovary. Follicles can undergo atresia at any time during development.

Follicular Development and the Monthly Menstrual Cycle

The first half of the monthly menstrual cycle is referred to as the **follicular phase** of the ovary and is characterized by the recruitment and growth of 15 to 20 large, antral follicles (2 to 5 mm in diameter), selection of one of these follicles as the dominant follicle, and growth of the dominant follicle until ovulation. The dominant follicle must contain a fully developed oocyte and also somatic follicle cells that secrete high levels of estrogen. It takes several months for a primordial follicle to reach the size of a large antral follicle that can be recruited (Figure 9-13). Therefore, it should be noted that much of follicular development occurs independently of the monthly menstrual cycle. The second half of the monthly menstrual cycle is referred to as the **luteal phase** of the ovary and is dominated by the hormonal secretions of the corpus luteum. Nevertheless, small follicles continue to develop within the ovarian stroma during the luteal phase.

REGULATION OF LATE FOLLICULAR DEVELOPMENT, OVULATION, AND LUTEINIZATION: THE HUMAN MENSTRUAL CYCLE

As stated earlier, late follicular development and luteal function are absolutely dependent on normal hypothalamic and pituitary function. As in the male, hypothalamic neurons secrete gonadotropin-releasing hormone (GnRH) in a pulsatile manner. GnRH, in turn, stimulates LH and FSH production by pituitary gonadotropes. A high frequency of GnRH pulses (1 pulse every 60 to 90 minutes) selectively promotes LH production, whereas a slow frequency promotes FSH production. A major difference between the male and the female reproductive axes is the midcycle gonadotropin surge in females, which is dependent on a superthreshold level of estrogen coming from the dominant follicle.

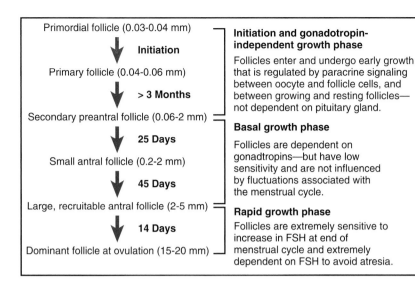

Primordial follicle (0.03-0.04 mm)

↓ **Initiation**

Primary follicle (0.04-0.06 mm)

↓ **> 3 Months**

Secondary preantral follicle (0.06-2 mm)

↓ **25 Days**

Small antral follicle (0.2-2 mm)

↓ **45 Days**

Large, recruitable antral follicle (2-5 mm)

↓ **14 Days**

Dominant follicle at ovulation (15-20 mm)

Initiation and gonadotropin-independent growth phase

Follicles enter and undergo early growth that is regulated by paracrine signaling between oocyte and follicle cells, and between growing and resting follicles—not dependent on pituitary gland.

Basal growth phase

Follicles are dependent on gonadtropins—but have low sensitivity and are not influenced by fluctuations associated with the menstrual cycle.

Rapid growth phase

Follicles are extremely sensitive to increase in FSH at end of menstrual cycle and extremely dependent on FSH to avoid atresia.

FIGURE 9-13 ■ Timing and phases of follicular growth.

A highly dynamic "conversation" occurs among the ovary, pituitary, and hypothalamus, which orchestrates the events of the menstrual cycle (Figure 9-14). This section outlines the main points of events involving the ovary and pituitary gonadotrope that regulate the menstrual cycle, with an overview of hypothalamic involvement. In the next section, the effects of the hormonal changes on the female reproductive tract, especially the uterus, are discussed.

The following outline of events, numbered as depicted in Figure 9-14, begins with the ovary at the end of the luteal phase of a previous, nonfertile cycle:

Ovary—Event 1: In the absence of fertilization and implantation, the corpus luteum regresses and dies (a phenomenon called **luteolysis**). This leads to a drastic decline in the levels of progesterone, estrogen, and inhibin A by day 24 of the menstrual cycle.

Pituitary gonadotrope—Event 2: The gonadotrope perceives the end of luteal function as a release from negative feedback. This permits a rise in FSH that occurs about 2 days before the onset of menstruation. The basis for the selective increase in FSH is incompletely understood, but may be due to the slow frequency of GnRH pulses during the luteal phase, which is due to high progesterone levels.

Ovary—Event 3: The rise in FSH levels recruits a crop of large (2- to 5-mm) antral follicles to begin rapid,

highly gonadotropin-dependent growth. These follicles produce low levels of estrogen and inhibin B.

Pituitary gonadotrope—Event 4: The gonadotrope responds to the slowly rising levels of estrogen and inhibin B by decreasing FSH secretion. Loss of high levels of progesterone and estrogen causes an increase in the frequency of GnRH pulses, thereby selectively increasing LH synthesis and secretion by the gonadotrope. Thus, the LH/FSH ratio slowly increases throughout the follicular phase.

Ovary—Event 5: The ovary's response to declining FSH levels is follicular atresia of all of the recruited follicles, except for one dominant follicle. Thus, the process of selection is driven by an extreme dependency of follicles on FSH in the face of declining FSH secretion. Usually, only the largest follicle with the most FSH receptors and best blood supply (i.e., most angiogenic) can survive. This follicle produces increasing amounts of estradiol-17β and inhibin B. FSH also induces the expression of LH receptors in the mural granulosa cells of the dominant follicle.

Pituitary gonadotrope—Event 6: Once the dominant follicle causes the circulating estrogen levels to exceed 200 pg/ml for about 50 hours in women, estrogen exerts a positive feedback on the gonadotrope, producing the midcycle LH surge. This is enhanced by the small amount of progesterone starting to be

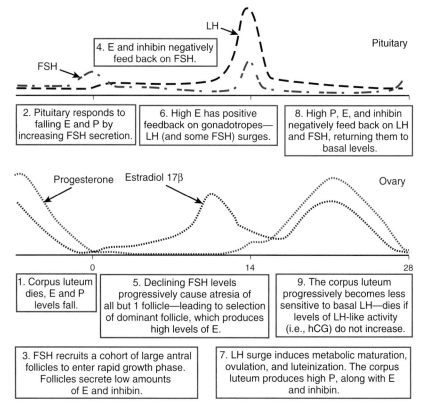

FIGURE 9-14 ■ The human menstrual cycle—a "conversation" between the ovary and the pituitary. See text for comments on the involvement of the hypothalamus. E, estrogen; FSH, follicle-stimulating hormone; hCG, human chorionic gonadotropin; LH, luteinizing hormone; P, progesterone.

made at midcycle. The exact mechanism of the positive feedback is unknown, but it occurs largely at the level of the pituitary. **GnRH receptors** and the sensitivity to GnRH signaling increase dramatically in the gonadotropes (Figure 9-15). The hypothalamus contributes to the gonadotropin surge by increasing the frequency of GnRH pulses, and a small amount of progesterone

Ovary—Event 7: The LH surge drives three general events in the ovary:

1. The primary oocyte completes meiosis I and arrests at metaphase of meiosis II. This is associated with **germinal vesicle breakdown (GVBD)**, which is the dissolution of the nuclear membrane and interphase nuclear structure. GVBD occurs around 30 hours after the onset of the LH surge.

2. The wall of the follicle and of the ovary at the stigma is broken down, and the free-floating

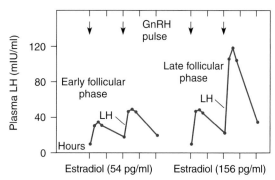

FIGURE 9-15 ■ Luteinizing hormone (LH) response to gonadotropin-releasing hormone (GnRH) administered either early in follicular phase when estrogen levels are relatively low or late in follicular phase when levels are high. *(Redrawn from Wang CF, et al: J Clin Endocrinol Metab 42:718, 1976.)*

cumulus-oocyte complex is extruded from the ovary (i.e., ovulation). This occurs about 32 to 36 hours after the onset of the LH surge.

3. The mural granulosa cells and theca cells are restructured to form the corpus luteum. This involves direct vascularization of the granulosa cells, and their differentiation into progesterone- and estrogen-producing cells. Note that estrogen production transiently drops for about 2 days after the onset of LH production, which may terminate the positive feedback. The granulosa cells also secrete inhibin A. The process of luteinization continues for several days after the onset of the LH surge. The small amount of progesterone secreted during the periovulatory period contributes to the magnitude of the LH surge.

Pituitary gonadotrope—Event 8: Rising levels of progesterone, estrogen and inhibin A by the mature corpus luteum negatively feedback on the pituitary gonadotrope. Even though estrogen levels exceed the 200 pg/ml threshold for positive feedback, the high progesterone levels block any positive feedback. Consequently, both FSH and LH levels decline to basal levels.

Ovary—Event 9: Basal levels of LH (but not FSH) are absolutely required for normal corpus luteum function. The corpus luteum becomes progressively insensitive to LH signaling, however, and will die unless LH-like activity (i.e., hCG from an implanted embryo) increases. In a nonfertile cycle, the corpus luteum of menstruation will regress in 14 days, and progesterone and estrogen levels will start to decline by about 10 days.

Pituitary gonadotrope—Event 1: Removal of negative feedback causes an increase in FSH at the end of the cycle, and the entire process begins again.

From this sequence of events, it is evident that the ovary is the primary clock for the menstrual cycle. The timing of the two main pituitary-based events—the transient rise in FSH that recruits large antral follicles and the LH surge that induces ovulation—is determined by two respective ovarian events: (1) the highly regular lifespan of a corpus luteum and its demise after 14 days and (2) the growth of the dominant follicle to a point where it can maintain a sustained high production of estrogen that induces a switch to positive feedback at the pituitary.

THE FEMALE REPRODUCTIVE TRACT

The Oviduct

Structure/Function (see Figures 9-16 and 9-17) The **oviducts** (also called the **uterine tubes** or **fallopian tubes**), are muscular tubes with the distal end close to the surface of the each ovary, and the proximal end traversing the wall of the uterus. The oviducts can de divided into four sections (going from distal to proximal): (1) the **infundibulum**, or open end of the oviduct, which has finger-like projections called **fimbriae** that sweep over the surface of the ovary; (2) the **ampulla**, which has a relatively wide lumen and extensive folding of the mucosa; (3) the **isthmus**, which has a relatively narrow lumen and less mucosal folding; and (4) the **intramural** or **uterine segment**, which extends through the uterine wall at the superior corners of the uterus.

The main functions of the oviducts are as follows:

1. Capture of the cumulus-oocyte complex at ovulation and transfer of the cumulus-oocyte complex to a midway point (the **ampullary-isthmus junction**), where fertilization takes place. Oviductal secretions coat and infuse the cumulus-oocyte complex and may be required for viability and fertilizability.

2. Provision of a site for sperm storage. Women who ovulate up to 5 days after sexual intercourse can become pregnant. Sperm remain viable by adhering to the epithelial cells lining the isthmus. The secretions of the oviduct also induce capacitation and hyperactivity of sperm (see Chapter 10).

3. Provision of nutritional support to the preimplantation embryo by the oviductal secretions. Also, the timing of the movement of the embryo into the uterus is critical, because the uterus has an implantation window of approximately 3 days. The oviduct needs to contain the early embryo until it reaches the blastocyst stage (5 days after fertilization); then it allows the embryo to move into the uterine cavity (see Chapter 10).

The wall of the oviduct is composed of a mucosa called the **endosalpinx,** a two-layered muscularis called the **myosalpinx**, and outerlying connective tissue, the **perisalpinx**. The endosalpinx is lined by a simple

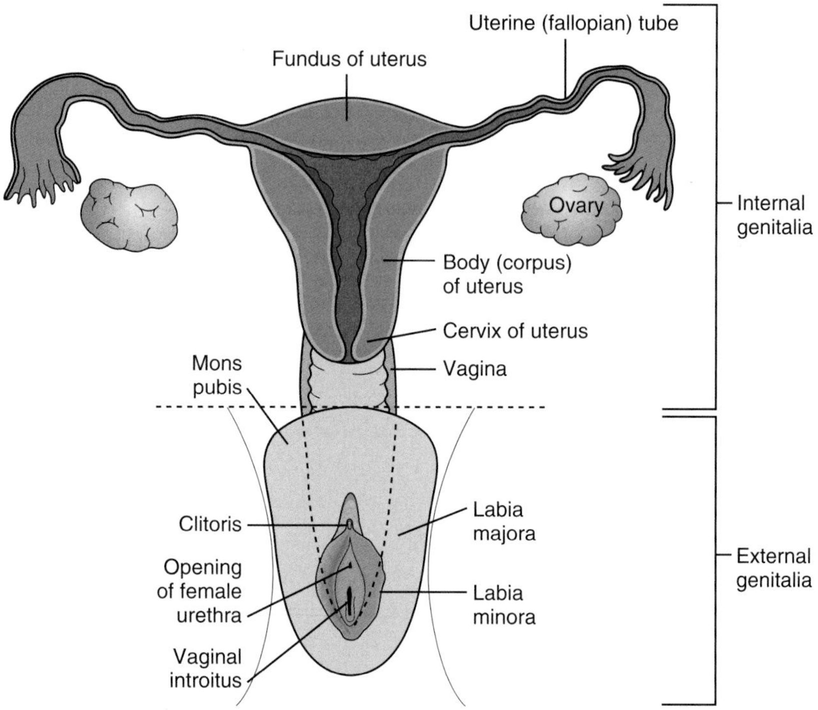

FIGURE 9-16 ■ The internal and external genitalia of the female reproductive tract. *(Modified from Drake RL, Vogl W, Mitchell AWM: Gray's anatomy for students, Philadelphia, 2005, Churchill Livingstone.)*

epithelium made up of two cell types: **ciliated cells** and **secretory cells** (Figure 9-18). The cilia are most numerous at the infundibular end and beat toward the uterus. The cilia on the fimbriae are the sole mechanism for transport of the ovulated cumulus-oocyte complex. Once the complex passes through the ostium of the oviduct and enters the ampulla, it is moved by both cilia and peristaltic contractions of the muscularis. The importance of ciliary transport is indicated by the finding that women with **immotile cilia syndrome** (also called **Kartagener syndrome**) are infertile or subfertile.

The secretory cells produce a protein-rich mucus that is conveyed along the oviduct to the uterus by the cilia. This ciliary-mucus escalator maintains a healthy epithelium, moves the cumulus-oocyte complex toward the uterus, and may provide directional cues for swimming sperm. The movement of the cumulus-oocyte complex slows at the ampullary-isthmus junction, where fertilization normally takes place. This appears to be due in part to a thick mucus that is produced by the human isthmus and to increased tone of the muscularis of the isthmus.

The composition of oviductal secretions is complex and includes growth factors, enzymes, and oviduct-specific glycoproteins. Note that in vitro fertilization has shown that the secretions of the oviduct are not absolutely necessary for fertility by in vitro techniques. However, normal oviductal function is absolutely required for both fertilization and implantation from in vivo insemination, and to minimize the risk of **ectopic implantation** (i.e., implantation outside of the uterus).

Hormonal Regulation During the Menstrual Cycle In general, estrogen secreted during the follicular phase increases endosalpinx epithelial cell size and height. Estrogen increases blood flow to the lamina propria of the oviducts, increases the production of oviduct-specific glycoproteins (whose functions are poorly understood), and increases ciliogenesis throughout the oviduct. Estrogen promotes the secretion of a thick mucus in the isthmus and increases tone of the muscularis of the isthmus, thereby keeping the cumulus-oocyte complex at the ampullary-isthmus junction for fertilization. High progesterone, along with estrogen,

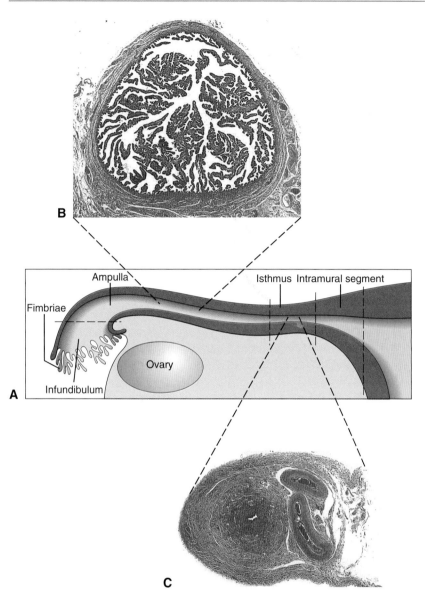

FIGURE 9-17 ■ **A,** Structures of the oviduct. **B,** Cross-section of the oviduct at the ampulla. **C,** Cross-section of the oviduct at the isthmus, showing a much smaller lumen. *(Modified from Stevens A, Lowe J: Human histology, ed 3, Philadelphia, 2005, Mosby.)*

during the early to midluteal phase decreases epithelial cell size and function. Progesterone promotes deciliation. Progesterone also decreases the secretion of thick mucus and relaxes the tone in the isthmus. It also should be noted that oviductal epithelial cells express the LH receptor, which may synergize with estrogen to optimize oviductal function during the periovulatory period.

The Uterus

Structure/Function The **uterus** is a single organ that sits in the midline of the pelvic cavity between the bladder and the rectum. The mucosa of the uterus is called the **endometrium**, the three-layered, thick muscularis is called the **myometrium**, and the outer connective tissue and serosa are called the **perimetrium**. The parts of the uterus are the **fundus**, which is that

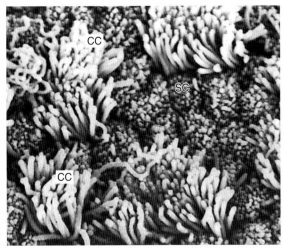

FIGURE 9-18 ■ Scanning electron micrograph of the surface of the ampullary endosalpinx, showing ciliated cells (CC) and secretory cells (SC). *(From Stevens A, Lowe J: Human histology, ed 3, Philadelphia, 2005, Mosby.)*

portion that rises superiorly from the entrance of the oviducts; the **body**, which makes up most of the uterus; the **isthmus**, a short narrowed part of the body at its inferior end; and the **cervix**, which extends into the **vagina** (Figure 9-16). Because the cervical mucosa is distinct from the rest of the uterus and does not undergo the process of menstruation, it is discussed separately later on.

The established functions of the uterus all are related to pregnancy (see Chapter 10). The main functions of the uterus are as follows:

1. To provide a suitable site for attachment and implantation of the blastocyst, including a thick, nutrient-rich stroma.
2. To limit the invasiveness of the implanting embryo, so that it stays in the endometrium and does not reach the myometrium.
3. To provide a maternal side of the mature placental architecture. This includes the basal plate, to which the fetal side attaches, and large, intervillous spaces that become filled with maternal blood after the first trimester.
4. To grow and expand with the growing fetus, so that the fetus develops within an aqueous, nonadhesive environment.

5. To provide strong muscular contractions to expel the fetus and placenta at term.

An understanding of the function of the uterus and uterine changes during nonfertile menstrual cycles requires a basic knowledge of the fine structure of the endometrium, and of the relationship of the uterine blood supply to the endometrium (Figure 9-19). The luminal surface of the endometrium is covered by a simple cuboidal/columnar epithelium. The epithelium is continuous with mucosal glands (called **uterine glands**) that extend deep into the endometrium. The mucosa is vascularized by **spiral arteries**, which are branches of the **uterine artery** that runs through the myometrium. The terminal arterioles of the spiral arteries project to a position just beneath the surface epithelium. These arterioles give rise to a subepithelial plexus of capillaries and venules, which have ballooned, thin-walled segments called **venous lakes** or **lacunae**. The lamina propria itself is densely cellular. The stromal cells of the lamina propria play important roles both during pregnancy and menstruation.

About two thirds of the luminal side of the endometrium is lost during menstruation, and is called the **functional zone** (also called the **stratum functionalis**) (see Figure 9-19). The basal one third of endometrium that remains after menstruation is called the **basal zone** (also called the **stratum basale**). The basal zone is fed by straight arteries that are separate from the spiral arteries, and contains all of the cell types of the endometrium (i.e., epithelial cells from the remaining tips of glands, stromal cells, and endothelial cells).

Hormonal Regulation of the Uterine Endometrium During the Menstrual Cycle

The Proliferative Phase (Figure 9-20) Monthly oscillations in ovarian steroids induce the uterine endometrium to enter different stages. At the time of selection of the dominant follicle and its production of estrogen, the uterine endometrium is just ending menstruation. The stratum functionalis has been shed, and only the stratum basale remains. The rising levels of estrogen during the mid- to late- follicular phase of the ovary induce the **proliferative phase** of the uterine endometrium. Estrogen induces all cell types in the stratum basale to growth and divide. In fact, the

UTERINE LUMEN

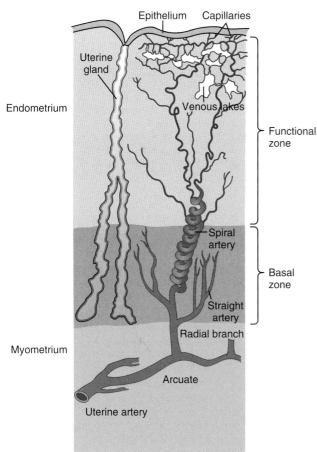

FIGURE 9-19 ■ Structure of the uterine endometrium. *(Modified from Strauss J III, Coutifaris C: The endometrium and myometrium: regulation and dysfunction. In Yen SSC, Jaffe RB, Barbieri RL, editors: Reproductive endocrinology, ed 4, Philadelphia, 1999, WB Saunders, pp 191-217.)*

definition of an *estrogenic compound* has historically been one that is "uterotrophic." It is not clear whether estrogen stimulates the growth and differentiation of pluripotential stem cells, or stimulates the growth of cells that are already defined as endothelial, epithelial, and stromal. Estrogen increases cell proliferation directly through its cognate receptors (ER-α and ER-β), and indirectly through the production of growth factors, such as insulin-like growth factor-I (IGF-I) and vascular endothelial growth factor (VEGF). Estrogen also induces the expression of progesterone receptors, thereby "priming" the uterine endometrium so that it can respond to progesterone during the luteal phase of the ovary.

The Secretory Phase By ovulation, the thickness of stratum functionalis has been reestablished under the proliferative actions of estradiol-17β. After ovulation, the corpus luteum produces high levels of progesterone, along with estradiol-17β. The luteal phase of the ovary switches the proliferative phase of the uterine endometrium to the **secretory phase**. In general, progesterone inhibits further endometrial growth and induces the differentiation of epithelial and stromal cells. Progesterone induces the uterine glands to secrete a nutrient-rich product, which will support blastocyst viability. As the secretory phase proceeds, the mucosal uterine glands become corkscrewed and sacculated. Progesterone also induces changes in the

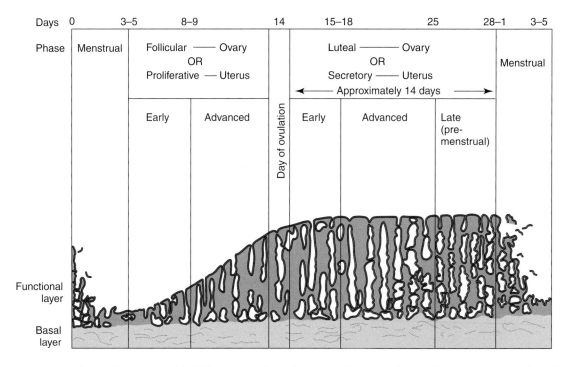

FIGURE 9-20 ■ Changes in endometrial thickness, glands, and arteries relative to phases of ovarian cycle. *(Redrawn from Cunningham FG, et al, editors: Williams' obstetrics, Norwalk, Conn, 1993, Appleton & Lange.)*

adhesivity of the surface epithelium, thereby generating the "window of receptivity" for implantation. Progesterone also promotes the differentiation of the stromal cells into "**predecidual cells**," which must be prepared to form the decidua of pregnancy, or to orchestrate menstruation in the absence of pregnancy.

Of importance, progesterone opposes the proliferative actions of estradiol-17β. Progesterone down-regulates the estrogen receptor. Progesterone also induces **inactivating isoforms of 17β-hydroxysteroid dehydrogenase**, thereby converting the active estradiol-17β into the inactive estrone. This opposition of the mitogenic actions of estradiol-17β by progesterone is extremely important in protecting the uterine endometrium from estrogen-induced uterine cancer. By contrast, the administration of **unopposed estrogen** significantly increases the risk of uterine cancer in women.

The Menstrual Phase In a nonfertile cycle, death of the corpus luteum leads to a sudden withdrawal of progesterone, which leads to changes in the uterine endometrium that result in the loss of the lamina functionalis. **Menstruation** normally lasts for 4 or 5 days (called a **period**), and the volume of blood loss ranges from 25 to 35 ml. Menstruation coincides with the early follicular phase of the ovary.

Disorders of menstruation are relatively common, and include **menorrhagia** (loss of more than 80 ml of blood), and **dysmenorrhea** (painful periods). The existence of few, irregular periods, called **oligomenorrhea**, and the absence of periods, called **amenorrhea**, often are due to dysfunction of the hypothalamus-pituitary-ovarian axis, as opposed to local pelvic pathophysiology.

The breakdown of the stratum functionalis is due to the up-regulation of hydrolytic enzymes, called **matrix metalloproteases**, which destroy the extracellular matrix and basal lamina of the endometrium. These enzymes are produced by the three resident cell types of the endometrium: the epithelial cell, the stromal cell, and the endothelial cell. Matrix metalloproteases also are produced by **leukocytes**, which infiltrate into the endometrium just before menstruation. The other major component that leads to menstruation is the production of **prostaglandins**. The inducible enzyme required for prostaglandin synthesis, **cyclooxygenase-2 (COX-2),** is increased in endothelial cells on progesterone withdrawal. This increases production of inflammatory prostaglandins, especially **PGF2α,** which, in turn, promotes contraction of the smooth muscle cells of the myometrium, and the vascular smooth muscle cells of the spiral arteries. Intermittent spiral artery contraction and dilation causes hypoxic necrosis, followed by reperfusion injury of weakened tissue. The degree of tissue loss and the onset of tissue repair appear to be dependent on increasing estrogen levels during the early to midfollicular phase.

Hormonal Regulation of the Myometrium The smooth muscle cells of the myometrium also are responsive to changes in steroid hormones. Peristaltic contractions of the myometrium favor movement of luminal contents from the cervix to the fundus at ovulation, and these contractions may play a role in rapid bulk transport of ejaculated sperm from the cervix to the oviducts. During menstruation, contractions propagate from the fundus to the cervix, thereby promoting expulsion of sloughed stratum functionalis. The size and number of smooth muscle cells are determined by estrogen and progesterone. Healthy, cycling women maintain a robust myometrium, whereas the myometrium progressively thins in postmenopausal women. The most drastic changes are seen during pregnancy, when the smooth muscle cells increase from 50 to 500 μm in length. The pregnant myometrium also has a greater number of smooth muscle cells and more extracellular matrix. The myometrium gives rise to the most common benign tumors, called **uterine fibroids** or **leiomyomas**. Uterine fibroids retain their sensitivity to ovarian steroids, progressively growing in size during the reproductive years and then regressing after menopause.

The Cervix

Structure/Function The cervix represents the inferior extension of the uterus that projects into the vagina (see Figure 9-16). It has a mucosa that lines the **endocervical canal**, which has a highly elastic lamina propria, and a muscularis that is continuous with the myometrium. The part of the cervix that extends into

the vaginal vault is called the **ectocervix**; the part surrounding the endocervical canal is called the **endocervix**. The openings of the endocervical canal at the uterus and vagina are called the **internal cervical os** and the **external cervical os**, respectively. The cervix acts as a gateway to the upper female tract—at midcycle, the endocervical canal facilitates sperm viability and entry. During the luteal phase, changes in the endocervical canal serve to impede the passage of sperm and microbes, thereby minimizing the chance of **superimplantation** of a second embryo, as well as inhibiting ascending infections into the placenta, fetal membranes, and fetus. The cervix physically supports the weight of the growing fetus. At term, **cervical softening and dilation** allow passage of the newborn and placenta from the uterus into the vagina.

Hormonal Regulation of Cervical Mucus During the Menstrual Cycle The endocervical canal is lined by a simple columnar epithelium that secretes **cervical mucus** in a hormonally responsive manner. Estrogen stimulates production of a copious quantity of thin, watery, slightly alkaline mucus that is an ideal environment for sperm. It is described as stringy because when the mucus is dropped on a slide and a stick is touched to it and then elevated, a long "string" of mucus can be formed. This characteristic is termed **spinnbarkeit** (Figure 9-21). This occurs because macromolecules in the mucus align themselves in parallel chains when the mucus is "pulled." These macromolecules are thought to facilitate sperm movement through the mucus. When the mucus is allowed to dry on a slide, a fernlike pattern (**ferning**) is formed as a

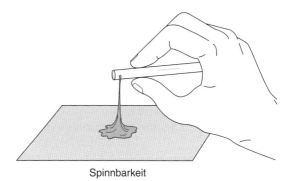

Spinnbarkeit

FIGURE 9-21 ■ Spinnbarkeit. Cervical mucus from a periovulatory woman is stringy.

result of the high electrolyte content of the mucus. Progesterone stimulates production of a scant, viscous, slightly acidic mucus that is hostile to sperm and does not "fern." During the normal menstrual cycle, the conditions of the cervical mucus are ideal for sperm penetration and viability at the time of ovulation.

The Vagina

Structure/Function The vagina represents one of the copulatory structures in women, and acts as the birth canal (see Figure 9-16). Its mucosa is lined by a nonkeratinized, stratified squamous epithelium. The mucosa has a thick lamina propria enriched with elastic fibers and is well vascularized. There are no glands in the vagina, so that lubrication during intercourse comes from (1) cervical mucus (especially during midcycle) and (2) a transudate (i.e., ultrafiltrate) from the blood vessels of the lamina propria and (3) from the vestibular glands (see later). The mucosa is surrounded by a relatively thin (i.e., relative to the uterus and cervix) two-layered muscularis and an outer connective tissue. The vaginal wall is innervated by branches of the pudendal nerve, which contributes to sexual pleasure and orgasm during intercourse.

Hormonal Regulation During the Menstrual Cycle The superficial cells of the vaginal epithelium are continually desquamating and the nature of these cells is influenced by the hormonal environment. Estrogen stimulates proliferation of the vaginal epithelium and increases their glycogen content. Progesterone increases the desquamation of the epithelial cells. The glycogen is metabolized to lactic acid by commensal lactobacilli, thereby maintaining an acidic environment. This relative acidity inhibits infections by noncommensal bacteria and fungi.

The External Genitalia

Structure/Function The female external genitals are surrounded by the **labia majora** (homologs of the scrotum) laterally and the **mons pubis** anteriorly (Figure 9-22). The **vulva** collectively refers to an area that includes the labia majora and the mons pubis, plus the **labia minora**, the **clitoris**, the **vestibule of the vagina**, the **vestibular bulbs** (glands), and the **external urethral orifice**. The vulva also is referred to

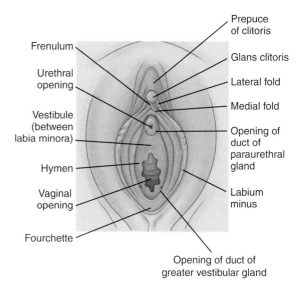

FIGURE 9-22 ■ External genitalia in women. *(From Drake RL, Vogl W, Mitchell AWM: Gray's anatomy for students, Philadelphia, 2005, Elsevier/Churchill Livingstone.)*

as the **pudendum** by clinicians. The structures of the vulva serve the functions of sexual arousal and climax and of directing the flow of urine and also partially cover the opening of the vagina, thereby inhibiting the entry of pathogens.

The clitoris is the homolog of the penis and is composed of two **corpora cavernosa**, which attach the clitoris to the ischiopubic rami, and a **glans**. These structures are composed of erectile tissue and undergo the process of erection in essentially the same manner as for the penis. Unlike the penis, clitoral tissue is completely separate from the urethra. Thus, the only function of the clitoris is involved with sexual arousal and climax at orgasm. The clitoris performs this function (in conjunction with sensory innervation from the vaginal wall) through its innervation by the deep dorsal branch of the pudendal nerve.

Hormonal Regulation During the Menstrual Cycle The structures of the vulva do not show marked changes during the menstrual cycle. The health and function of these structures, however, are dependent on hormonal support. The external genitalia and vagina appear to be responsive to androgens (testosterone and dihydrotestosterone), as well as estrogen. Androgens also act on the central nervous sytem (CNS) to increase libido in women.

BIOLOGY OF ESTRADIOL-17β AND PROGESTERONE

Mechanisms of Estrogen and Progesterone Hormone Action

Estrogen and progesterone are steroid hormones; accordingly, their cognate receptors belong to the nuclear hormone receptor superfamily. In the absence of ligand, the **estrogen receptor (ER)** (two separate genes encode two related estrogen receptors, ER-α and ER-β) and the **progesterone receptor (PR)** (three splicing variants are produced from one gene) are complexed with chaperone proteins (e.g., heat-shock proteins, cyclophilins). Ligand binding induces dissociation of chaperones and dimerization (Figure 9-23), nuclear translocation, and binding to an **estrogen-response element (ERE)** or a **progesterone-response element (PRE)**. DNA-bound hormone-receptor complexes recruit **co-activator proteins**, which induce an "open" chromatin structure, thereby allowing the assembly of transcriptional factors on the promoter of a nearby gene (see Chapter 1).

Of all of the steroid hormone receptors, the estrogen receptor has been studied the most in terms of manipulation by agonists and antagonists. These drugs, called **selective estrogen receptor modulators (SERMs)**, include **tamoxifen** and **raloxifene** (see Figure 9-23). Tamoxifen currently is used as an estrogen receptor antagonist for the treatment of breast cancer (whose early progression is promoted by estrogen). SERM binding to the ER can induce conformational changes that allow co-repressors to bind to the ER, or promote the degradation of the ER. The effect of SERMs are cell context specific—for example, tamoxifen acts as an **ER antagonist** in breast ductal tissue but as an **ER agonist** in uterine endometrial tissue.

The estrogen signaling pathway is also the best studied in terms of **"nongenomic" signaling** (also called **"membrane-initiated" signaling**). For example, estrogen has very rapid effects on nitric oxide production in endothelial cells—too rapid to be explained by the classical pathway of gene regulation (i.e., the "genomic" signaling pathway). Membrane-initiated signaling by estrogen is mediated by either the classic ER associated with other membrane signaling proteins or possibly by the GPCR, **GPR30**, which is coupled to Gs and Gq pathways (or by both).

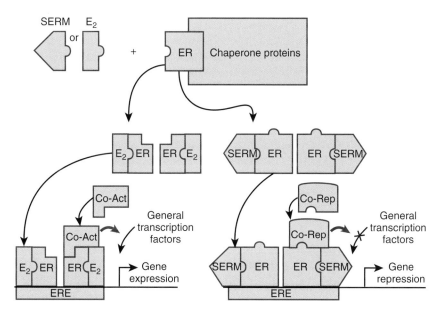

FIGURE 9-23 ■ "Genomic" mechanism of action of estradiol-17β (E_2) and selective estrogen receptor modulators (SERMs), as mediated by the estrogen receptor (ER). Co-Act, co-activator proteins; Co-Rep, co-repressor proteins; ERE, estrogen response element.

Biological Effects of Estrogen and Progesterone

Although the levels of estradiol-17β and progesterone fluctuate during the menstrual cycle, estrogen and progesterone levels are always higher in women than in men. Estradiol-17β and progesterone have multiple effects that can be categorized according to whether or not they are directly related to the reproductive system. As discussed previously, both steroid hormones have profound effects on the ovary, oviduct, uterus, cervix, vagina, and external genitalia, and on the hypothalamus and pituitary. Estrogen and progesterone also have important effects on nonreproductive tissues:

Bone: Estrogen is required for closure of the epiphyseal plates of long bones in both sexes. Estradiol-17β has a **bone anabolic effect** and a **calciotropic effect** at several sites. E_2 stimulates intestinal calcium absorption and renal tubular calcium reabsorption. E_2 also is one of the most potent regulators of osteoblast and osteoclast function. Estrogen promotes survival of osteoblasts and apoptosis of osteoclasts, thereby favoring bone formation over resorption.

Liver: The overall effect of estradiol-17β on the liver is to improve **circulating lipoprotein profiles**. Estrogen increases expression of the LDL receptor, thereby increasing clearance of cholesterol-rich LDL particles by the liver. Estrogen also increases circulating levels of high density lipoprotein (HDL) levels. Estrogen regulates hepatic production of several transport proteins, including cortisol-binding protein, thyroid hormone–binding protein, and sex hormone–binding protein.

Cardiovascular organs: Premenopausal women have significantly lower cardiovascular disease than men or postmenopausal women. Estrogen promotes **vasodilation** through increased production of **nitric oxide**, which relaxes vascular smooth muscle and inhibits platelet activation. **ER single-nucleotide polymorphisms** are associated with an increased incidence of cardiovascular disease.

Integument: Overall, estrogen and progesterone maintain a healthy, smooth skin with normal epidermal and dermal thickness. Estrogen stimulates proliferation and inhibits apoptosis of keratinocytes. In the dermis, estrogen and progesterone increases collagen synthesis and inhibits(along with progesterone the breakdown of collagen by suppressing matrix metalloproteases. Estrogen also increases glycosaminoglycan production and deposition in the dermis. Estrogen also promotes wound healing.

CNS: In general, estrogen is **neuroprotective**—that is, it inhibits neuronal cell death in response to hypoxia or other insults. Estrogen's positive effects on angiogenesis may account for some of the beneficial and stimulant-like actions of estrogen on the CNS. Currently, the proposed benefits of estrogen for the onset and severity of Parkinson disease and Alzheimer disease are controversial. Progesterone acts on the hypothalamus to increase the set-point for thermoregulation, thereby elevating **body temperature** by approximately 0.5° F. This is the basis for using body temperature measurements to determine whether ovulation has occurred. Progesterone generally acts as a depressant on the CNS. Loss of progesterone on demise of the corpus luteum of menstruation is the basis for **premenstrual dysphoria**—experienced by some women as **premenstrual syndrome (PMS)**. Progesterone acts at the brain stem to sensitize the ventilatory response to carbon dioxide levels, so that ventilation increases and the partial pressure of carbon dioxide (P_{CO_2}) decreases.

Kidney: Progesterone is a competitive inhibitor of aldosterone; at the kidney, it has a **natriuretic action**.

Adipose tissue: Estrogen decreases adipose tissue by decreasing lipoprotein lipase activity and increasing hormone-sensitive lipase (i.e., it has a **lipolytic effect**). Loss of estrogen results in an accumulation of adipose tissue, especially in the abdomen.

Transport and Metabolism of Ovarian Steroids

Steroid hormones are sparingly soluble in blood and are carried primarily associated with plasma proteins. Approximately 60% of the estrogen is transported bound to **sex hormone–binding globulin (SHBG)**, 20% is bound to albumin, and 20% is in the free form.

Progesterone binds primarily to **cortisol-binding globulin (CBG) (i.e., transcortin)** and albumin. Because it has a relatively low binding affinity for these proteins, its circulating half-life ($t_{1/2}$) is approximately 5 minutes.

Although the ovary is the primary site of estrogen production, it is important to understand that **peripheral aromatization of androgens** to estrogens can generate locally high levels of estradiol-17β in specific tissues. For example, the fact that CYP19 (aromatase) is expressed in the breast is the basis for the use of **aromatase inhibitors** in the treatment of estrogen-dependent breast cancer.

Estrogens and progestins are degraded in the liver to inactive metabolites, **conjugated with sulfate or glucuronide**, and excreted in the urine. Major metabolites of estradiol include estrone, estriol, and catecholestrogens (2-hydroxyestrone and 2-methoxyestrone). The major metabolite of progesterone is pregnanediol, which is conjugated with glucuronide and excreted in the urine.

THE ONTOGENY OF THE FEMALE REPRODUCTIVE SYSTEM

Development of the Female Reproductive Tract

If the testis-determining gene *SRY* is absent, ovaries develop from the genital ridge. Although the fetal testis begins to develop at 6 weeks of gestation, the fetal ovary remains undifferentiated until after 9 weeks of gestation (Figure 9-24). By this time, the fetal testis is already producing testosterone. By contrast, the fetal ovary remains quiescent during fetal development, and in the absence of testicular anti-müllerian hormone and testosterone, the **müllerian ducts** become the fallopian tubes, uterus, and upper vagina; the **urogenital sinus** gives rise to the lower vagina; and the **genital folds**, **genital swelling**, and **genital tubercle** become the labia (majora and minora) and the clitoris. Ovaries are not necessary for the fetal development of female internal and external genitalia.

The female fetus, like the male, shows a peak in LH and FSH secretion in utero, followed by a second peak 2 to 3 months postpartum. Subsequently, LH and FSH secretion remain relatively low until adolescence.

Puberty

Pubertal changes in the female in many ways resemble those in the male (Figure 9-25) (see Chapter 8).

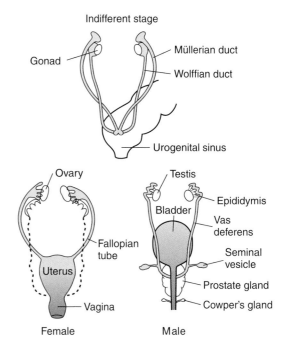

FIGURE 9-24 ■ Differentiation of internal genitalia and primordial ducts. *(Redrawn from George FW, Wilson JD: Embryology of the genital tract. In Walsh PC, et al, editors: Campbell's urology, ed 6, Philadelphia, 1992, WB Saunders.)*

The timing of puberty in females is influenced by the level of body fat. Lean girls tend to enter puberty later. Female athletes with low body fat levels often have amenorrhea. This may be due in part to the fact that adipose tissue expresses significant levels of CYP19 (aromatase), which aromatizes androgens to estrogens. Growing evidence, however, suggests that **leptin**, which also is produced by adipose tissue, plays a permissive role in hypothalamic maturation at puberty. Several years before **menarche** (onset of menstrual cycles), **adrenarche** occurs. This is manifested by the development of **pubic hair** and **axillary hair**.

A landmark of puberty in women is breast growth with some limited development. **Mammary glands** are composed of about 15 to 20 lobes, which are made up of smaller lobules (see Chapter 10). The termini of lobules are secretory alveoli. Ducts of increasing size emanate from the secretory **lobuloalveolar structures** to give rise to one duct for each lobe that opens at the **nipple**. The lobules and lobes are surrounded and supported by connective tissue. The superficial fascia

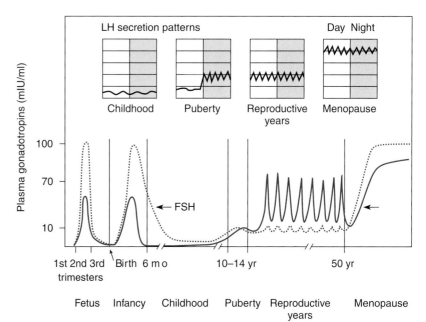

FIGURE 9-25 ■ Relative serum luteinizing hormone (LH) and follicle-stimulating hormone (FSH) levels across the life span in women. *(Redrawn from Braunwald E, et al: Harrison's principles of internal medicine, ed 4, New York, 1987, McGraw-Hill.)*

of the breasts is infiltrated with adipose tissue, called the **fat pads**, which make up most of the volume of the breasts in nonpregnant women. At puberty, the increase in estrogen induces an enlargement and darkening of the **areola**, which is the pigmented, hairless circle surrounding the nipple, and some limited ductal growth beneath the areola and nipple. The onset of these mammary gland changes is referred to as **thelarche**. Once ovulatory cycles begin, progesterone stimulates further growth and maturation of the mammary glands. Progesterone also increases stromal edema and vacuolation of the epithelia, thereby inducing a sensation of fullness or tenderness during the late luteal phase. Both estrogen and progesterone stimulate mammary gland growth, but the primary action of estrogen is on the development of the ductile system and the primary action of progesterone is on the lobular-alveolar system. Table 9-1 shows the Tanner stages of pubertal development for women, and Figure 9-26 shows the ages at which these changes occur.

Menopause

Menopause generally is thought to result from primary ovarian deficiency due to depletion of functional follicles. The observation that some morphologically normal oocytes can be present in the postmenopausal ovary, however, suggests that oocyte depletion is not the sole cause of menopause. These remaining follicles are hypothesized to be less sensitive to gonadotropins. It has been proposed recently that age-related changes in the central nervous system, including critical patterns

TABLE 9-1		
Tanner Pubertal Stages in Female		
STAGE	BREAST	PUBIC HAIR
1	Prepubertal	Prepubertal—no pubic hair
2	Breast bud and papilla elevated, small mound present	Slight growth of fine downy hair
3	Enlargement of breast mound, palpable glandular tissue	Hair darker, coiled, denser
4	Areola and nipple elevated	Adult-type hair, but area covered is less than in adult
5	Adult breast	Adult-type hair with triangular-shaped distribution

Data from Marshall WA, Tanner JM: *Arch Dis Child* 44:291, 1969.

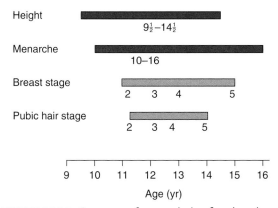

FIGURE 9-26 ■ Sequence of events during female puberty indicating ranges of ages at which each event normally occurs. Numbers 2 to 5 refer to Tanner stages. *(Data from Marshall WA, Tanner JM: Arch Dis Child 45:13, 1970.)*

of GnRH secretion, precede follicular depletion and may play an important role in menopause. Because follicles do not develop in response to LH and FSH secretion, estrogen and progesterone levels drop. Loss of the negative feedback inhibition of estrogen on GnRH and LH/FSH results in a marked rise in serum LH and FSH. FSH levels rise more than LH levels. This may result from ovarian inhibin loss.

Menopause typically occurs between 45 and 55 years of age. It extends over several years. Initially the cycles become irregular and are periodically anovulatory. The cycles tend to shorten, primarily in the follicular phase. Eventually, the woman ceases to cycle altogether. The serum estradiol levels drop to about one sixth the mean levels in younger cycling women, and progesterone levels drop to about one third those in the follicular phase in younger women. Production of these hormones does not cease entirely, but the primary source of these hormones in the postmenopausal woman becomes the adrenal, although interstitial cells of the ovarian stroma continue to produce some steroids. Most circulating estrogens are now produced peripherally from androgens. Because estrone is the primary estrogen produced in adipose tissue, it becomes the predominant estrogen in postmenopausal women.

Most of the signs and symptoms associated with menopause result from **estrogen deficiency**. The vaginal epithelium atrophies and becomes dry, and **bone loss** is accelerated, potentially leading to **osteoporosis**. The incidence of **cardiovascular disease** increases markedly after menopause. **Hot flashes** result from periodic increases in core temperature, which produce peripheral vasodilation and sweating. Hot flashes are now thought to be linked to increases in LH release and are probably associated not with the pulsatile rise in LH secretion but rather with central mechanisms controlling GnRH release. Hot flashes typically subside within 1 to 5 years of the onset of menopausal symptoms. Estrogen therapy generally provides relief from hot flashes, decreases the rate of bone loss, and decreases vaginal atrophy and dryness. Results from the **Women's Health Initiative** and other studies, however, have provided conflicting findings on the safety of estrogens and progestins (which often are not in the form of bioidentical estradiol-17β and progesterone) for **hormone replacement therapy** in postmenopausal women, emphasizing the need for physicians to fully consider each woman's individual medical and family history before deciding on the course of therapy for the alleviation of postmenopausal symptoms.

OVARIAN PATHOPHYSIOLOGY

Turner Syndrome

Turner syndrome, or **gonadal dysgenesis**, is the most common cause of congenital hypogonadism. In about 50% of cases, it results from the complete absence of the second X chromosome, so that the karyotype of the affected person is 45,XO. The germ cells do not develop, and each gonad consists of a connective tissue–filled streak. The major clinical characteristics include short stature, a characteristic webbed neck, low-set ears, a shield-shaped chest, short fourth metacarpals, and sexual infantilism resulting from gonadal dysgenesis (Figure 9-27). Internal and external genitalia typically are female.

Polycystic Ovarian Syndrome

Chronically anovulatory women with high circulating androgen, estrogen, and LH levels often have the disorder called **polycystic ovarian syndrome (PCOS)**. This syndrome may be caused by any of a broad array of underlying problems, and PCOS accounts for 75%

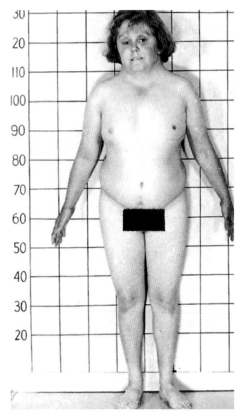

FIGURE 9-27 ■ Female with Turner syndrome. Note the characteristically broad, "webbed" neck. Stature is reduced, and sexual secondary characteristics are poorly developed. *(From Goodman RM, Gorlin RJ: Atlas of the face in genetic disorders, ed 2, St. Louis, 1977, Mosby.)*

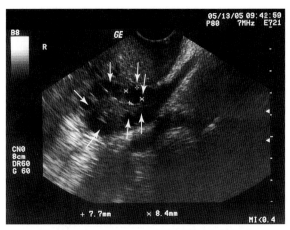

FIGURE 9-28 ■ Sonogram of polycystic ovary. Cysts *(arrows)* are due to large antral follicles in the cortex that failed to ovulate. *(Courtesy of Dr. Andrea DiLuigi, Reproductive Endocrinology and Infertility Fellow, Department of Obstetrics and Gynecology, UConn Health Center, Farmington, Conn.)*

of anovulatory infertility. Currently, the diagnosis of PCOS requires two of the following three conditions: **amenorrhea**, evidence of **excessive androgen secretion** (i.e., acne, hirsutism), and **polycystic ovaries**, as usually detected by **sonogram** (Figure 9-28). The ovarian cysts represent large antral follicles that have failed to ovulate and luteinize. The continuous gonadotropin secretion leads to ovarian enlargement, and the ovaries typically show a thickened capsule and numerous follicles, many of which are undergoing atresia. FSH levels are low, which inhibits granulosa cell function, and the high intrafollicular androgen level inhibits follicular maturation. A significant proportion of the circulating estrogen, present in high levels, is estrone formed from peripheral aromatization of androstenedione. These high androgen levels can produce **hirsutism** and **acne**. Hirsutism is the abnormal formation of coarse sexual hair in regions atypical for a woman, such as the face, back, and chest. The exact cause of PCOS is not well understood, but the primary defect appears to be inappropriate signals between the hypothalamic-pituitary axis and the ovary. A significant subset of patients with PCOS are obese and have insulin resistance and hyperinsulinemia. Insulin promotes ovarian androgen production, and hyperinsulinism may account for increased androgen production. Reduction of insulin levels (such as by weight loss, exercise, or metformin administration) ameliorates the hyperandrogenism and PCOS in these patients. Alternatively, an inadequate response of the follicle to FSH may be due to impaired IGF-I or insulin signaling.

SUMMARY

1. The female reproductive system includes the ovary, oviducts, uterus, cervix, vagina, and external genitalia, along with the pituitary gonadotropes and the hypothalamic GnRH neurons. The mammary glands (breasts) also can be considered a part of the female reproductive system.

2. The ovarian phases of the human menstrual cycle are the follicular phase, the periovulatory period and the luteal phase.

3. The ovarian follicle contains a primary oocyte arrested in meiotic prophase and variable layers of granulosa and thecal cells. Preantral and early antral follicular growth is gonadotropin-independent. Intermediate antral follicular growth is dependent on a basal level of FSH, but not affected by fluctuations in FSH associated with the menstrual cycle. Large antral follicular development is exquisitely dependent on fluctuations of FSH. Follicles can degenerate at any phase during the process of atresia.

4. The dominant follicle is selected based on its size, number of FSH receptors, aromatase activity, and blood supply. The dominant follicle is the endocrine structure of the follicular phase. The thecal cells express the LH receptor, and LH stimulates the production of androgens (primarily androstenedione). The granulosa cells express the FSH receptor, and FSH promotes the aromatization of androgens to estrogens (primarily estradiol-17β). FSH also induces the expression of the LH receptor in granulosa cells of the dominant follicle.

5. The dominant follicle signals that it is ready to ovulate by its estrogen production. High sustained levels of estrogen induce the midcycle LH surge through a positive feedback mechanism. This is due, in part, to a marked increase in the sensitivity of the pituitary gonadotropes to GnRH pulses.

6. The periovulatory period involves the meiotic maturation of the primary oocyte to a secondary oocyte (egg) arrested at metaphase II. Ovulation involves the rupture of the follicular wall at the stigma, release of the cumulus-oocyte complex, and differentiation of the remaining follicular cells into a corpus luteum.

7. The luteal phase is characterized by high progesterone production. The corpus luteum is programmed to die in 14 days, unless rescued by human chorionic gonadotropin (hCG).

8. The oviduct functions to capture the cumulus-oocyte complex, transport and nurture both male and female gametes, promote fertilization and early embryonic development, and determines the timing of the movement of the blastocyst into the uterine cavity.

9. The mucosa of the uterus is called the endometrium. The function of the endometrium is to allow implantation and placentation. Estrogen produced during the mid- to late- follicular phase of the ovary drives the proliferative phase of the uterus, during which the endometrium grows in thickness. The progesterone produced by the luteal phase of the ovary drives the secretory phase of the uterus. Loss of progesterone after the death of the corpus luteum causes the endometrium to break down. This represents the menstrual phase of the uterus.

10. The cyclic changes in ovarian steroids also alter cervical mucus and vaginal epithelium. The external genitalia are responsive to estrogen and androgens.

11. Estrogen and progesterone regulate numerous processes directly associated with reproduction. However, these steroids also regulate nonreproductive aspects of physiology, including bone growth and health, cardiovascular function, hepatic functions, and others. Estrogen and progesterone act primarily through interaction with classical ERs and PRs, which belong to the family of nuclear hormone receptors. Estrogen and progesterone also have rapid, membrane-initiated actions.

12. Puberty involves activation of the hypothalamic-pituitary-gonadal axis. Adrenarche is the first menstrual period. Thelarche represents the first growth of breast tissue. Estrogen and progesterone stimulate breast growth. Menopause represents the cessation of menstrual periods, and is due largely to a depletion of ovarian follicles.

13. Turner syndrome (gonadal dysgenesis) is the most common cause of congenital hypogonadism. It typically results from the absence of the second X chromosome, so that the karyotype of the affected person is 45,XO.

14. Polycystic ovarian syndrome produces chronic anovulation. Circulating androgen, estrogen, and LH levels typically are high.

KEY WORDS AND CONCEPTS

- Endocrine function (of ovaries)
- Gametogenic function (of ovaries)
- Secondary oocytes
- Eggs
- Ovulation
- Human menstrual cycle
- Oogonium
- Ovum
- Menopause
- Follicular phase
- Ovarian follicle
- Midcycle gonadotropin surge
- Corpus luteum
- Luteal phase
- Hypothalamus-pituitary-ovary axis
- Negative feedback by low levels of estrogen
- Positive feedback by high levels of estrogen
- Infertility
- Female reproductive tract
- Uterine endometrium
- Proliferative phase
- Secretory phase
- Menstruation
- Fertilization
- Implantation
- Placentation
- Parturition
- Mammary glands (breasts)
- Broad ligament
- Ovarian follicles
- Ovarian surface epithelial cells
- Ovarian cancer
- Resting primordial follicles
- Primary oocytes
- Follicle cells
- Pregranulosa cells

- Gap junctions
- Ovarian reserve
- Follicular atresia
- Premature ovarian failure
- Kit ligand
- c-Kit
- Growth differentiation factor-9 (GDF-9)
- Bone morphogenetic protein-15 (BMP-15)
- Anti-müllerian hormone (AMH)
- Diplotene
- Germinal vesicle
- Preantral
- Antral cavity
- Primary follicle
- Secondary follicle
- Thecal cells
- Mature preantral follicle
- Zona pellucida
- ZP1, ZP2, ZP3 (glycoproteins)
- LH receptor
- FSH receptor
- Androgens
- Androstenedione
- Early antral follicles
- Antrum
- Mural granulosa cells
- Cumulus cells
- Cumulus oophorus
- Cumulus-oocyte complex
- Recruited
- Meiotic competence
- Meiotic arrest
- GPR3
- Inhibin B
- Ovulatory quota
- Selection
- Dominant follicle
- Preovulatory follicle
- LDL receptor
- HDL receptor
- CYP11A1 (side-chain cleavage enzyme)
- StAR protein
- 3β-hydroxysteroid dehydrogenase (3β-HSD)
- CYP17
- CYP19 (aromatase)
- Testosterone
- Estrone

- Estradiol-17β
- 17β-hydroxysteroid dehydrogenase (17β-HSD)
- Periovulatory period
- Luteinization
- Progesterone
- Stigma
- Cumulus expansion
- Membrane hyaluronidase
- Angiogenic factors
- Epidermal growth factor (EGF)-related paracrine factors
- Maturation-promoting factor (MPF)
- Cyclin-dependent kinase
- CDK1
- Cyclin B
- Metaphase II
- Cytostatic factor (CSF)
- c-Mos
- Mitogen-activated kinase kinase (MAPKK)
- MEP1
- MAPK
- In vitro fertilization (IVF)
- StAR protein
- Corpus hemorrhagicum
- Granulosa lutein cells
- Corpus luteum of menstruation
- Human chorionic gonadotropin (hCG)
- Corpus luteum of pregnancy
- Prostaglandin
- PGF$_{2\alpha}$
- Corpus albicans
- Inhibin A
- Luteal phase deficiency (LPD)
- Relaxin
- Follicular atresia
- Apoptosis
- Interstitial gland
- Luteal phase
- Luteolysis
- GnRH receptors
- Germinal vesicle breakdown (GVBD)
- Oviducts
- Uterine tubes
- Fallopian tubes
- Infundibulum (of oviduct)
- Fimbriae
- Ampulla (of oviduct)

- Isthmus (of oviduct)
- Intramural (uterine) segment (of oviduct)
- Ampullary-isthmus junction
- Endosalpinx
- Myosalpinx
- Perisalpinx
- Ciliated cells (of oviduct)
- Secretory cells (of oviduct)
- Immotile cilia syndrome
- Kartagener syndrome
- Ectopic implantation
- Uterus
- Endometrium
- Myometrium
- Perimetrium
- Fundus (of uterus)
- Body (of uterus)
- Isthmus (of uterus)
- Cervix
- Vagina
- Uterine glands
- Spiral arteries
- Uterine artery
- Venous lakes (lacunae)
- Functional zone (stratum functionalis)
- Basal zone (stratum basale)
- Predecidual cells
- Inactivating isoforms of 17β-hydroxysteroid dehydrogenase
- Unopposed estrogen
- Period
- Menorrhagia
- Dysmenorrhea
- Oligomenorrhea
- Amenorrhea
- Matrix metalloproteases
- Leukocytes
- Cyclooxygenase-2 (COX-2)
- Uterine fibroids
- Leiomyoma
- Endocervical canal
- Ectocervix
- Endocervix
- Internal cervical os
- External cervical os
- Superimplantation
- Cervical softening and dilation

- Cervical mucus
- Spinnbarkeit
- Ferning
- Labia majora
- Mons pubis
- Vulva
- Labia minora
- Clitoris
- Vestibule of the vagina
- Vestibular bulbs
- External urethral orifice
- Corpora cavernosa (of clitoris)
- Glans (of clitoris)
- Estrogen receptor (ER)
- Progesterone receptor (PR)
- Estrogen-response element (ERE)
- Progesterone-response element (PRE)
- Co-activator proteins
- Selective estrogen receptor modulators (SERMs)
- Tamoxifen
- Raloxifene
- ER antagonist
- ER agonist
- "Nongenomic" signaling
- "Membrane-initiated" signaling
- GPR30
- Bone anabolic effect
- Calciotropic effect
- Circulating lipoprotein profiles
- Vasodilation
- Nitric oxide
- ER single-nucleotide polymorphisms
- Neuroprotective
- Body temperature
- Premenstrual dysphoria
- Premenstrual syndrome (PMS)
- Natriuretic action
- Lipolytic effect
- Sex hormone–binding globulin (SHBG)
- Cortisol-binding globulin (CBG)
- Transcortin
- Peripheral aromatization of androgens
- Aromatase inhibitors
- Sulfate/glucuronide conjugation
- Müllerian ducts
- Urogenital sinus
- Genital folds
- Genital swelling
- Genital tubercle
- Leptin
- Menarche
- Adrenarche
- Pubic hair
- Axillary hair
- Lobuloalveolar structures
- Nipple
- Fat pads
- Areola
- Thelarche
- Estrogen deficiency
- Bone loss
- Osteoporosis
- Cardiovascular disease
- Hot flashes
- Women's Health Initiative
- Hormone replacement therapy
- Turner syndrome
- Gonadal dysgenesis
- Polycystic ovarian syndrome (PCOS)
- Excessive androgen secretion
- Polycystic ovaries
- Sonogram
- Hirsutism
- Acne

SELF-STUDY PROBLEMS

1. During treatment for in vitro fertilization, the patient receives a daily injection of FSH for 8 to 10 days, followed by one injection of hCG. Cumulus-oocyte complexes are retrieved 35 hours after the hCG injection from ovarian follicles just before they ovulate. Because oocytes are retrieved *before* ovulation, and patients are treated with *progesterone after retrieval*, what is the purpose of the hCG injection?

2. When and in what cells is the LH receptor expressed during the menstrual cycle? How may a defect in FSH signaling that failed to up-regulate LH receptor expression affect ovarian function?

3. Describe the major ovarian processes that occur during the periovulatory period.

4. What is meant by the "two-cell model" of ovarian steroidogenesis?

5. Name three effects of estrogen on reproductive tissue, and three effects on nonreproductive tissue.

6. What would be the outcome of luteal phase deficiency (with early death of the corpus luteum) on the uterine endometrium?

7. What is the relationship of the ovarian reserve to the ovulatory quota in humans?

8. What organs would be affected in dysgenesis of the müllerian ducts before female differentiation?

9. What is the response of the pituitary gonadotropes to the death of a corpus luteum of menstruation?

10. What is the response of the ovary to declining FSH levels during the early folliclular phase?

BIBLIOGRAPHY

Deroso BJ, Korach KS: Estrogen receptors and human disease, *J Clin Invest* 116:561-570, 2006.

Eppig JJ, et al: Regulation of mammalian oocyte maturation. In Leung PCK, Adashi EY, editors: *The ovary*, ed 2, San Diego, 2004, Elsevier/Academic Press, pp 113-143.

Gougeon A: Dynamics of human follicular growth: morphologic, dynamic and functional aspects. In Leung PCK, Adashi EY, editors: *The ovary*, ed 2, San Diego, 2004, Elsevier/ Academic Press, pp 25-43.

Jabbour HN, Kelly RW, Fraser HM, Critchley HOD: Endocrine regulation of menstruation, *Endocr Rev* 27:17-46, 2006.

Lewis JS, Jordan VC: Selective estrogen receptor modulators (SERMs): mechanisms of anticarcinogenesis and drug resistance, *Mutation Res* 591:247-263, 2005.

Mehlmann L: Stops and starts in mammalian oocytes: recent advances in understanding the regulation of meiotic arrest and oocyte maturation, *Reproduction* 130:791-799, 2005.

Murphy BD: Luteinization. In Leung PCK, Adashi EY, editors: *The ovary*, ed 2, San Diego, 2004, Elsevier/Academic Press, pp 185-199.

Reproductive endocrine female, UpToDate Online 14.1. Available at: *www.uptodate.com*

Strauss J III, Coutifaris C: The endometrium and myometrium: regulation and dysfunction. In Yen SSC, Jaffe RB, Barbieri RL, editors: *Reproductive endocrinology*, ed 4, Philadelphia, 1999, WB Saunders, pp 218-256.

Yen SSC: The human menstrual cycle: neuroendocrine regulation. In Yen SSC, Jaffe RB, Barbieri RL, editors: *Reproductive endocrinology*, ed 4, Philadelphia, 1999, WB Saunders, pp 191-217.

10 FERTILIZATION AND PREGNANCY

OBJECTIVES

1. Describe the synchronization among fertilization, early embryonic events, and the human menstrual cycle.
2. Describe the events involved in fertilization.
3. Explain how implantation and placentation occur.
4. Discuss the endocrine and transport functions of the placenta.
5. Describe the development of the fetal endocrine system.
6. Discuss maternal endocrine changes during pregnancy.
7. Discuss the current models for the initiation and progression of labor (parturition) in humans.
8. Describe the development and regulation of the mammary glands.
9. Discuss the endocrine basis for contraception, the "morning after" pill, the abortion pill, and in vitro fertilization technology.

Human reproduction involves internal insemination, internal fertilization, and internal gestation, all within the female tract. Internal gestation also involves the development of a transient organ, the **placenta.** The placenta is remarkable in that it is composed of tissues from two organisms: (1) an extraembryonic membrane (called the **chorion**) of the fetus and (2) endometrial tissue (called **decidua**) of the mother. From an endocrine point of view, pregnancy represents a state in which three separate endocrine systems—maternal, fetal, and placental—interact to promote adequate growth and nutrition of the fetus, the timing of parturition, and preparation of the maternal mammary glands to support extrauterine life of the fetus.

FERTILIZATION, EARLY EMBRYOGENESIS, IMPLANTATION, AND PLACENTATION

Synchronization with Maternal Ovarian and Reproductive Tract Function

Fertilization, early embryogenesis, implantation, and early gestation all are synchronized with the human menstrual cycle (Figure 10-1). Just before ovulation, the ovary is in the late follicular stage and produces high levels of estrogen. Estrogen promotes growth of the uterine endometrium and induces expression of the progesterone receptor. Estrogen ultimately induces the luteininzing hormone (LH) surge, which in turn induces meiotic maturation of the oocyte and ovulation of the cumulus-oocyte complex.

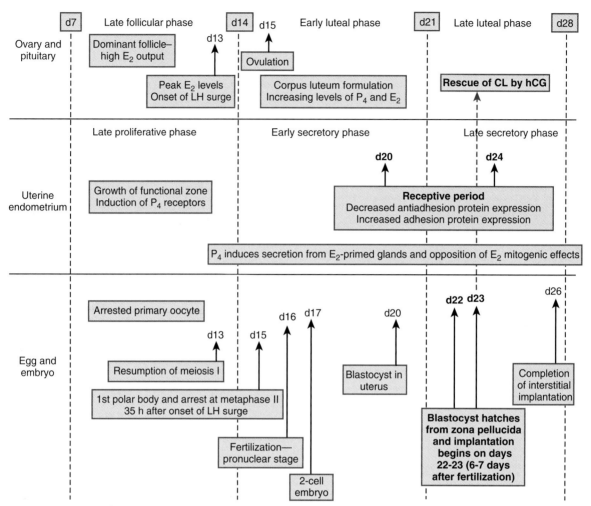

FIGURE 10-1 ■ Synchronization of the human menstrual cycle with fertilization and early embryogenesis. CL, corpus luteum; E, estrogen; E_2, estrone; hCG, human chorionic gonadotropin; LH, luteinizing hormone; P_4, progesterone.

The events between fertilization and implantation take about 6 days to complete, so that implantation occurs at about day 22 of the menstrual cycle. At this time, the ovary is in the mid luteal phase, secreting large amounts of progesterone. Progesterone stimulates secretion from uterine glands, which provide nutrients to the embryo. This is referred to as **histiotrophic nutrition** and is an important mode of maternal-to-fetal transfer of nutrients for about the first trimester of pregnancy, after which it is replaced by **hemotropic nutrition** (see later). Progesterone inhibits myometrial contraction and prevents the release of paracrine

factors (e.g., cytokines, prostaglandins, chemokines, vasoconstrictors) that lead to menstruation. Progesterone induces the "**window of receptivity**" in the uterine endometrium, which exists from about day 20 to 24 of the menstrual cycle. This receptive phase is associated with increased adhesivity of the endometrial epithelium and involves the formation of cellular extensions, called pinopodes, on the apical surface of endometrial epithelia, along with increased expression of adhesive proteins (e.g., integrins, cadherins) and decreased expression of antiadhesive proteins (e.g., mucins) in the apical cell membrane.

Thus, during the time it takes a fertilized egg to implant in the uterus, the uterine endometrium is at its full thickness, actively secretory, and capable of tightly adhering to the implanting embryo. It also should be noted that the uterine endometrium is well vascularized at the time of implantation. **Spiral arteries** extend to the basal lamina of the surface epithelium (see Figure 9-19) and give rise to rich capillary beds and postcapillary **venous lakes** (also called **lacunae**). Apart from its nutrient supply to all cells of the endometrium, the extensive blood supply immediately adjacent to the surface epithelium plays a critical role in capturing embryonic **human chorionic gonadotropin (hCG)** and transporting hCG to the ovary, where it "rescues" the corpus luteum. The rich endometrial blood supply also is important for efficient delivery of progesterone to the endometrium.

Fertilization

Fertilization accomplishes both the recombination of genetic material to form a new, genetically distinct organism and the initiation of events that begin embryonic development. There are several steps that must occur for successful fertilization to be achieved. The sperm must find its way to the egg, and the sperm and the egg must contact, recognize one another, and fuse. After sperm-egg fusion, an intracellular signaling cascade occurs within the egg that has two major consequences. First, it allows the egg to regulate sperm entry such that only one sperm can fuse with the egg. This prevention of **polyspermy** is critical for further development, because the fusion of more than one sperm with the egg is lethal. Second, it "wakes up" the metabolically quiescent egg so that it can resume meiosis and begin embryonic development. This process is called **egg activation**.

Spermatozoa present in the male ejaculate enter the vagina near the cervix and must reach the ampulla of the oviduct, or fallopian tube, where fertilization occurs. Sperm transport is largely dependent on the female reproductive tract and, while the sperm are still in the uterus, is independent of swimming. In fact, sperm can be found in the oviduct within several minutes after ejaculation, and this would be physically impossible if transport through the uterus depended on sperm swimming alone. Large numbers of sperm

in the ejaculate generally are required for successful fertilization of the egg by one sperm—of the 300 million sperm typically ejaculated, only about 200 reach the oviduct. Clinically, males with fewer than 20 million sperm per milliliter of ejaculate are considered to be infertile. The requirement for so many sperm is due to the large area that needs to be covered and the fact that a large proportion of sperm do not even make it through the cervix; of those that do, many are lost along the way.

The female reproductive tract is an important regulator of sperm transport. Toward the end of the follicular phase of the menstrual cycle, before ovulation, estrogen levels are high. Estrogen causes the cervix to produce a watery mucus, often called "egg white cervical mucus" because of its consistency (see Figure 9-21). This mucus forms channels to aid the passage of sperm through the cervix, and only motile sperm can pass through this barrier. Estrogen also causes contractions of the myometrium to help propel sperm upward toward the oviduct (i.e., cervical-to-fundal contractions). In addition to hormonal regulation of sperm transport, the state of sexual arousal in the woman can aid in the process of sperm transport. Increased blood flow to the genitals during arousal produces a vaginal transudate that neutralizes the acidic pH of the vagina and increases oxygen tension, which is beneficial for sperm metabolism. Vaginal tenting occurs during sexual arousal, which draws the cervix away from the vagina, creating a localized reservoir for sperm.

Sperm must undergo a process called **capacitation** in the female reproductive tract before they are able to fertilize the egg. Sperm capacitation is an incompletely understood, transient event that occurs largely in the oviduct and modifies the spermatozoan in several ways so that it becomes capable of fertilizing the egg. These changes include the following:

1. An altered membrane fluidity due to the removal of cholesterol from the sperm membrane
2. The removal of proteins and/or carbohydrates from the membrane that may otherwise block sites that bind to the egg
3. A change in membrane potential that may permit Ca^{2+} to enter the sperm and thereby facilitate the acrosome reaction (see later)
4. Numerous protein phosphorylations

Uncapacitated sperm bind actively to the epithelial cells of the oviductal isthmus and become unbound when they are capacitated. This binding slows down the capacitation process, extends the sperm life span, prevents too many sperm from reaching the egg, and increases the probability that sperm will be in the oviduct when the egg is ovulated. Sperm can therefore survive in the female reproductive tract for several days. **Hyperactivation** is another phenomenon associated with sperm capacitation. Hyperactivation involves a change in flagellar motion from a wavelike to a whip-like motion. This type of flagellar movement is necessary for the sperm to detach from the oviductal epithelium, is well suited to swimming through the thick oviductal fluid, and helps propel the sperm through the outer layers of the egg to reach the egg's plasma membrane.

Capacitated sperm reach the egg, surrounded by its expanded cumulus cells, in the ampulla of the oviduct. Fertilization involves the penetration of the egg by the entire sperm. To do this, the sperm must breach three barriers (refer to Figure 10-2): the expanded cumulus, the zona pellucida, and the plasma membrane of the egg (called the oolemma). The cumulus cell matrix is composed predominantly of hyaluronic acid, and the sperm are able to digest through this layer with a membrane-bound **hyaluronidase** called **PH-20**. The next obstacle the sperm encounters is the **zona pellucida**, an extracellular coat made up of three glycoproteins called **ZP1**, **ZP2**, and **ZP3**. The sperm contains a receptor(s) that binds to ZP3. This binding triggers the **acrosome reaction**, in which the inner sperm plasma membrane fuses with the outer acrosomal membrane to release the contents of the acrosomal vesicle (see Figure 10-2). The enzymes released from the acrosomal vesicle then digest the zona pellucida. The acrosome reaction is a complex, Ca^{2+}-dependent secretory event. After the acrosome reaction, the sperm loses the receptors that bind to ZP3, and it undergoes a secondary binding instead to ZP2. The sperm is thus held in place as the enzymes from the acrosome digest a hole in the zona pellucida and the still-swimming sperm can go through to reach the egg plasma membrane. The molecular mechanisms involved in the interactions of the sperm and egg plasma membranes are not completely understood. Sperm-egg binding precedes membrane fusion, but so far no definitive candidates have been identified that mediate this process.

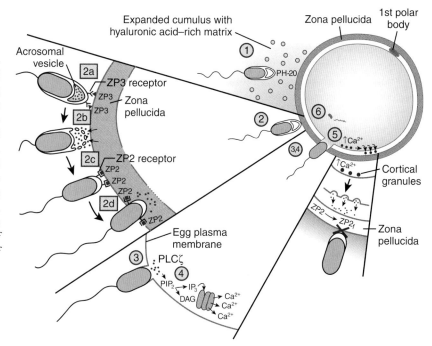

FIGURE 10-2 ■ Events of fertilization: 1, penetration of expanded cumulus; 2, acrosome reaction; 3, fusion of sperm membrane with egg membrane and 4, egg activation; 5, exocytosis of cortical granules and block to polyspermy. DAG, diacylglycerol; IP_3, inositol 1,4,5-triphosphate; PIP_3, phosphatidylinositol 4,5-biphosphate; PLCζ, phospholipase Cζ; ZP2, ZP3, zona pellucida glycoproteins 2 and 3; $ZP2_f$. *(Courtesy of Dr. Lisa Mehlmann, Department of Cell Biology, UConn Health Center, Farmington, Conn.)*

Sperm-egg fusion is likely to resemble a **viral fusion event** and involves the **tetraspanin proteins** CD9 and CD81 in the egg that bind to a sperm protein called **Izumo** (see Figure 10-2).

The entire sperm enters the egg during fusion. The flagellum and mitochondria disintegrate, so most of the mitochondrial DNA in cells is maternally derived. Once the sperm is inside the egg, protamines associated with the tightly condensed sperm DNA are uncoiled by the highly reducing egg cytoplasm, causing **decondensation** of the sperm DNA. A membrane called the **pronucleus** forms around the sperm DNA as the newly activated egg completes the second meiotic division.

The egg is a metabolically quiescent cell that is "woken up" as a result of sperm-egg fusion, in a process called egg activation. Egg activation allows the egg to prevent **polyspermy**, initiates the completion of meiosis so that it finally becomes a truly haploid cell, and stimulates the recruitment of maternal RNAs necessary for embryonic development. All of these events depend on intracellular release of Ca^{2+} in the egg, which occurs soon after sperm-egg fusion. Although the earliest molecular events that stimulate the signaling cascade leading to Ca^{2+} release are not completely understood, ultimately Ca^{2+} release is stimulated by the production of inositol 1,4,5-triphosphate (IP_3). It is currently thought that the sperm contains a specialized phospholipase C enzyme, called PLCζ, that is released into the egg cytoplasm following sperm-egg fusion. PLCζ hydrolyzes phosphatidylinositol 4,5-biphosphate (PIP_3) in the egg's plasma membrane to produce diacylglycerol (DAG) and IP_3. IP_3 binds to a receptor on the egg's endoplasmic reticulum and opens Ca^{2+} channels, so that Ca^{2+} stored in the endoplasmic reticulum enters the cytoplasm (refer to Chapter 1 for discussion of this signaling pathway). In mammalian eggs, a large initial release of Ca^{2+} is followed by a series of subsequent, smaller Ca^{2+} oscillations that can last for hours. The events stimulated by Ca^{2+} release depend on the number of Ca^{2+} oscillations produced, with some events require only a few transients and others requiring several.

One of the earliest Ca^{2+}-dependent events that occurs at fertilization of mammalian eggs is the prevention of polyspermy. Enzyme-filled vesicles, called **cortical granules**, reside in the outermost, or cortical, region of the unfertilized egg. These vesicles translocate to the plasma membrane and are exocytosed shortly after fertilization. The exocytotic machinery responsible for granule exocytosis is complex but is dependent on fertilization-induced Ca^{2+} release; preventing Ca^{2+} release at fertilization experimentally completely blocks the release of cortical granules, and the eggs become polyspermic. The enzymes contained in the cortical granules are released to the outside of the egg on exocystosis. These enzymes modify both ZP2 and ZP3 of the zona pellucida, such that ZP2 can no longer bind acrosome-reacted sperm and ZP3 can no longer bind capacitated, acrosome-intact sperm. Thus, only one sperm usually enters the egg. Occasionally, more than one sperm does enter the egg. This results in a triploid cell, which is unable to develop further. Therefore, polyspermy prevention is critical for the normal development of the fertilized egg.

Ca^{2+} release also stimulates the egg to reenter the cell cycle, complete meiosis, and recruit maternal mRNAs following fertilization. The unfertilized egg is held in meiotic arrest at metaphase II by the cell cycle regulatory protein complex, **maturation-promoting factor (MPF)**, as well as cytostatic **factor (CSF)**, which contains components of the mitogen-activating protein kinase (MAPK) pathway. These proteins keep the metaphase II chromosomes tightly condensed and inactivate the anaphase-promoting complex that is necessary for the progression of meiosis from metaphase to anaphase. Ca^{2+} release at fertilization activates Ca^{2+}/calmodulin-dependent protein kinase II (CaMKII), which has downstream effects to inactivate both MPF and CSF such that the metaphase II chromosomes decondense, the anaphase-promoting complex becomes active, and the egg can form a pronucleus. The unfertilized egg is transcriptionally inactive, and Ca^{2+} release at fertilization also is needed for the recruitment of stored maternal mRNAs. Thus, the newly fertilized egg is able to synthesize proteins needed for early embryonic development.

The activated egg completes the second meiotic division as the sperm DNA decondenses and a pronucleus forms around it (Figure 10-3). Once the egg has completed meiosis, a pronucleus forms around the female chromosomes as well. A **centrosome**, contributed by the sperm, becomes a microtubule-organizing center from which microtubules extend until they contact the female pronucleus. The male and female DNAs replicate as the two pronuclei are

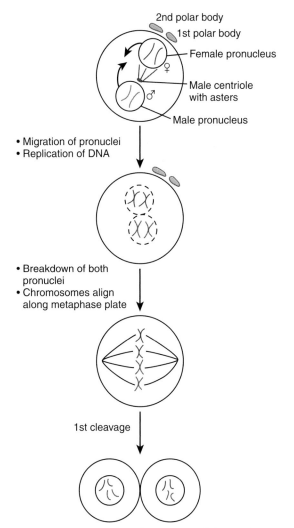

2nd polar body
1st polar body
Female pronucleus
♀
Male centriole
with asters
♂
Male pronucleus

• Migration of pronuclei
• Replication of DNA

• Breakdown of both
  pronuclei
• Chromosomes align
  along metaphase plate

1st cleavage

FIGURE 10-3 ■ Pronuclear formation and first embryonic cleavage.

pulled together. Once the pronuclei contact each other, the nuclear membranes break down, the chromosomes align on a common metaphase plate, and the first cleavage occurs.

Early Embryogenesis and Implantation

Fertilization typically occurs on day 16 or 17 of the menstrual cycle, and implantation occurs about 6 days later. Thus, the first week of embryogenesis occurs within the lumina of the oviduct and uterus (Figure 10-4).

For most of this time, the embryo remains encapsulated by the zona pellucida. The first two cleavages take about 2 days, and the embryo reaches a 16-cell **morula** by 3 days. The outer cells of the morula become tightly adhesive with each other and begin transporting fluid into the embryonic mass. During days 4 and 5, the transport of fluid generates a cavity, called the blastocyst cavity, and the embryo is now called a **blastocyst** (Figure 10-5). The blastocyst is composed of two subpopulations of cells: (1) the eccentric **inner cell mass** and (2) an outer, epithelial-like layer of **trophoblasts**. The region of trophoblast layer immediately adjacent to the inner cell mass is referred to as the **embryonic pole**, and it is this region that attaches to the uterine endometrium at implantation (see Figure 10-5).

The embryo resides within the oviduct during the first 3 days and then enters the uterus. By 5 to 6 days of development, the trophoblasts of the blastocyst secrete proteases that digest the outerlying zona pellucida. At this point, corresponding to about day 22 of the menstrual cycle, the "**hatched**" **blastocyst** is able to adhere to and implant into the receptive uterine endometrium (Figure 10-6).

At the time of attachment and implantation, the trophoblasts differentiate into two cell types: an inner layer of **cytotrophoblasts** and an outer layer of multinuclear/multicellular **syncytiotrophoblasts** (Figure 10-7). The cytotrophoblasts initially provide a feeder layer of continuously dividing cells. Syncytiotrophoblasts initially perform three general types of functions: adhesive, invasive, and endocrine. Syncytiotrophoblasts express adhesive surface proteins (i.e., cadherins and integrins) that bind to uterine surface epithelia and, as the embryo implants, to components of the uterine extracellular matrix. In humans, the embryo completely burrows into the superficial layer of the endometrium (see Figure 10-7). This mode of implantation, called **interstitial implantation**, is the most invasive among placental mammals. Invasive implantation involves adhesion-supported migration of syncytiotrophoblasts into the endometrium, along with the breakdown of extracellular matrix by the secretion of matrix metalloproteases and other hydrolytic enzymes.

The endocrine function begins with the onset of implantation, when syncytiotrophoblasts begin secreting the LH-like protein **human chorionic**

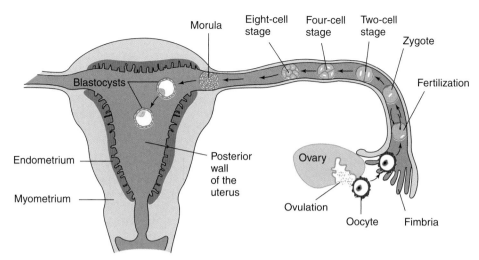

FIGURE 10-4 ■ Fertilization and human development during the first week.

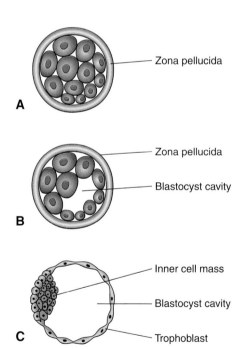

FIGURE 10-5 ■ Early cleavage stages in embryos. **A,** Morula. **B,** Early blastocyst with zona pellucida intact. **C,** Late blastocyst shows inner cell mass and blastocyst cavity.

gonadotropin (hCG) (see later), which maintains the viability of the corpus luteum and, thus, progesterone secretion. Syncytiotrophoblasts also become highly steroidogenic. By 10 weeks, the syncytiotrophoblasts acquire the ability to make progesterone at sufficient levels to maintain pregnancy independently of a corpus luteum. Syncytiotrophoblasts produce several other hormones (see later), as well as enzymes that modify hormones (e.g., 11β-hydroxysteroid dehydrogenase type 2) (see later).

As implantation and placentation progresses, syncytiotrophoblasts take on the important functions of phagocytosis (during histiotropic nutrition) and bidirectional placental transfer of gases, nutrients, and wastes (see later). Exchange across the syncytiotrophoblasts involves diffusion (e.g., gases), facilitated transport (e.g., GLUT-1–mediated transfer of glucose), active transport (e.g., amino acids by specific transporters), and pinocytosis/transcytosis (e.g., of iron-transferrin complexes).

There also is a maternal response to implantation, which involves the transformation of the endometrial stroma. This response, called **decidualization**, involves an enlargement of stromal cells as they become lipid- and glycogen-filled decidual cells (at this time, the endometrium is referred to as the **decidua**). The decidua forms an epithelial-like sheet with adhesive junctions that inhibit migration of the

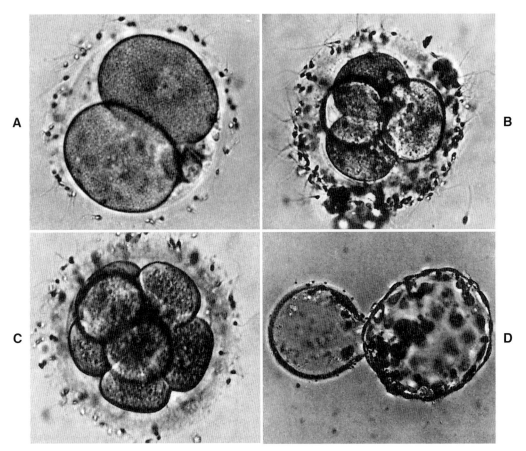

FIGURE 10-6 ■ Cleavage stages of human eggs fertilized in vitro. **A,** Two cells 39 hours after fertilization. Polar body is at right of boundary between the two cells. **B,** Four cells 42 hours after fertilization. **C,** Eight cells 49 hours after fertilization. **D,** Hatching blastocyst 123 hours after fertilization. In **A** to **C,** numerous spermatozoa can be seen clinging to zona pellucida. *(From Veeck LL: Atlas of the human oocyte and early conceptus, vol 2, Baltimore, 1991, Williams & Wilkins.)*

implanting embryo. The decidua also secretes factors, such as **tissue inhibitors of metalloproteases (TIMPs)**, that moderate the activity of syncytiotrophoblastic-derived hydrolytic enzymes in the endometrial matrix. Consequently, decidualization allows for regulated invasion during implantation. Normally, the implanting embryo and placenta do not extend to and involve the myometrium. **Placenta accreta** is the destruction of the endometrium and adherence of the placenta to the myometrium, a condition associated with potentially life-threatening postpartum hemorrhage. It is important to note that the decidual response occurs only in the uterus. Thus, the

highly invasive nature of the human embryo poses considerable risk to the mother in the case of **ectopic implantations**. The most common site of ectopic implantation is the oviduct (giving rise to a **tubal pregnancy**), but implantations also rarely occur in the ovary and cervix and within the abdominal cavity.

Structure of Mature Placenta

The progression of placental development is complicated, and the reader is referred to embryology texts for a more complete discussion than the one presented here (see Bibliography). It is useful to consider placental

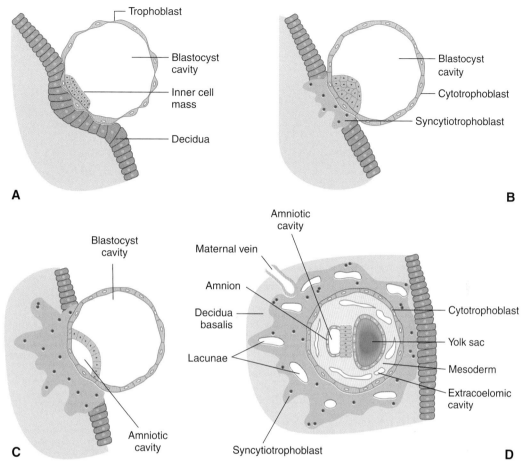

FIGURE 10-7 ■ Steps in implantation. **A,** Early implantation of blastocyst. **B,** Formation of cytotrophoblast and syncytiotrophoblast. **C,** Formation of amniotic cavity. **D,** Formation of lacunae with maternal venous penetration.

development with a focus first on the entire gravid uterus and then on the fine structure of the mature placenta.

Initially, the growing syncytiotrophoblasts extend evenly from the embryo into the outerlying decidua. At about 9 days, spaces appear within the syncytiotrophoblast layer, called **lacunae**. These spaces become filled with the secretions of endometrial glands, maternal blood, and the remnants of enzymatically digested matrix, referred to as the **embryotroph**, which provides for histiotropic nutrition. (Figure 10-8). By the end of the second week of development, the columns of syncytiotrophoblasts with a core of cytotrophoblasts are distinguishable as **primary villi** (Figure 10-9). By this time, a new extraembryonic layer, called **extraembryonic mesoderm**, becomes associated with the cytotrophoblast and syncytiotrophoblast layers. The three layers are now referred to as the **chorionic membrane**. Once primary villi gain a mesodermal core, they are referred to as **secondary villi**. The extraembryonic mesoderm provides a connection, called the **connecting stalk**, between the chorion and the embryo. It is within this mesoderm that the fetal (**umbilical**) circulation develops, carrying nutrients from the syncytiotrophoblast layer to the fetus, and wastes from the fetus to the maternal blood. Once villi

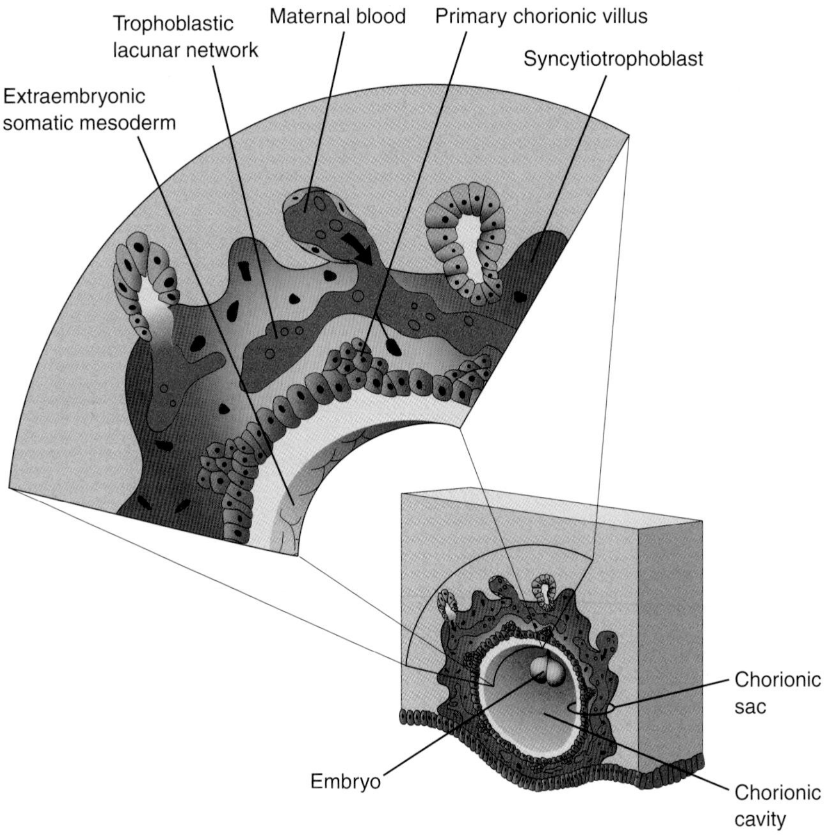

Trophoblastic
lacunar network   Maternal blood   Primary chorionic villus

Extraembryonic
somatic mesoderm   Syncytiotrophoblast

FIGURE 10-8 ■ Histiotropic nutrition (*arrows*) as the endometrial glands and spiral arteries are invaded and eroded by advancing syncytiotrophoblasts (at 14 days). (*Modified from Moore KL, Persaud TVN: The developing human: clinically oriented embryology, Philadelphia, 2003, Saunders.*)

Chorionic
sac

Embryo

Chorionic
cavity

FIGURE 10-9 ■ Development of primary (1°), secondary (2°), and tertiary (3°) villi. CTB, cytotrophoblast; FBVs, fetal blood vessels; STB, syncytiotrophoblast.

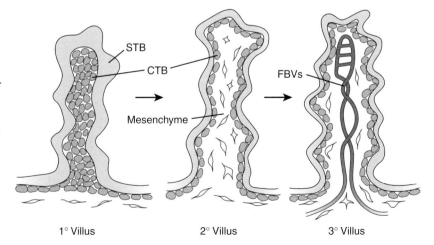

STB

CTB

FBVs

Mesenchyme

1° Villus   2° Villus   3° Villus

contain fetal blood vessels, they are referred to as **terti-ary villi** (see Figure 10-9). Chorionic villi only represent the functional unit of the placenta and, through extensive branching, greatly increase the surface area for maternal-fetal exchange. Although villi develop from the entire spherical chorionic membrane, they quickly degenerate around most of the chorion, forming a **smooth chorion**, or the **chorion laeve** (Figure 10-10). In the region of the original embryonic pole, however, the chorion develops into a highly branching **villous chorion**, called the **chorion frondosum** (see Figure 10-10). The chorion frondosum represents the fetal side of the mature placenta.

The uterine decidua immediately apposed to the chorion frondosum is called the **decidua basalis** and forms the maternal side of the mature placenta (see Figure 10-10). The decidua that is apposed to the chorion laeve is called the **decidua capsularis**.

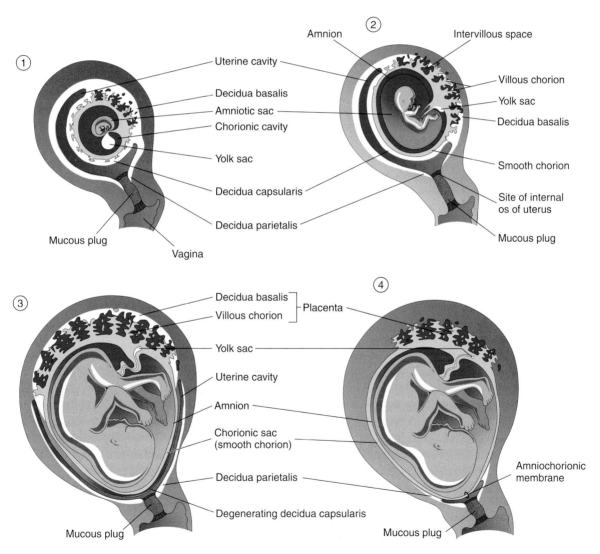

FIGURE 10-10 ■ Development and fusion of fetal membranes and decidua. *(From Moore KL, Persaud TVN: The developing human: clinically oriented embryology, Philadelphia, 2003, Saunders.)*

The decidua capsularis greatly increases in surface area as the fetus grows. With time, the decidua capsularis fuses with the **decidua parietalis**, which is the part of the uterine endometrium that is not directly associated with the chorionic membrane. This means that the original uterine lumen is obliterated. The decidua capsularis ultimately degenerates.

Another extraembryonic membrane, called the **amnion**, grows and surrounds the developing fetus. The amnion becomes a fluid-filled sac, allowing for a nonadhesive environment in which the fetus can develop. By the beginning of the third trimester, the amnion fuses with the chorion, forming the **amnio-chorionic membrane**, which in turn fuses with the decidua parietalis (see Figure 10-10). With the disappearance of the decidua capsularis, only the fetal amniochorionic membrane stretches across the internal opening of the cervical canal, and it is the amniochorionic membrane that ruptures during childbirth.

The mature placenta (Figure 10-11) is composed of three major structures:

1. The **chorionic villi**, which are lined externally by the syncytiotrophoblast layer and contain the termini of umbilical blood vessels within their core. As chorionic villi branch, they become increasingly smaller, thinner, and more involved in maternal-fetal exchange. The smallest villi, called **terminal villi**, are the predominant sites of maternal-fetal exchange (Figure 10-12). Terminal villi have an outer layer of syncytiotrophoblasts, which becomes extremely thin in certain regions. Subjacent to the thinnest regions of syncytiotrophoblasts, the cytotrophoblasts have disappeared, and a fetal capillary is pressed against the syncytiotrophoblast layer. Thus, nutrients from the maternal blood that bathes the terminal villi (see **intervillous space** in next entry) have to cross only a single, flat layer of syncytiotrophoblast, the fused

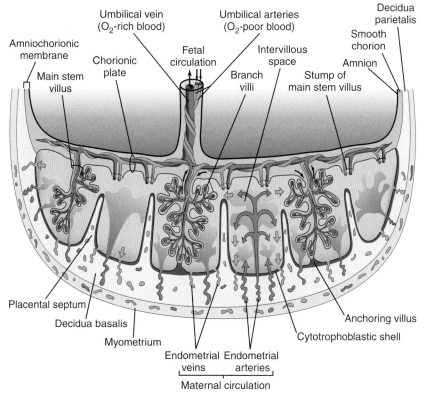

FIGURE 10-11 ■ Structure of the mature hemochorial placenta. Villi have been removed in some segments to show flow of maternal blood. *(From Moore KL, Persaud TVN: The developing human: clinically oriented embryology, Philadelphia, 2003, Saunders.)*

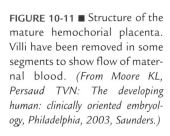

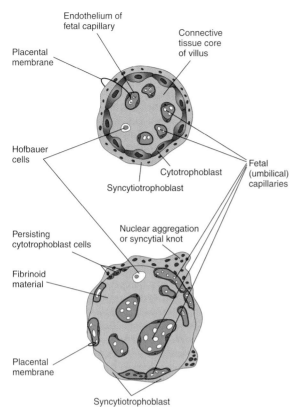

FIGURE 10-12 ■ Cross-section of an early (*upper*) and mature (*lower*) terminal villi. In the mature terminal villus, the cytotrophoblast layer becomes discontinuous, the fetal vessels assume an eccentric position subjacent to the syncytiotrophoblast layer, and the syncytiotrophoblast becomes very thinned out except for nuclear aggregations (also called syncytial knots). (*From Moore KL, Persaud TVN: The developing human: clinically oriented embryology, Philadelphia, 2003, Saunders.*)

basal lamina of the syncytiotrophoblast and capillary endothelium, and a flattened fetal endothelial cell. This barrier between maternal blood and the umbilical circulation is called the **placental membrane** (see Figure 10-12) and is called a **vasculosyncytial membrane**. It represents the thinnest barrier to maternal-fetal exchange among placental (i.e., **eutherian**) mammals.

2. The **intervillous space**, into which maternal blood flows from the open ends of spiral arteries (see Figure 10-11). This blood bathes the chorionic villi and returns to maternal circulation via endometrial veins. Because the maternal side of the placenta is represented by maternal blood within the intervillous space, and the fetal side is represented by the vasculosyncytial membrane, human placentation is referred to as **hemochorial placentation**.

3. The **decidua basalis**. Some villi, called anchoring villi, extend through the intervillous space and anchor onto the decidua. Columns of cytotrophoblasts migrate out of the end of the anchoring villi and spread across the decidua basalis. These extravillous cytotrophoblasts form an adhesive layer, called the **cytotrophoblastic shell**, that anchors the chorion frondosum to the decidua basalis (see Figure 10-11). Spiral arteries extend through the decidua basalis and open into the intervillous space through breaks in the cytotrophoblastic shell. During the first trimester, extravillous cytotrophoblasts migrate into the spiral arteries and plug them up. Thus, embryonic and early fetal development is supported primarily by histiotropic nutrition within a hypoxic environment. During this time, the cytotrophoblasts that have invaded the spiral arteries replace the tunica media and tunica intima, thereby converting the arteries into low-resistance, high-capacitance vessels. At the beginning of the second trimester, coincident with entry of the fetus into a rapid growth phase, the converted spiral arteries become unplugged, and hemotropic nutrition predominates until parturition. **Preeclampsia**, which is a form of **hypertension of pregnancy**, often is accompanied by a shallow invasion of the placenta and an inability of the cytotrophoblasts to convert the spiral arteries.

The Endocrine Function of the Placenta

The syncytiotrophoblasts of the placental produce several steroid and protein hormones. The general functions of these hormones in pregnancy include the following:

1. Maintain the pregnant state of the uterus
2. Stimulate lobuloalveolar growth and function of maternal breasts

3. Adapt aspects of maternal metabolism and physiology to support a growing fetus
4. Regulate aspects of fetal development
5. Regulate the timing and progression of parturition

Human Chorionic Gonadotropin

The first hormone produced by the syncytiotrophoblasts is **human chorionic gonadotropin (hCG)**. This hormone is structurally related to the pituitary glycoprotein hormones (see Chapter 5). As such, hCG is composed of a common **α-glycoprotein subunit (α-GSU)** and a **hormone-specific β subunit, β-hCG**. Antibodies used to detect hCG (as in laboratory assays and over-the-counter pregnancy tests) are designed to specifically detect the β subunit. Human chorionic gonadotropin is most similar to luteinizing hormone (LH) and binds with high affinity to the LH receptor. The β subunit of hCG is longer than that of LH and contains more sites for **glycosylation**, which greatly increases the half-life of hCG to 24 to 30 hours. The stability of hCG allows it to rapidly accumulate in the maternal circulation, so that hCG is detectable within maternal serum within 24 hours of implantation. Serum hCG levels double every 2 days for the first 6 weeks until they peak at about 10 weeks. Serum hCG then declines to a constant level at about 50% of the peak value (Figure 10-13).

The primary action of hCG is to stimulate LH receptors on the corpus luteum. This prevents luteolysis and maintains a high level of luteum-derived progesterone production during the first 10 weeks. The rapid increase in hCG is responsible for the nausea of "**morning sickness**" associated with early pregnancy. Human chorionic gonadotropin binds weakly to the thyrotropin (thyroid-stimulating hormone [TSH]) receptor, so that early pregnancy can be associated with a transient gestational hyperthyroidism. A small amount (i.e., 1% to 10%) of hCG enters into the fetal circulation. The hCG stimulates fetal Leydig cells to produce testosterone before the fetal gonadotropic axis is fully mature. It also stimulates the fetal adrenal cortex (see later) during the first trimester.

Human chorionic gonadotropin is produced in high levels by cancers derived from trophoblastic cells, such as **molar disease** and **choriocarcinoma**. Thus, hCG levels can be used as a measure of the efficacy of chemotherapy.

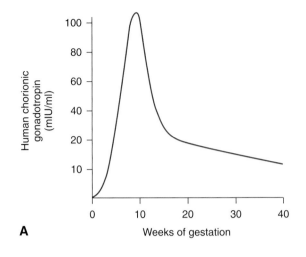

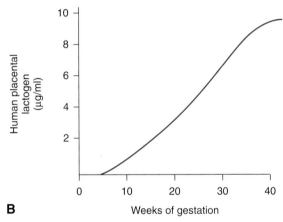

FIGURE 10-13 ■ Maternal serum human chorionic gonadotropin levels (**A**) and human placental lactogen levels (**B**) during pregnancy.

Progesterone

The syncytiotrophoblasts express high levels of CYP11A1 (side-chain cleavage enzyme) and a placenta-specific 3β-hydroxysteroid dehydrogenase (3β-HSD type 1) but do not express CYP17 (Figure 10-14). Syncytiotrophoblasts also express the receptors (e.g., low-density lipoprotein receptor) that import cholesterol from the maternal blood. Consequently, the placenta produces a high amount of **progesterone**, which is absolutely required to maintain a quiescent myometrium and a pregnant uterus. Progesterone production by the

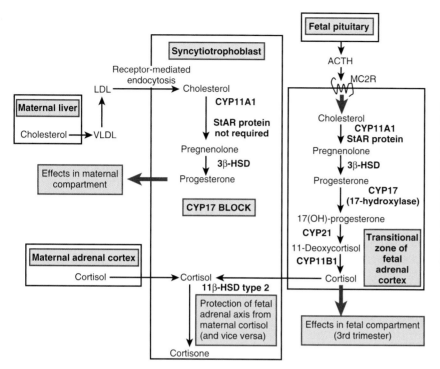

FIGURE 10-14 ■ Progesterone biosynthesis by the syncytiotrophoblast. ACTH, adrenocorticotropic hormone; 3β-HSD, 3β-hydroxysteroid dehydrogenase; 11β-HSD, 11β-hydroxysteroid dehydrogenase; LDL, low-density lipoprotein; MC2R, melanocortin-2 receptor (ACTH receptor); StAR protein, steroidogenic acute regulatory protein; VLDL, very-low-density lipoprotein.

placenta is largely unregulated—the placenta produces as much progesterone as the supply of cholesterol and the levels of CYP11A1 and 3β-HSD will allow. Of note, placental steroidogenesis differs from that in the adrenal cortex, ovaries, and testis, in that cholesterol is transported into the placental mitochondria by a mechanism that is independent of the labile steroidogenic acute regulatory (**StAR**) **protein**. Thus, this first step in steroidogenesis is not a regulated, rate-limiting step in the placenta as it is in other steroidogenic glands. This means that fetuses with an inactivating mutation in StAR protein will develop lipoid congenital adrenal hyperplasia (see Chapter 7) and hypogonadism, but will have normal progesterone levels produced by their placenta. It also should be noted that progesterone production by the placenta does not require fetal tissue. Consequently, progesterone levels are largely independent of fetal health status and cannot be used as a measure of fetal well-being. Maternal progesterone levels continue to increase throughout pregnancy (Figure 10-15).

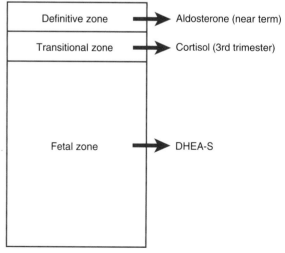

FIGURE 10-15 ■ The zones of the fetal adrenal cortex.

Progesterone is released primarily into the maternal circulation and is required for implantation and the maintenance of pregnancy. Progesterone also has several effects on maternal physiology and induces breast growth and differentiation (discussed later on). The switch from corpus luteum–derived progesterone to placenta-derived progesterone (referred to as the **luteal-placental shift**) is complete at about the eighth week of pregnancy. Progesterone, and also pregnenolone, are used by the transitional zone of the fetal cortex (see later) to make cortisol late in pregnancy.

Estrogen

Estrogens also are produced by the syncytiotrophoblasts. Syncytiotrophoblasts are similar to ovarian granulosa cells in that they lack CYP17 and are dependent on another cell type to provide 19-carbon androgens for aromatization. The ancillary, androgen-producing cell resides in the **fetal adrenal cortex**.

The fetal adrenal cortex contains an outer **definitive zone**, a middle **transitional zone**, and an inner **fetal zone** (see Figure 10-15). The definitive and transitional zones give rise to the zona glomerulosa and zona fasciculata, respectively. Aldosterone synthesis is initiated close to parturition. Cortisol synthesis begins at about 6 months and increases during late gestation. The fetal zone is the predominant portion of the adrenal cortex in the fetus, constituting as much as 80% of the bulk of the large fetal adrenal, and is the site of most fetal adrenal steroidogenesis. The fetal zone strongly resembles the zona reticularis, in that it expresses little or no 3β-hydroxysteroid dehydrogenase (Figure 10-16). The fetal zone releases primarily the sulfated form of the inactive androgen, **dehydroepiandrosterone sulfate (DHEA-S)**, throughout most of gestation. The production of DHEA-S from the fetal adrenal is absolutely dependent on fetal adrenocorticotropic hormone (ACTH) from the fetal pituitary by the end of the first trimester.

The DHEA-S released from the fetal zone has two fates. First, DHEA-S can go directly to the syncytiotrophoblast, where it is desulfated by a placental **steroid sulfatase** and used as a 19-carbon substrate for the synthesis of estradiol-17β and estrone (see Figure 10-16). The second fate of DHEA-S is **16-hydroxylation** in the fetal liver by the enzyme CYP3A7. 16-Hydroxyl-DHEA-S is then converted by the syncytiotrophoblasts

to the major estrogen of pregnancy, called **estriol** (see Figure 10-16).

Because estrogen production is dependent on a healthy fetus, estriol levels can be used to assess fetal well-being. The collective term used for the placental syncytiotrophoblasts and fetal organs in the context of estrogen production is the **fetoplacental unit**. Estrogens increase uteroplacental blood flow, enhance low-density lipoprotein (LDL) receptor expression in syncytiotrophoblasts, and induce several components (e.g., prostaglandins, oxytocin receptors) involved in parturition. Estrogens increase breast growth directly, and also indirectly through the stimulation of maternal pituitary prolactin production. Estrogens also increase lactotrope size and number, thereby increasing the overall pituitary mass more than twofold by term. Estrogens also affect several aspects of maternal physiology. Of note, in male fetuses with X-linked **steroid sulfatase deficiency**, the fetoplacental unit cannot make estrogens. This results in maternal estrogen levels that are an order of magnitude less than those in normal pregnancies. These babies typically are delivered by cesarean section, because the absence of estrogen results in a quiescent myometrium and a pregnancy that goes several weeks beyond the due date. Nevertheless, the pregnancy proceeds normally, and the newborn is normal except for the phenotype associated with sulfatase deficiency (ichthyosis).

Human Placental Lactogen

Human placental lactogen (hPL), also called **human chorionic somatomammotropin (hCS)**, is a 191-amino acid protein hormone produced in the syncytiotrophoblast that is structurally similar to growth hormone (GH) and prolactin (PRL). Its function overlaps those of both GH and PRL (Box 10-1). It can be detected within the syncytiotrophoblast by 10 days after conception and in maternal serum by 3 weeks of gestation (Figure 10-13). Maternal serum levels rise progressively throughout the remainder of the pregnancy. The quantity of hormone produced is directly related to the size of the placenta, so that as the placenta grows during gestation, hPL secretion increases. As much as 1 g/day of hPL can be secreted late in gestation.

Like GH, hPL is protein anabolic and lipolytic. Its antagonistic action to insulin is the major basis for the

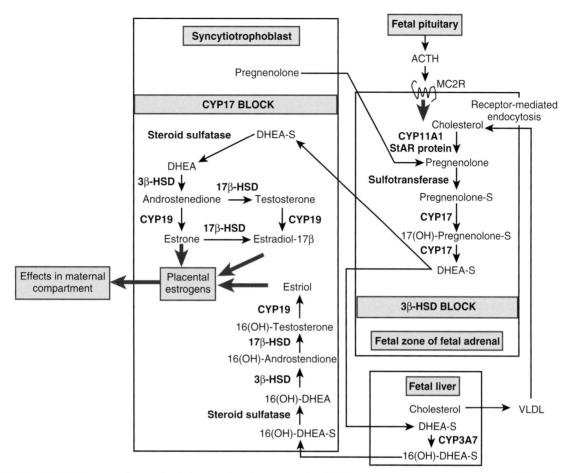

FIGURE 10-16 ■ Estrogen biosynthesis by the fetoplacental unit. ACTH, adrenocorticotropic hormone; DHEA, dehydroepiandrostenedione; DHEA-S, dehydroepiandrostenedione sulfate; 3β-HSD, 3β-hydroxysteroid dehydrogenase; 17β-HSD, 17β-hydroxysteroid dehydrogenase; MC2R, melanocortin-2 receptor (ACTH receptor); 16(OH)-, 16-hydroxy-; StAR protein, steroidogenic acute regulatory protein; VLDL, very-low-density lipoprotein.

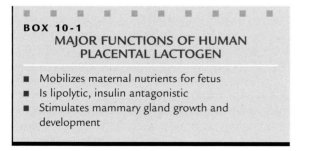

BOX 10-1

MAJOR FUNCTIONS OF HUMAN PLACENTAL LACTOGEN

- Mobilizes maternal nutrients for fetus
- Is lipolytic, insulin antagonistic
- Stimulates mammary gland growth and development

diabetogenicity of pregnancy. Like PRL, it stimulates mammary gland growth and development. Mammary gland development in pregnancy results from the actions of hPL, PRL, estrogens, and progestins. The hPL inhibits maternal glucose uptake and use, thereby increasing serum glucose levels. Glucose is a major energy substrate for the fetus, and hPL increases fetal glucose availability (Figure 10-17).

As with hCG, far less hPL is found in fetal circulation than in maternal circulation. This suggests that the hormones may play a more important role in the mother than in the fetus. Human placental lactogen is not essential for the pregnancy.

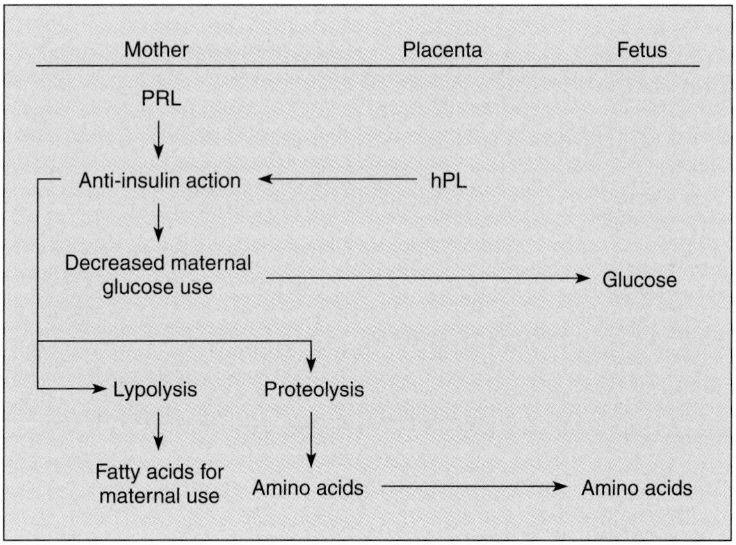

FIGURE 10-17 ■ Role of human placental lactogen (hPL) and prolactin (PRL) in altering maternal metabolism to provide amino acids and glucose to fetus.

Both hPL and PRL act as fetal growth hormones and stimulate production of the fetal growth-promoting hormones: insulin-like growth factors (IGF-I and IGF-II). Ironically, fetal GH does not appear to regulate growth, and anencephalic infants and GH-deficient children typically have normal birth weights.

Other Placental Hormones

The placenta is a source of many other hormones, including placental ACTH, placental thyroid–stimulating hormone (TSH), and relaxin. The role of placental ACTH and TSH is not understood. The placenta produces **parathyroid hormone–related protein (PTHrP)**, which increases placental calcium transport. Cytotrophoblastic PTHrP production increases in response to decreased extracellular calcium concentration. All the hypothalamic-releasing and -inhibiting hormones have homologs produced in the placenta, and placental gonadotropin–releasing hormone (GnRH) may regulate hCG secretion. The exact role of these placental releasing and inhibiting hormones remains to be conclusively established.

PLACENTAL TRANSPORT

As placental development continues, the cytotrophoblast becomes discontinuous so that the minimal placental barrier (**placental membrane**, described earlier) to transport consists of the syncytiotrophoblast, fetal capillary endothelium, and their fused basal laminae (see Figure 10-12). The complexity of the mature placental villi markedly increases the surface area for transport between maternal and fetal blood. Depending on the substance involved, transport can occur by simple diffusion, facilitated diffusion, active transport, or endocytosis.

Gases, water, and many electrolytes cross the placenta by simple diffusion. Because the placental membrane is considerably thicker than the diffusional surface of the lungs, placental gas transport efficiency is only about 1/50th that of the lung on a per unit weight basis. A sizable gradient exists for oxygen between maternal and fetal blood. It is debatable whether the steep gradient results from lack of oxygen equilibration or high placental oxygen consumption, or both. The partial pressure of oxygen (P_{O_2}) in placental venous blood (oxygenated blood) is approximately 30 mm Hg (maternal arterial P_{O_2} is approximately 105 mm Hg). Fetal compensation for the low P_{O_2} is aided by a high fetal blood flow rate and the high oxygen affinity of fetal hemoglobin.

Carbon dioxide, on the other hand, is more soluble in body tissues, and the diffusion capacity is greater. The partial pressure of carbon dioxide (P_{CO_2}) in placental venous blood is about 43 mm Hg (maternal arterial blood P_{CO_2} is approximately 32 mm Hg).

Amino acids are transported by carrier-mediated secondary active transport (Box 10-2). Glucose is transported by carrier-mediated facilitated diffusion and is a major substrate for energy metabolism in the fetus. Although there is limited fatty acid transport, neutral fats do not cross the placenta, and LDLs are transported into the placenta by LDL receptor–mediated endocytosis.

The fat-soluble steroid hormones cross relatively readily, but protein hormone transport is minimal. Limited thyroid hormone transport occurs, and carrier-mediated systems may be involved.

THE FETAL ENDOCRINE SYSTEM

Pancreas

The fetal pancreas can secrete insulin and glucagon by 15 weeks after conception. However, in the fetus, blood glucose is determined more by the glucose transported across the placenta than by fetal metabolism or fetal insulin production. The ability of the fetal pancreas to respond to chronically elevated glucose levels in the latter half of gestation is demonstrated by pancreatic hyperplasia and hyperinsulinemia that develop in neonates of diabetic mothers with poor hyperglycemic control.

Parathyroid Gland

Fetal serum calcium levels typically are higher than maternal levels because placental PTHrP increases placental calcium transport. Although the fetal parathyroid is functional by the end of the first trimester, the high fetal serum calcium levels resulting from the transport of calcium across the placenta suppress fetal parathyroid function. The placenta produces 1,25-dihydroxyvitamin D, which increases maternal intestinal Ca^{2+} absorption. Maternal PTH levels are suppressed by both increased 1,25-dihydroxyvitamin D and Ca^{2+}, so that maternal serum calcium remains normal and very little or no maternal bone is utilized for fetal Ca^{2+} requirements.

Pituitary Gland

The fetal anterior pituitary develops relatively early in gestation. Typically the pituitary hormones are present and secreted before establishment of the feedback control systems mediated through the hypothalamus. By 12 weeks after conception, all of the anterior pituitary hormones can be detected in the gland, and hypothalamic-releasing or -inhibiting hormones are present in the hypothalamus. The hypophyseal portal system is not functional until approximately 18 weeks of gestation. Typically, at midgestation, anterior pituitary hormone levels are high because of immature feedback control systems. The fetal pituitary is not necessary for the early development and secretion of the endocrine target organs. Although fetal serum GH levels are high late in gestation, GH is not thought to be an important regulator of fetal growth, and the high serum levels probably reflect the immaturity of the control systems for GH regulation. Fetal PRL is secreted early in development, and by birth, fetal levels exceed maternal levels. In addition, PRL levels are particularly high in amnionic fluid; much of this PRL is produced by the decidua. Both fetal and decidual PRL may be important in osmoregulation of amnionic fluid. PRL and hPL have been proposed as fetal growth regulators.

The fetal posterior pituitary secretes oxytocin and antidiuretic hormone (ADH) by midgestation. Fetal oxytocin has been proposed to play a role in parturition.

Thyroid Gland

The fetal thyroid is capable of producing thyroid hormones between 10 and 12 weeks after fertilization, and fetal serum levels of thyroxine (T_4) increase rapidly in midgestation. The initial function of the thyroid does not depend on fetal TSH secretion. During the first half of gestation, fetal T_4 is derived mainly from the maternal compartment, and placental transport of maternal T_4 remains an important source of thyroid hormone throughout gestation. Very little triiodothyronine (T_3) can be detected in fetal serum up to midgestation. The increase in T_3 after 30 weeks of gestation is due to the expression of type I monodeiodinase in the fetus.

Thyroid hormone is crucial for normal neurologic development. A congenitally hypothyroid fetus is protected somewhat by the maternal source of thyroid hormones but nevertheless has severe neurologic deficits, which typically manifest during the early years of life. Alternatively, maternal hypothyroidism can impair full neurologic development in a normal fetus. The fetus is protected from maternal hyperthyroidism by the presence of a placental type III inner ring deiodinase that converts T_4 to reverse T_3 (rT_3) (see Chapter 6).

Adrenal Gland

As mentioned earlier, the fetal adrenal cortex is essential for key steps in placental hormone synthesis. The fetal adrenal cortex becomes large during prenatal development, and the greatest portion of the adrenal cortex consists of the fetal zone. Fetal adrenal production of DHEA-S is present by 7 weeks after conception. During the first few postnatal months, the fetal zone regresses and the definitive and transitional zones enlarge.

A major role of fetal cortisol is the induction of **surfactant** production in the fetal lungs. The fetal type II pneumocyte begins production of surfactant late in gestation. Surfactant contains multiple compounds, but the primary constituent is phospholipids, of which phosphatidylcholine (60%) and phosphatidylglycerol (10%) are the most prevalent. Phosphatidylglycerol production does not occur until about 35 weeks of gestation, and the progressive rise in the surfactant phosphatidylglycerol level is used as an index of lung maturation. Surfactant reduces alveolar surface tension in the postnatal lung. Both corticosteroids and thyroid hormones accelerate fetal lung surfactant production in vivo and in vitro. Consequently, one or both of the groups of compounds have been used to prevent anticipated **respiratory distress syndrome (RDS)** in premature deliveries. Corticosteroids induce lung structural maturation, resulting in increased

---

BOX 10-3
CONTROL OF FETAL SURFACTANT PRODUCTION

Increased Production
- Corticosteroids
- Thyrotropin-releasing hormone (TRH), thyroid hormones

Decreased Production
- Insulin
- Transforming growth factor-β (TGF-β)

---

diffusional surface area, and stimulate synthesis of enzymes regulating surfactant production. Other hormones, such as insulin and transforming growth factor-β, can block lung maturation (Box 10-3).

Testes and Ovaries

Fetal testicular development and function are regulated primarily by hCG, rather than fetal LH, during midgestation. The presence of a functional feedback system for the control of gonadal steroidogenesis is demonstrated by the rise in LH secretion in the immediate postnatal period, when maternal steroids are no longer present. The endocrine role of the ovaries during fetal development is minimal—although primordial follicles undergo development, they do not reach the large antral stage required for significant steroidogenesis.

MATERNAL ENDOCRINE CHANGES DURING PREGNANCY

Pituitary Gland

PRL levels rise during pregnancy because estrogen stimulates PRL synthesis and secretion (see later). Pituitary enlargement in pregnancy reflects growth of PRL-secreting lactotropes. Secretion of other anterior pituitary hormones decreases or remains relatively constant. Pituitary enlargement during pregnancy makes the pituitary susceptible to vascular insult and necrosis at parturition (Sheehan's syndrome; see Chapter 5).

Pituitary production of LH and FSH decreases during pregnancy because of negative feedback inhibition by the high levels of placentally produced estrogen and progestin.

Maternal GH levels are comparable with, or slightly lower than, those in nonpregnant women.

Thyroid Gland

Thyroid size increases during pregnancy, and serum total T_4 and T_3 levels can double. The primary basis for the increase in serum thyroid hormone levels is an estrogen-induced increase in liver **thyroxine-binding globulin (TBG)** production, which leads to an increase in hormone binding. Serum *free* T_4 and T_3 levels do not increase markedly during gestation, however, because hormone turnover rate is increased. The increased thyroidal growth and hormone synthesis during pregnancy are not caused predominantly by placental TSH. Instead, thyroidal stimulation is thought to reflect the actions of hCG. The increased thyroid function parallels the first-trimester serum hCG rise. Late in the first trimester, when maternal serum hCG levels peak, maternal thyroid size and hormone synthesis also peak and maternal serum TSH levels are at their lowest. Because the α chains of hCG are identical to those of TSH and the β chains are similar, hCG can cross-react with TSH receptors when hCG levels are high. There is a transient drop in serum TSH levels at this time because of the rise in serum T_4 and T_3 levels. Free thyroid hormone levels do increase slightly at this time.

Adrenal Gland

Estrogens not only stimulate liver TBG production but also nonspecifically stimulate liver production of many other serum proteins, such as **cortisol-binding globulin (CBG)** (also called **transcortin**). Consequently, total serum cortisol levels rise. Although maternal serum ACTH levels increase slightly during pregnancy, they typically remain within the normal nonpregnant range. Late in pregnancy, however, serum free cortisol levels rise steadily to a peak at parturition that is about twice nonpregnancy levels. This surge in cortisol production is important for the initiation of lactation.

Estrogen stimulates liver angiotensinogen production and renal renin production. Consequently, synthesis of angiotensin II and aldosterone increases. Estrogens potentiate the adrenal action of angiotensin II but inhibit the vascular actions. Although aldosterone secretion in pregnancy increases, clinical signs of hyperaldosteronism typically are not present in pregnancy because progesterone is antagonistic to the action of aldosterone on the kidney.

MATERNAL PHYSIOLOGIC CHANGES DURING PREGNANCY

Physiologic changes occur in the pregnant woman both as a consequence of the size of the developing fetus and as a result of the endocrine and cardiovascular changes associated with the pregnancy (Box 10-4).

Cardiovascular Changes

Both heart rate and stroke volume, and therefore cardiac output, increase in pregnancy to approximately 40% more than preconception levels, with most of this

---

BOX 10-4
PHYSIOLOGIC CHANGES IN PREGNANCY

Cardiovascular Changes
- ↑Vascular volume
- ↓Peripheral resistance
- ↑Stroke volume
- ↑Heart rate
- ↑Contractility
- ↑Cardiac output

Respiratory Changes
- ↑Minute volume
- ↑Tidal volume
- ↓P_{CO_2}
- ↓Functional residual capacity
- ↓Inspiratory reserve volume

Renal Changes
- ↑Antidiuretic hormone, renin, angiotensin II, aldosterone secretion
- Respiratory alkalosis

increase occurring by 8 weeks of gestation. Blood volume increases 50% during pregnancy.

As the pregnancy progresses, the placental circulation requires a progressively larger portion of the maternal cardiac output. The additional vasculature of the maternal side of the placenta produces a large increase in the capacity of the vascular system. Uteroplacental blood flow near term is estimated to be as much as 900 ml/min. Much of the increase in blood volume occurs between 6 and 32 weeks of gestation. It is in part a result of the estrogen-stimulated increase in renin-angiotensin-aldosterone secretion. Progesterone, hPL, and PRL stimulate erythropoiesis; late in pregnancy, however, blood volume expands faster than increased red blood cell synthesis, so the hematocrit value drops slightly.

Because the placenta is essentially an arteriovenous shunt, vascular resistance is low. Therefore, total peripheral resistance drops and diastolic pressure tends to drop. Blood pressure typically does not rise until late in pregnancy unless preeclampsia develops. Because the growing uterus exerts pressure on the veins of the legs where these veins enter the abdomen, venous pressure in the lower extremities rises on standing, and edema and venous damage can occur.

In part, these changes can be attributed to the need for increased blood flow to the growing uterus and placenta; however, significant cardiovascular changes occur relatively early in gestation when the uterus and placenta are still small. Although the arteriovenous shunt through the placenta is the basis for some of the cardiovascular changes, the basis for the early development of the cardiovascular changes has not been definitively established.

Respiratory Changes

As pregnancy proceeds, the functional residual capacity (volume of air in the lungs at the end of a quiet expiration) and the residual volume (volume remaining at the end of a maximal expiration) decrease, and respiratory rate remains unchanged. Minute volume increases and tidal volume increases, so P_{CO_2} decreases.

There are three major causes of the respiratory changes associated with pregnancy. The bulk of the growing fetus and uterus increases intra-abdominal

pressure and forces the diaphragm upward. The high metabolic rate of the growing fetus increases maternal oxygen consumption and carbon dioxide production. In addition, progesterone acts directly on the central nervous system (CNS) to lower the set-point for regulation of respiration by carbon dioxide, thereby increasing ventilation. Consequently, P_{CO_2} decreases from 40 to approximately 32 mm Hg. The increased need for fetal oxygen and release of carbon dioxide and the direct CNS actions of progesterone all act to alter respiration during pregnancy. The progesterone-induced hyperventilation of pregnancy produces a mild, compensated respiratory alkalosis with a decrease in serum P_{CO_2} and therefore a drop in serum HCO_3^-.

Renal Changes

Water retention occurs in normal pregnancies. This is caused in part by changes in the set-points for regulation of ADH secretion and thirst so that both increase, with a resultant decrease in serum osmolality. The cause of this change is not known, but it may be related to actions of hCG.

The glomerular filtration rate (GFR) increases approximately 60% over nonpregnant levels. The exact cause of the increased GFR is not known. As GFR increases, the filtered load of filtered substances increases, and the increased filtered loads of glucose and amino acids can lead to glucosuria and aminoaciduria in pregnancy. Glucosuria in pregnancy also results from impaired distal tubule glucose absorption. The mechanisms underlying this change are not known.

Plasma renin, angiotensin II, and aldosterone increase, at least in part because of the decrease in blood pressure resulting from the decreased vascular resistance. Because "effective circulating blood volume" tends to decrease with growth of the placental circulation, mean arterial pressure drops, resulting in increased renin release. The uterus also produces renin in pregnancy. Angiotensin II stimulates aldosterone production, and aldosterone increases renal salt and water retention. In addition, estrogen stimulates liver synthesis of angiotensinogen, the precursor of angiotensin I. Estrogen and progesterone both directly increase the secretion of renin, the enzyme converting angiotensinogen to angiotensin I. Consequently, as placental estrogen and progesterone production increases, angiotensin II formation increases. Although angiotensin II stimulates aldosterone synthesis, the vasculature appears refractory to its vasopressive actions.

Maternal serum levels of the mineralocorticoid **deoxycorticosterone (DOC)** increase during pregnancy. This increase in circulating DOC levels results not from increased adrenal secretion but from renal conversion of placental progesterone to DOC. DOC stimulates renal salt and water retention. Maternal aldosterone secretion increases to levels about 20 times those of nonpregnant women. The increased secretion of the mineralocorticoids aldosterone and DOC is important for the volume expansion seen in the mother during pregnancy.

Gastrointestinal Changes

Gastric emptying rate and intestinal transit times are decreased in pregnancy. These changes might be a result of progesterone actions decreasing smooth muscle motility. Heartburn, or reflux of acidic gastric secretions into the esophagus, occurs for multiple reasons. The increased intraabdominal pressure increases intragastric pressure, which increases the likelihood of reflux into the esophagus. Progesterone also decreases lower esophageal sphincter tone, thereby increasing reflux tendency.

Diabetogenicity of Pregnancy

Pregnancy represents an **insulin-resistant state**. During the last half of pregnancy, when hPL levels are highest, maternal energy metabolism shifts from an anabolic state in which nutrients are stored, to a catabolic state, sometimes described as **accelerated starvation**, in which maternal energy metabolism shifts toward fat utilization with glucose sparing. As maternal glucose use for energy decreases, lipolysis increases and fatty acids become a major energy source. The peripheral responsiveness to insulin decreases and pancreatic insulin secretion increases. Beta cell hyperplasia occurs in pregnancy. Although this usually does not lead to any clinical condition, pregnancy aggravates existing diabetes mellitus, and diabetes mellitus can develop for the first time in pregnancy. If the diabetes resolves spontaneously with delivery, the condition is referred to as **gestational diabetes**. Other hormones contributing to the diabetogenicity of pregnancy are estrogens and progestins, because both of these hormones decrease insulin sensitivity.

PARTURITION

Human pregnancy lasts an average of 40 weeks from the beginning of the last menstrual period (gestational age). This corresponds to an average fetal age of 38 weeks. **Parturition** is the process whereby uterine contractions lead to childbirth. **Labor** consists of three stages: (1) strong uterine contractions that force the fetus against the cervix, with dilation and thinning of the cervix (several hours); (2) delivery of the fetus (less than 1 hour); and (3) delivery of the placenta, along with contractions of the myometrium, which serve to halt bleeding (less than 10 minutes).

Parturition control in humans is complex, and the exact mechanisms underlying parturition control are not well understood. In many species, such as sheep, the timing of parturition is controlled by fetus-derived signals, and fetal regulation is at least a factor in humans.

Placental Corticotropin–releasing Hormone and the Fetal Adrenal Axis

The placenta produces **corticotropin-releasing hormone (CRH)**, which is identical to the 41-amino acid peptide produced by the hypothalamus. Placental CRH production, and maternal serum CRH levels, increase rapidly during late pregnancy and labor. Moreover, circulating CRH is either in the form of free CRH, which is bioactive, or complexed to a CRH-binding protein. Maternal levels of CRH-binding protein plummet during late pregnancy and labor, so that free CRH levels increase. Placental CRH also accumulates in the fetal circulation and stimulates fetal ACTH secretion. ACTH stimulates both fetal adrenal cortisol production and fetoplacental estrogen production. In contrast with the inhibitory effect of cortisol on hypothalamic CRH production, cortisol stimulates placental CRH production. This establishes a self-amplifying positive feedback. CRH itself promotes myometrial contractions through sensitizing the uterus to prostaglandins and oxytocin (see later). Estrogens also directly and indirectly stimulate myometrial contractility (see later). This model also correlates with the onset of parturition with cortisol-induced maturation of fetal systems, including the lungs and gastrointestinal system.

Estrogen and Progesterone Secretion

Although a rise in maternal serum estrogen and a drop in progesterone levels are seen late in gestation in some species, no change in the ratio of the two hormones is seen in human serum. "Functional" progesterone withdrawal, involving changes in uterine progesterone receptor and in progesterone metabolism, has been proposed, however.

Oxytocin

Oxytocin, which stimulates powerful uterine contractions, plays a major role in parturition (Figure 10-18). It is released in response to stretch of the cervix, and it stimulates uterine contractions, thereby facilitating delivery. Oxytocin can be used to induce parturition, and uterine sensitivity to oxytocin increases before parturition. Because maternal serum oxytocin levels do not increase until after parturition has begun, oxytocin is not thought to initiate parturition. However, progesterone inhibits and estrogen stimulates synthesis of oxytocin receptors, and, although maternal serum progesterone levels do not decrease immediately before human parturition, estrogen levels rise and oxytocin receptor synthesis increases.

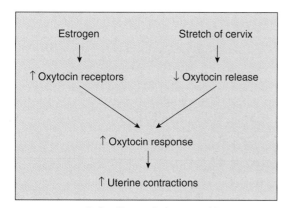

FIGURE 10-18 ■ Role of oxytocin in parturition.

Prostaglandins

Prostaglandins and other cytokines increase uterine motility, and levels of these compounds increase during parturition, thereby facilitating delivery. Their exact role in the initiation of parturition is not known. Prostaglandin levels in amnionic fluid, fetal membranes, and uterine decidua increase before the onset of labor. The prostaglandins $PGF_{2\alpha}$ and PGE_2 increase uterine motility. Large doses of these compounds have been used to induce labor. Because estrogens stimulate prostaglandin synthesis in the uterus, amnion, and chorion, the rising estrogen levels late in gestation can increase uterine prostaglandin formation before parturition.

Uterine Size

Uterine size is thought to be a factor regulating parturition because stretch of smooth muscle, including the uterus, increases muscle contraction. In addition, uterine stretch stimulates uterine prostaglandin production. Multiple births generally occur prematurely. The tendency for early delivery can be a result of increased uterine size, increased fetal production of chemicals stimulating delivery, or both.

MAMMOGENESIS AND LACTATION

Structure of the Mammary Gland

The **mammary gland** is composed of about 20 lobes, each with an excretory **lactiferous duct** that opens at the nipple. Lobes, in turn, are composed of several lobules, which contain secretory structures called **alveoli**, and the terminal portions of the ducts. The epithelium of the alveoli and ducts is a simple one, except for the presence of a **myoepithelial cell** layer on the basal side of the epithelium (but apical to the basal lamina). Myoepithelial cells are stellate, smooth muscle–like cells, and contraction of these cells in response to a stimulus (see later) expels milk from the lumina of the alveoli and ducts. Lobes and lobules are supported within a connective tissue matrix. The other major tissue component of the breast is adipose tissue. The lactiferous ducts empty at the **nipple**, which is a highly innervated, hairless protrusion of the breast designed for suckling by an infant. The nipple is surrounded by a pigmentated, hairless areola, which is

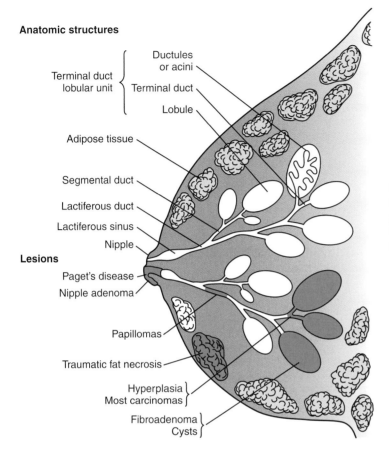

Anatomic structures

- Terminal duct lobular unit
  - Ductules or acini
  - Terminal duct
  - Lobule
- Adipose tissue
- Segmental duct
- Lactiferous duct
- Lactiferous sinus
- Nipple

Lesions

- Paget's disease
- Nipple adenoma
- Papillomas
- Traumatic fat necrosis
- Hyperplasia / Most carcinomas
- Fibroadenoma / Cysts

FIGURE 10-19 ■ Anatomy of the breast and major lesions at each site within the breast. *(From Cotran RS, Kumar V, Robbins SL: Pathologic basis of disease, ed 5, Philadelphia, 1994, WB Saunders.)*

lubricated by sebaceous glands. Protusion of the nipple, called **erection**, is mediated by sympathetic stimulation of smooth muscle fibers in response to suckling and other mechanical stimulation, erotic stimulation, and cold.

Hormonal Regulation of Mammary Gland Development

The mammary glands develop in utero as rudimentary mammary buds of invaginated epithelia in the thoracic region, along with limited ductal and lobuloalveolar development. After parturition, the alveolar development largely regresses, and the breasts remain as rudimentary ductal buds until puberty. At puberty, estrogen increases ductal growth and branching. With the onset of luteal phases of the ovary, progesterone and estrogen induce further ductal growth and the formation of rudimentary alveoli. During nonpregnant cycles, the breasts develop somewhat and then regress. Estrogen also increases the deposition of adipose tissue, which makes a major contribution to the size and overall form of the breasts. Adipose tissue expresses CYP19, so that accumulation of this tissue in the breast increases the local production of estrogens from circulating androgens.

The greatest degree of breast development occurs during pregnancy, during which extensive ductal growth and branching and lobuloalveolar development occur. The parenchymal growth of the breast during development occurs at the expense of stroma, which is degraded to make room for enlarging lobuloalveolar structures. Several placental hormones stimulate breast development, including **estrogen**, **progesterone**, **placental lactogen**, and the **growth hormone variant GH-V**. Estrogen acts on the breast directly and also indirectly through maternal pituitary prolactin. Estrogen increases prolactin gene expression and secretion from pituitary lactotropes. Estrogen also stimulates lactotrope hypertrophy and proliferation, which accounts for the twofold increase in pituitary volume during pregnancy in humans. Although epithelial cells express genes encoding milk protein and enzymes involved in milk production, progesterone inhibits the onset of milk production and secretion (called **lactogenesis**).

After parturition, the human breast produces **colostrum**, which is enriched with antimicrobial and anti-inflammatory proteins. In the absence of placental progesterone, normal breast milk production occurs within a few days. The lobuloalveolar structures produce milk, which is subsequently modified by the ductal epithelium. Lactogenesis and the maintenance of milk production (**galactopoiesis**) require stimulation by pituitary prolactin, in the presence of normal levels of other hormones, including insulin, cortisol and thyroid hormone. Whereas placental

estrogen stimulates prolactin secretion during pregnancy, the stimulus for prolactin secretion during the nursing period is suckling by the infant (Figure 10-20). The levels of prolactin are directly correlated with the frequency and duration of sucking at the nipple. The link between suckling at the nipple and prolactin secretion involves a neuroendocrine reflex, in which dopamine (the prolactin-release inhibitory factor— see Chapter 5) secretion at the median eminence is inhibited. It also is possible that suckling increases the secretion of unidentified prolactin-releasing hormones.

Prolactin also inhibits GnRH release; consequently, nursing can be associated with **lactational amenorrhea** (see Figure 10-20). This effect of prolactin has been called "nature's contraceptive" and may play a role in spacing out pregnancies. Only very regular nursing over a 24-hour period, however, is sufficient to allow for a prolactin-induced anovulatory state in the mother. Thus, lactational amenorrhea is not an effective or reliable form of birth control for most women.

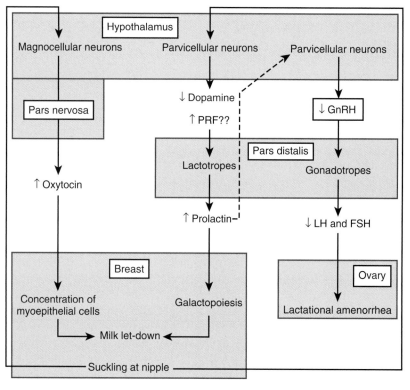

FIGURE 10-20 ■ The neuroendocrine reflex linking suckling at the nipple to oxytocin and prolactin release. FSH, follicle-stimulating hormone; GnRH, gonadotropin-releasing hormone; LH, luteinizing hormone; PRL, prolactin.

The inhibition of GnRH by high levels of prolactin is important clinically. The **prolactinoma** is the most common form of hormone-secreting pituitary tumor, and **hyperprolactinemia** is a significant cause of infertility in both sexes. Hyperprolactinemia can also be associated with **galactorrhea**, or the inappropriate flow of breast milk, in men and women.

Suckling at the nipple also stimulates the release of **oxytocin** from the pars nervosa (see Chapter 5) through a neuroendocrine reflex (see Figure 10-20). Oxytocin receptors on the myoepithelial cells cause contraction through a Gq-phospholipase C signaling pathway that ultimately increases intracellular Ca^{2+}. Contraction of myoepithelial cells induces **milk let-down**, or the expulsion of milk from alveolar and ductal lumina. Thus, the nursing infant does not gain milk by applying negative pressure to the breast from suckling. Rather, milk is actively ejected through a neuroendocrine reflex. Oxytocin release and milk let-down can be induced by psychogenic stimuli, such as the sound of a baby crying on a television program or thinking about the baby. Such psychogenic stimuli do not affect prolactin release.

The breast epithelium represents a hormonally responsive, highly mitogenic population of cells. Breast cancer arises from breast epithelium (primarily ductal epithelium). This tumor is the most common cancer in women in the United States and is a major cause of death among women 45 to 55 years of age. Although hormones do not initiate carcinogenesis, estrogen plays a major role in the progression of breast cancer. Less-transformed breast cancer cells express the estrogen receptor and respond better to treatment (surgical, radiation, chemotherapy) than do estrogen receptor–negative cancers. Also, selective estrogen receptor modulators (SERMs) such as tamoxifen and also aromatase (CYP19) inhibitors further increase efficacy of initial localized treatment when used for subsequent systemic adjuvant therapy.

CONTRACEPTION

Behavioral and Mechanical Approaches

There are multiple methods of **contraception**. These methods include the age-old rhythm method, which relies on abstinence from sexual intercourse during fertile periods around the time of ovulation. (The fertile period is considered to be the period extending from 3 to 4 days before the time of ovulation until 3 to 4 days afterward.) A second method is withdrawal before ejaculation, **coitus interruptus**. Both of these methods have higher failure rates (20% to 30%) than the **barrier methods** (2% to 12%), **intrauterine devices (IUDs)** (<2%), and **oral contraceptives** (<1%).

Barriers such as condoms or diaphragms are more effective as contraceptives when used with spermicidal jellies.

Among the various methods of contraception, IUDs are the most effective except for oral contraceptives. These devices are thought to prevent implantation by producing a local inflammatory response in the endometrium. Some forms of IUDs contain copper, zinc, or progestins, which inhibit sperm transport or viability in the female reproductive tract.

Oral Contraceptives

Oral contraceptives have been marketed in the United States since the early 1960s. The doses of steroids used today are many-fold lower than those used in the initial preparations. Properly used, oral contraceptives have a low failure rate.

Many forms of oral contraceptives are marketed today. The trend over the years has been to decrease the dosage of steroids used because the side effects are dose dependent. All oral steroidal contraceptives contain a progestin. Five Food and Drug Administration (FDA)–approved **synthetic progestins** are used in oral contraceptives. These are norgestrel, norethindrone, norethindrone acetate, ethynodiol diacetate, and norethynodrel. These compounds have some androgenic activity. In addition, all oral contraceptives except the **mini-pill** contain an estrogenic compound. The two commercially approved estrogens are ethinyl estradiol and mestranol. Therefore, all oral steroidal contraceptives contain either a combination of an estrogen and a progestin or a progestin alone. The differences between the various pills are a result of varying patterns and doses of hormone administration or variation among the five progestins and two estrogens used. The treatment regimens include **fixed-dose combination pills**, progestin-only mini-pills, and **biphasic** or **triphasic pills**, in which the estrogen level typically remains constant but the progestin levels vary during the cycle. The dose of steroids can be decreased by use of the more complicated biphasic and triphasic regimens.

Oral contraceptives work through multiple mechanisms. Most block the LH surge that triggers ovulation. However, some pills, such as the progestin-only mini-pill, do not prevent LH surges. Fertility also is blocked by changing the nature of cervical mucus, by altering endometrial development, and by regulating fallopian tube motility. Because these contraceptives suppress FSH, they impair early follicular development.

Hormonal Treatment for Emergency Contraception and Abortion

Emergency contraception involves hormonal treatment designed to inhibit or delay ovulation, inhibit corpus luteum function, and/or disrupt the function of the oviducts and uterus. For example, candidates for emergency contraception include women who have been sexually assaulted or who experienced a failure of a barrier method (e.g., ruptured condom). More than 20 types of "morning after" pills are commercially available. The currently preferred medication is **levonorgestrel (Plan B)**, which is a synthetic progestin-only pill. The efficacy of the pill is inversely correlated with the time taken after intercourse. The exact mechanism of action is not known. Treatment has no effect if implantation has occurred.

Medical (hormonal) termination of pregnancy (**abortion**) can be achieved up to 49 days of gestation by administration of **mifepristone (RU-486)**. Mifepristone is a **progesterone receptor antagonist** (i.e., an **antiprogestin**), which induces collapse of the pregnant endometrium. Mifepristine is followed 48 hours later by ingestion or vaginal insertion of a synthetic **prostaglandin E** (e.g., misoprostol), which induces myometrial contractions.

IN VITRO FERTILIZATION

In many cases, a couple of reproductive age are unable to conceive a child. Infertility has a wide range of causes and can be associated with problems with either the male or the female reproductive system. For example, male infertility can be due to low numbers of sperm (fewer than 20 million sperm/ml)

or to abnormal sperm morphology or motility. Female infertility can be due to anovulatory disorders, endometriosis, polycystic ovarian syndrome, or problems with the fallopian tubes, or may be unexplained. **In vitro fertilization (IVF)**, a procedure in which eggs are retrieved from the woman, fertilized outside the body, and then transferred back into the uterus, can, in many cases, circumvent the aforementioned problems and allow a couple to achieve a successful pregnancy.

IVF takes advantage of current understanding of female reproductive endocrinology, in that the woman's cycle can be tightly controlled and eggs retrieved from the ovaries at the optimal stage for fertilization. Women undergoing a typical IVF regimen often are given a GnRH agonist or antagonist to shut down the biologic cycle for about a week. Next, daily injections of a high dose of FSH are given to stimulate the growth of many (sometimes as many as 30 or more) large, antral follicles. The patient's ovaries are subsequently monitored in a clinic using ultrasound to assess follicular growth. Estrogen levels in the blood also are monitored. Generally, when several follicles of about 18 mm in diameter are observed, the patient is given an injection of hCG to initiate oocyte maturation. Although hCG, acting through LH receptors, can trigger ovulation, mature eggs are retrieved from the ovaries just before ovulation.

Eggs are retrieved from both ovaries using a large needle that is guided through the vaginal wall, on each side, with the aid of ultrasound. The woman must be given a general anesthetic for this procedure. Cumulus-enclosed eggs are aspirated from the largest antral follicles. After collection, cumulus-enclosed eggs are sometimes fertilized directly by mixing them with sperm. In many cases, however, the cumulus cells are enzymatically stripped from the eggs, and the isolated eggs are injected with sperm. This procedure, called **intracytoplasmic sperm injection (ICSI)**, must be used in cases of male factor infertility and is now used for a majority of in vitro fertilization procedures in many clinics.

Newly fertilized eggs are incubated for approximately 3 days, developing into 2- to 8-cell embryos. During this time, the woman begins daily injections of progesterone to prepare the uterus for pregnancy. Embryos are then transferred into the uterus. The number of embryos transferred depends on their perceived quality, the woman's age, and the number of previous failed IVF treatments she has undergone. Generally, 1 to 3 embryos are transferred. After the transfer, pregnancy is confirmed by a blood test, and later by observing a heartbeat using ultrasound.

Success rates for IVF vary from clinic to clinic, ranging from about 30% to 50%. The associated costs are quite high, averaging $10,000 to $15,000 per treatment regimen. In addition, although IVF generally is safe, it is not without risks. One serious complication, particularly for women presenting with polycystic ovarian syndrome, is that of **ovarian hyperstimulation syndrome**

(**OHSS**), in which the ovary responds to follicle stimulation by producing exceptionally high levels of estrogen. This can result in enlarged ovaries, free fluid in the pelvis, electrolyte abnormalities, and intravascular depletion of fluid. Hospitalization is required, and the cycle must be canceled. Another risk is the successful implantation of two or more embryos. Indeed, **multiple births**, especially twins, are more common among women receiving IVF treatments than in the general population. Multiple fetuses and births increase the risk of morbidity and mortality for both mother and fetuses.

SUMMARY

1. The events of fertilization, early embryogenesis, and implantation are synchronized with the hormonal changes of the human menstrual cycle, ultimately ensuring a receptive uterus at the time of implantation.

2. Spermatozoa bind to the epithelium of the oviductal isthmus, which secretes factors that capacitate the sperm. Hyperactivation allows the sperm to detach and swim to the cumulus-oocyte complex in the ampulla. Fertilization involves the penetration by a spermatozoon of the expanded cumulus as mediated by a membrane hyaluronidase, penetration of the zona pellucida as mediated by the acrosome reaction, and fusion with the oocyte membrane as mediated by specific membrane fusion proteins. The egg is activated, completes the second meiotic division, and releases cortical granule enzymes that prevent polyspermy. The female and male pronuclei are drawn together, line up on a metaphase plate, and undergo the first cleavage.

3. The embryo undergoes cleavage and formation of a morula within the oviduct. The embryo enters the uterus on day 3, forms a blastocyst, degrades the zona pellucida (hatches), and implants on day 6 or 7.

4. The trophoblast layer differentiates into the cytotrophoblastic layer and an outer syncytiotrophoblastic layer. The syncytiotrophoblasts secrete invasive enzymes, express adhesion molecules, produce protein and steroid hormones, and ultimately become the primary cell involved in maternal-fetal

exchange. With the addition of an extraembryonic mesoderm, the trophoblast layers become the chorion. The fetal (umbilical) blood vessels develop within the mesenchyme of the extraembryonic mesoderm. The chorion ultimately gives rise to protrusions, the chorionic villi, which constitute the functional unit of the placenta.

5. The uterine endometrium decidualizes in response to implantation. The decidua impose restraint on the invading embryo.

6. The intervillous spaces become filled with maternal blood from eroded spiral arteries. This gives rise to a hemochorial placenta. Spiral arteries are plugged up by extravillous cytotrophoblasts for the first trimester, so that the embryo/early fetus develops in a relatively hypoxic environment and receives histiotropic nutrition. The cytotrophoblasts convert the spiral arteries to low-resistance, high-capacitance vessels that supply blood to the placenta during the second and third trimesters.

7. The first hormone produced by the placenta is hCG. This hormone is structurally similar to LH but has a longer half-life. Its function is to rescue the corpus luteum, which is needed to produce progesterone for the first 10 weeks. Human chorionic gonadotropin also stimulates male fetal gonadal production of testosterone and stimulates the early fetal adrenal.

8. Progesterone production is taken over by the placenta. Syncytiotrophoblasts utilize maternal

cholesterol to make progesterone. Because no fetal tissues are involved in progesterone synthesis, progesterone levels are not a measure of fetal health. Progesterone is required for pregnancy. Progesterone maintains a quiescent uterus and affects several aspects of maternal physiology. Progesterone is utilized by the fetal adrenal cortex for cortisol synthesis.

9. The fetal adrenal cortex is different from the adult. The large inner zone is called the fetal zone. The fetal zone produces DHEA-S, which is then converted by the syncytiotrophoblasts to estradiol-17β and estrone. DHEA-S also is converted to 16-hydroxy-DHEA-S by the fetal liver, and this steroid is further converted to estriol by the syncytiotrophoblasts. This multiorgan pathway for estrogen synthesis is referred to as the fetoplacental unit. Maternal serum estriol levels can be used as an indicator of fetal health. Estrogen is not required for pregnancy. The primary function of estrogen is to prepare the uterus for parturition. Both estrogen and progesterone play important roles in mammary gland development during pregnancy.

10. Two other zones exist within the fetal adrenal cortex. The outer definitive zone begins to make aldosterone close to term. The middle transitional zone begins to make cortisol at midgestation. Cortisol production increases toward late pregnancy, playing a role in fetal lung surfactant synthesis, fetal gastrointestinal tract maturation, and other aspects of late fetal development.

11. Human placental lactogen (hPL) is structurally and functionally similar to both GH and PRL. It stimulates mammary gland development during pregnancy and mobilizes maternal nutrients for the fetus. It is an insulin antagonist and is lipolytic.

12. Glucose crosses the placenta by carrier-mediated facilitated diffusion. Amino acid transport is by carrier-mediated secondary active transport, and LDL transport is by receptor-mediated endocytosis. Gas transport is by simple diffusion.

13. Cardiovascular changes in pregnancy include increased vascular volume; decreased peripheral resistance; and increased heart rate, cardiac contractility, and cardiac output.

14. Respiratory changes in pregnancy include increased minute volume and increased tidal volume. The hyperventilation of pregnancy produces a mild compensated respiratory alkalosis.

15. During pregnancy, ADH, renin, angiotensin II, and aldosterone secretion all increase. These changes produce water retention. GFR increases, thereby increasing the filtered load of filtered substances. This increased load can result in a greater tendency for aminoaciduria and glucosuria in pregnancy.

16. The exact mechanism underlying initiation of parturition in humans has not been defined. Possible stimuli include increased uterine size, increased placental CRH and fetal ACTH production, increased oxytocin receptor concentration, and increased uterine prostaglandin production. Parturition requires estrogen, which stimulates prostaglandin synthesis and oxytocin receptor expression.

17. Corticosteroids and thyroid hormones can accelerate surfactant production in late-gestational fetuses.

18. Mammary glands are lobuloalveolar structures. Estrogen and progesterone promote ductal and alveolar growth, whereas progesterone and prolactin stimulate alveolar development. Progesterone development in pregnancy is regulated by hPL, PRL, estrogens, and progestogens. Copious milk production in pregnancy is blocked by progestogerone. After parturition, sucking at the nipple is required for prolactin and oxytocin secretion. Prolactin maintains milk production (galactopoiesis), and oxytocin causes the myoepithelial cells to contract. Prolactin inhibits GnRH secretion—the basis for lactational amenorrhea and for both male and female infertility due to a prolactinoma with associated hyperprolactinemia. Breast cancer is a hormonally responsive cancer in the earlier stages, so antiestrogens and aromatase inhibitors are effective as adjuvant therapy.

19. Elucidation of the basic science of reproductive endocrinology has led to the development of oral contraceptives, emergency contraceptives, medical abortion pills, and in vitro fertilization procedures.

KEYWORDS AND CONCEPTS

- Placenta
- Chorion
- Decidua

- Histiotropic nutrition
- Hemotropic nutrition
- Window of receptivity
- Spiral arteries
- Venous lakes (lacunae)
- Human chorionic gonadotropin (hCG)
- Polyspermy
- Egg activation
- Capacitation
- Hyperactivation
- Hyaluronidase
- PH-20
- Zona pellucida
- ZP1, ZP2, ZP3 (zona pellucida glycoproteins)
- Acrosome reaction
- Viral fusion event
- Tetraspanin proteins
- Izumo
- Decondensation (of sperm DNA)
- Pronucleus
- Cortical granules
- Maturation-promoting factor (MPF)
- Cytostatic factor (CSF)
- Morula
- Centrosome
- Blastocyst
- Inner cell mass
- Trophoblasts
- Embryonic pole
- "Hatched" blastocyst
- Cytotrophoblasts
- Syncytiotrophoblasts
- Interstitial implantation
- Decidualization
- Tissue inhibitors of metalloproteases (TIMPs)
- Placenta accreta
- Ectopic implantations
- Tubal pregnancy
- Embryotroph
- Primary villi
- Extraembryonic mesoderm
- Chorionic membrane
- Secondary villi
- Connecting stalk
- Umbilical
- Tertiary villi
- Smooth chorion

- Chorion laeve
- Villous chorion
- Chorion frondosum
- Decidua basalis
- Decidua capsularis
- Decidua parietalis
- Amnion
- Amniochorionic membrane
- Chorionic villi
- Terminal villi
- Intervillous space
- Placental membrane
- Vasculosyncytial membrane
- Eutherian
- Hemochorial placentation
- Cytotrophoblastic shell
- Preeclampsia
- Hypertension of pregnancy
- α-glycoprotein subunit (α-GSU)
- Hormone-specific β subunit (β-hCG)
- Hlycosylation
- Morning sickness
- Molar disease
- Choriocarcinoma
- Progesterone
- StAR protein
- Luteal-placental shift
- Fetal adrenal cortex
- Definitive zone
- Transitional zone
- Fetal zone
- Dehydroepiandrostenedione sulfate (DHEA-S)
- Steroid sulfatase
- 16-hydroxylation
- Estriol
- Fetoplacental unit
- Steroid sulfatase deficiency
- Human placental lactogen (hPL)
- Human chorionic somatomammotropin (hCS)
- Parathyroid hormone–related protein (PTHrP)
- Surfactant
- Respiratory distress syndrome (RDS)
- Thyroxine-binding globulin (TBG)
- Cortisol-binding globulin (CBG)
- Transcortin
- Deoxycorticosterone (DOC)
- Insulin-resistant state

- Accelerated starvation
- Gestational diabetes
- Parturition
- Corticotropin-releasing hormone (CRH)
- Mammary gland
- Lactiferous duct
- Alveoli
- Myoepithelial cell
- Nipple
- Erection (of nipple)
- Estrogen
- Placental lactogen
- Placental growth hormone variant (GH-V)
- Lactogenesis
- Colostrum
- Galactopoiesis
- Lactational amenorrhea
- Prolactinoma
- Hyperprolactinemia
- Glactorrhea
- Milk let-down
- Contraception
- Coitus interruptus
- Barrier methods
- Intrauterine devices (IUDs)
- Oral contraceptives
- Synthetic progestins
- Mini-pill
- Fixed-dose combination pills
- Biphasic/triphasic pills
- Emergency contraception
- Levonorgestrel (Plan B)
- Abortion
- Mifepristone (RU-486)
- Progesterone receptor antagonist
- Antiprogestin
- In vitro fertilization (IVF)
- Intracytoplasmic sperm injection (ICSI)
- Ovarian hyperstimulation syndrome (OHSS)
- Multiple births

2. How does placental progesterone synthesis differ from placental estriol synthesis?
3. What is the role of estrogen in pregnancy and parturition?
4. What would be the effect of a deficiency in CYP17 in the fetal adrenal cortex? Would this affect fetal ACTH?
5. What is the basis for hyperthyroidism during the first trimester of pregnancy Why is it transient?
6. How does progesterone affect maternal respiration?
7. What is the relationship between infertility and PRL in a physiologic situation? in a pathologic condition?
8. Why is hCG given during an IVF Regimen?

BIBLIOGRAPHY

Cross JC: How to make a placenta: mechanisms of trophoblast cell differentiation in mice—a review, *Placenta* 26:S3-S9, 2005.

Erkkola R, Landgren BM: Role of progestins in contraception, *Acta Obstet Gynecol Scand* 84:207-216, 2005.

Fazleabas AT, Kim JJ, Strakova Z: Implantation: embryonic signals and the modulation of the uterine environment—a review, *Placenta* 25:S26-S31, 2004.

Frantz AG, Wilson JD: Endocrine disorders of the breast. In Larsen PR, Kronenberg HM, Melmed S, Polonsky KS, editors: *Williams' textbook of endocrinology*, ed 9, Philadelphia, 1998, WB Saunders.

Killian GJ: Evidence for the role of oviduct secretions in sperm function, fertilization and embryo development, *Anim Reprod Sci* 82-83:141-153, 2004.

Lyall F: Priming and remodeling of human placental bed spiral arteries during pregnancy—a review, *Placenta* 26:S31-S36, 2005.

Macklon NS, Stouffer RL, Giudice LC, Fauser BCJM: The science behind 25 years of ovarian stimulation for in vitro fertilization, *Endocr Rev* 27:170-207, 2006.

Pollheimer J, Knofler M: Signalling pathways regulating the invasive differentiation of human trophoblasts: a review, *Placenta* 26, S21-S30, 2005.

Staun-Ram E, Shalev E: Human trophoblast function during the implantation process, *Reprod Biol Endocrinol* 3:56-67, 2005.

Weissgerber TL, Wolfe LA: Physiological adaptation in early human pregnancy: adaptation to balance maternal-fetal demands, *Appl Physiol Nutr Metab* 31:1-11, 2006.

SELF-STUDY PROBLEMS

1. Describe the events that are involved in implantation, including differentiation of the trphoblast, uterine receptivity, and decidualization.

APPENDIX A
List of Abbreviations and Symbols

αGSU	alpha glycoprotein subunit
β/TSH	beta thyroid-stimulating hormone
3β-HSD	3β-hydroxysteroid dehydrogenase
11β-HSD2	11β-hydroxysteroid dehydrogenase
AAs	amino acids
ABP	androgen-binding protein
ACE	angiotensin-converting enzyme
Ach	acetylcholine
ACTH	adrenocorticotropic hormone (corticotropin)
ADH	antidiuretic hormone
AIS	androgen insensitivity syndrome
ALS	acid labile subunit
AMH	antimüllerian hormone
ANP	atrial natriuretic peptide
APOs	apoproteins
AR	androgen receptor
ARE	androgen-response elements
ATP	adenosine triphosphate
BAT	brown adipose tissue
bFGF	basic fibroblast growth factor
BMP-15	bone morphogenetic protein-15
BMR	basal metabolic rate
Ca^{2+}	calcium phosphate
CaMKII	Ca^{2+}/calmodulin-dependent protein kinase II
cAMP	cyclic adenosine monophosphate
CaSR	Ca^{2+} sensing receptor
CBG	corticosteroid-binding globulin (also transcortin)
CCK	cholecystokinin
CDK1	cyclin-dependent kinase-1
CETP	cholesterol ester transfer protein
cGMP	cyclic guanosine monophosphate
CGRP	calcitonin gene-related peptide
CNS	central nervous system

COMT	catechol-O-methyltransferase
COX-2	cyclooxygenase-2
CPT-1/CPT-2	carnitine palmitoyl-transferase
CREB protein	cAMP response element binding protein
CRH	corticotropin-releasing hormone
CSF	cytostatic factor
CYP-11β	11β-hydroxylase
CYP-21β	21β-hydroxylase
CYPs	cytochrome p450 mono-oxidase gene
DAG	diacylglycerol
DBP	vitamin D-binding protein
DHEAS	dehydroepiandrosterone sulfate
DHT	dihydrotestosterone
DI	diabetes insipidus
DIT	diiodotyrosine
DM	diabetes mellitus
DNA	deoxyribonucleic acid
DOC	deoxycorticosterone
DOPA	dihydroxyphenylalanine
ECL	enterochromaffin-like (cells)
ED	erectile dysfunction
EGF	epidermal growth factor
EnaC	epithelial Na^+ channel
ENS	enteric nervous system
ER	estrogen receptor
ERE	estrogen-response elements
FAS	fatty acid synthase (complex)
FBHH	familial benign hypocalciuric hypercalcemia
FDA	Food and Drug Administration
FFAs	free fatty acids
FGF-23	fibroblast growth factor 23
FSH	follicle-stimulating hormone
α-GSU	α glycoprotein subunit (of hCG)

Gα	G alpha subunit	IRS	insulin-receptor substrate
Gβ/γ	G beta subunit dimer	IUDs	intrauterine devices
G-6-P	glucose-6-phosphate	IVF	in vitro fertilization
GAGs	glycosaminoglycans	LDL	low-density lipoprotein
GDF-9	growth differentiation factor-9	LH	luteinizing hormone
GEFs	guanine nucleotide exchange factors	LPD	luteal phase deficiency
GFR	glomerular filtration rate	LPL	lipoprotein lipase
GH	growth hormone	MAO	monoamine oxidase
GHRH	growth hormone-releasing hormone	MAP	kinase mitogen-activated protein kinase (also ERKs)
GHS	growth hormone secretogogue		
GH-V	growth hormone variant-V	MAPK	mitogen-activated kinase
GI	gastrointestinal	MC2R	melanocortin 2 receptor
GIP	gastroinhibitory peptide	MCsF	monocyte colony-stimulating factor
GLUTs	glucose transporters		
GnRH	gonadotropin-releasing hormone	MIT	monoiodotyrosine
GPCRs	G protein–coupled receptors	MMC	migrating myoelectric complex
GPCR3	G protein–coupled receptor-3	MODY	mature onset of diabetes of the young
GR	glucocorticoid receptor		
GREs	glucocorticoid-response elements	MPF	maturation-promoting factor
GRKs/RTKs	GPCR kinases	MR	mineralocorticoid receptor
GRP	gastrin-releasing peptide	MREs	mineralocorticoid-response elements
GTP	guanosine nucleotide triphosphate		
GVBD	germinal vesicle breakdown	MIS	müllerian-inhibiting substance
β-hCG	hormone-specific β subunit of hCG	MPF	maturation-promoting factor
17β-HSD	17β-hydroxysteroid dehydrogenase	mRNA	messenger RNA
HAD	histone diacetylase	NCX	sodium/calcium exchanger
HAT	histone acetyltransferase	NO	nitric oxide
HbA$_{1c}$	hemoglobin A$_{1c}$	OHSS	ovarian hyperstimulation syndrome
hCG	human chorionic gonadotropin		
HCO$_3^-$	bicarbonate ion	OPG	osteoprotegerin
hCS	human chorionic somatomammotropin	OxPhos	oxidative phosphorylation
		PCO$_2$	partial pressure of carbon dioxide
HDL	high-density lipoprotein	PCOS	polycystic ovarian syndrome
HPA	hypothalamus-pituitary-adrenal	PEPCK\t	PEP carboxykinase (phospho-enolpyruvate carboxykinase)
hPL	human placental lactogen		
HREs	hormone-response elements	PFK-1	phosphofructokinase-1
HSD	hydroxysteroid dehydrogenase	PGE$_2$	prostaglandin E$_2$
HSL	hormone-sensitive lipase	PGF$_{2\alpha}$	prostaglandin F$_{2\alpha}$
ICSI	intracytoplasmic sperm injection	PHEX	phosphate-regulating gene with homologies to endopeptidases on the X chromosome
IDL	intermediate-density lipoprotein (particles)		
IGF	insulin-like growth factors	Pi	phosphate
IGF-1	insulin-like growth factor-1	PI3K	phosphatidylinositol-3-kinase
IGFBPs	insulin-like growth factor–binding proteins	PIP$_3$	phosphatidylinositol 3,4,5-triphosphate
IP$_3$	inositol 1,4,5-triphosphate	PKA	protein kinase A
IR	insulin receptor	PKB	protein kinase B

PKG	protein kinase G		*SRY*	sex-determining region Y
PLCζ	phospholipase Cζ		StAR protein	steroidogenic acute regulatory protein
PMCA	plasma membrane calcium ATPase		STAT	signal transducers and activator of transcription
PMS	premenstrual syndrome			
PNMT	phenylethanolamine-*N*-methyl transferase		SUR	ATP-binding subunit
			$t_{1/2}$	half-life
PO_2	partial pressure of oxygen		T1DM	type 1 diabetes mellitus
POMC	pro-opiomelanocortin		T2DM	type 2 diabetes mellitus
PPARγ	peroxisome proliferator-activated receptor gamma		T_3	triiodothyronine
			T_4	thyroxine
PR	progesterone receptor		TBG	thyroxine-binding globulin
PREs	progesterone-response elements		TCA	tricarboxylic acid (cycle)
PRF	prolactin-releasing factor		TGF	transforming growth factor
PRL	prolactin		TGF-β	transforming growth factor-β
PSA	prostate-specific antigen		TG	thyroglobulin
PTH	parathyroid hormone		TGs	triglycerides
PTHrP	parathyroid hormone-related peptide		TNF-α	tumor necrosis factor-alpha
			TPO	thyroid peroxidase
PTU	propylthiouracil		TR	thyroid hormone receptor
PVH	paraventricular hypothalamus		TREs	thyroid hormone response elements
PVN	paraventricular nuclei			
RAIU	radioactive iodide uptake		TRH	thyrotropin-releasing hormone (also thyroid-releasing hormone)
RANKL	receptor activator of NF-KB ligand			
RAS	renin-angiotensin system			
RDS	respiratory distress syndrome		T/S	thyroid/serum (ratio)
RGS	regulators of G protein signaling		T/S[I]	thyroid/serum (measured with radioactive iodide)
RIAs	radioimmunoassays			
RNA	ribonucleic acid		TSA	thyroid-stimulating antibodies
ROMK channel	renal outer medullary K^+ channel		TSAb	thyroid-stimulating antibodies (abnormal)
ROS	reactive oxygen species			
rT_3	reverse T_3		TSH	thyroid stimulating hormone (also called thyrotropin)
RTK	receptor tyrosine kinase			
SERMs	selective estrogen receptor modulators		TTR	thyroxine-binding prealbumin
			TZDs	thiazolidinediones
SHBG	sex-hormone binding globulin		VDR	vitamin D receptor
SIADH	syndrome of inappropriate secretion of antidiuretic hormone		VEGF	vascular endothelial growth factor
			VLDL	very low-density lipoprotein
SOCS	suppressor of cytokine signaling		VMA	vanillylmandelic acid
SON	supraoptic nuclei		WAT	white adipose tissue
SRBEP-1C	sterol regulatory binding element protein 1C			

APPENDIX B
Answers to Self-Study Problems

CHAPTER 1

1. Cellular response to a hormone is determined primarily by 1, whether that cell type expresses the receptor to the hormone, and the level of receptor expression; 2, the relative levels of signaling components that are linked to the receptor; 3, the differentiated phenotype of that cell type.

2. Protein hormones are stored within secretory vesicles, and are secreted in response to a stimulus. Steroid hormones freely diffuse out of cells.

3. Hormone-binding proteins in the serum generally increase the circulating half-life of a hormone. However, it is the "free" fraction (i.e., unbound) that is considered to be active. Recent studies have indicated that in some cases, steroid hormones enter cells as hormone-transport protein complexes through the process of receptor-mediated endocytosis, in which the transport protein acts as the ligand for endocytosis.

4. Increasing the GTPase activity of Gs would result in a more rapid inactivation of Gs, thereby decreasing adenylate cyclase activity and cAMP levels.

5. The IRS protein is recruited to and phosphorylated by the insulin receptor. The phosphotyrosines recruit and activate the Ras-Raf-MAPK pathway, which transduces insulin receptor binding into a growth response. Other phosphotyrosines on IRS protein activate the PI3 kinase-PKB pathway, which is linked primarily to metabolic actions of insulin (including Glut-4 translocation to the membrane).

6. Cytokines and TGF-β–related hormones (e.g., inhibin) signal by phosphorylating a transcription factor (cytokines use STATs; TGF-β–related hormones use SMADs). The transcription factors then translocate to the nucleus (as dimers) and activate the expression of specific genes.

7. When estrogen binds to the ER, it promotes dimerization, DNA binding at an estrogen-response element, and the recruitment of co-activator proteins. The TR binds to DNA at a thyroid hormone-response element in the absence of hormone. The unliganded TR recruits co-repressor proteins. Thyroid hormone binding to the receptor induces dissociation of the co-repressors from the TR, and recruitment of co-activators.

CHAPTER 2

1. Cephalic, gastric, and intestinal. The greatest release of gastrin occurs during the gastric phase. This occurs because 1) the presence of amino acids in the stomach directly stimulates gastrin release from G cells; 2) the presence of food promotes gastrin release through pressor receptors in the stomach wall; 3) the presence of food buffers acidity, thereby decreasing inhibitory somatostatin release; and 4) there is minimal inhibitory signaling from the small intestine and colon.

2. a, stimulation; b, stimulation; c, inhibition; d, stimulation; e, stimulation

3. S cells secrete secretin, I cells secrete CCK. CCK inhibits gastric motility. Secretin may act as an enterogastrone to inhibit gastrin secretion, but has a minimal effect on gastric emptying.

4. a, some stimulation; b, strong stimulation; c, no effect; d, increase; e, decrease

5. Both glucagon-like peptide-1 (GRP-1) and glucagon are encoded within the same gene that encodes the

preproglucagon prohormone. Glucagon is secreted by alpha cells of the endocrine pancreas and binds to the glucagon receptor. GLP-1 is released by intestinal L cells and acts through the GLP-1 receptor.

6. An incretin is a hormone (peptide) that is released in response to food (especially glucose) in the intestine, and enhances the ability of glucose to promote insulin release from the pancreatic beta cells. Two incretins are GIP and GLP-1.

7. Hypertrophy and hyperplasia of the gastric mucosa and rugae (submucosal folds). Enterochromaffin-like cells (ECL cells) show the greatest degree of proliferation.

8. Erythromycin binds to and activates the motilin receptor.

CHAPTER 3

1. In the fed state, glycolysis in the liver leads to de novo fatty acid and triglyceride synthesis. In the adipose tissue, glycolysis generates glycerol-3-phosphate, which is utilized to reesterify fatty acids (from the digestion of chylomicrons by LPL) into triglycerides.

2. Glycogen is a storage form of glucose. In the liver, glycogenolysis contributes directly to blood glucose, because the liver can dephosphorylate glucose-6-phosphate to glucose. In the muscle, glycogen is utilized during exercise to provide ATP by glycolysis. Skeletal muscle cannot dephosphorylate glucose-6-phosphate, and thus cannot directly contribute to blood glucose levels. However, the lactate that is formed by glycolysis can be converted to glucose by the liver through the process of gluconeogenesis.

3. Ketone bodies. The liver produces ketone bodies from free fatty acids.

4. Accumulation of mitochondrial citrate (in times of plentiful ATP) can be transferred to the cytoplasm, where it can generate cytoplasmic acetyl CoA used for lipogenesis.

5. Lipoprotein lipase (insulin-dependent activation) and hormone-sensitive lipase (insulin-dependent inhibition).

6. Lipoprotein lipase (LPL) digests chylomicrons after a meal, generating chylomicron remnants.

Chylomicron remnants are internalized by the liver and contribute components to the synthesis of VLDL. VLDL are also digested by LPL, especially within skeletal muscle capillary beds during the interdigestive period. This generates VLDL remnants or IDLs. IDLs are further digested by hepatic lase into a relatively high cholesterol, low TG particles, the LDLs.

7. LDL particles lose apoprotein E, and bind to LDL receptors via apoprotein B100. LDL receptors remove these high cholesterol particles from the blood by receptor-mediated endocytosis. The liver plays the major role in LDL receptor–mediated removal of LDL particles, although steroidogenic cells and proliferating cells (i.e., cells that need cholesterol) also take up LDL particles by the LDL receptor. Loss of LDL receptor results in a high LDL concentration in the blood and, therefore, high cholesterol content in the blood.

8. Malonyl CoA inhibits the carnitine-palmitoyl transferase I transporter. This prevents the futile cycle of synthesizing fatty acids only to have them transported into the mitochondria for β-oxidation.

9. Early phase insulin represents stored insulin in secretory vesicles. Later phase insulin represents newly synthesized insulin.

10. Decreased glucokinase activity would inhibit glycolysis and therefore ATP production in β cells. Lower ATP would result in less insulin secreted.

11. Glucokinase insulin increases gene expression; fructose-1,6-bisphosphatase insulin represses gene expression, and indirectly inhibits enzyme by increasing the allosteric inhibitor, fructose-2, 6-bisphosphate; insulin increases pyruvate kinase and pyruvate dehydrogenase by protein phosphatase-mediated dephosphorylation; insulin stimulates acetyl CoA carboxylase gene expression and increases activity by phosphatase-mediated dephosphorylation; insulin represses PEPCK gene expression.

12. A hormone that acts to lower blood glucose concentration.

13. In the presence of a low I/G ratio, more fatty acids are released from adipose tissue. These fatty acids

are transported to the liver where they are metabolized. Beta oxidation increases. The low I/G ratio inhibits glycolysis and hence production of malonyl CoA. Malonyl CoA is a competitive inhibitor of carnitine palmitoyl–transferase I, therefore, as malonyl CoA levels drop, carnitine palmitoyl–transferase I activity increases. This enzyme transesterifies fatty acyl CoA to fatty acylcarnitine, the form in which it traverses the inner mitochondrial membrane. Mitochondria contain the enzymes for beta oxidation and ketogenesis. The elevated acetyl CoA production from beta oxidation along with the decreased TCA cycle activity caused by NAD depletion results in increased ketone body production.

14. Obesity is associated with the accumulation of TGs in skeletal muscle and liver. By-products of TG synthesis and turnover (especially diacylglycerol and ceramide) activate signaling pathways (serine-threonine kinases) that phosphorylate and desensitize the insulin receptor and insulin-receptor substrate.

15. Advanced glycation end products (AGEs) accumulate by intracellular **nonenzymatic glycation** of proteins in response to extended hyperglycemia. Intracellular AGEs have altered function, whereas secreted AGEs in the extracellular matrix interact abnormally with other matrix components and matrix receptors on cells. Finally, some secreted AGEs interact with receptors on macrophages and endothelial cells. Endothelial receptors for AGEs (RAGEs) lead to pro-inflammatory gene expression. Endothelial cells in specific capillary beds (retina, kidney, peripheral nerves) are susceptible to glucotoxicity. **Glucotoxicity** alters cell function in several ways that may contribute to pathological changes. These include increased synthesis of **polyols**, **hexosamines**, and **diacylglycerol** (which activates protein kinase C). Although the exact mechanisms by which intracellular accumulation of these molecules causes abnormal cell function remain unclear, current thinking indicates that these changes lead to increased oxidative stress within the cell. Increased oxidative stress and AGE accumulation impair endothelial function, leading to increased vascular resistance and cell death.

16. TNF-α opposes insulin's action in the liver.

CHAPTER 4

1. 1,25-dihydroxyvitamin D directly represses PTH gene expression. 1,25-dihydroxyvitamin D also increases gene expression of the Ca^{2+} sensing receptor, which represses PTH in response to elevated serum calcium. Therefore, loss of 1,25-dihydroxyvitamin D would lead to an increase of PTH secretion. PTH would also increase in response to lowered Ca^{2+}, primarily due to less absorption by the GI tract.

2. Osteoclasts perform the bone resorption phase of bone remodeling. Osteoblasts promote the differentiation of monocyte/macrophage lineage cells into pre-osteoclasts (via secretion of M-CSF) and the maturation of pre-osteoclasts into actively resorbing osteoclasts (via membrane expression and secretion of RANKL). Note that PTH/PTHrP receptors are expressed by osteoblasts, not osteoclasts.

3. PTH-related peptide (PTHrP) binds to the same receptor as PTH (the PTH/PTHrP receptor). PTHrP normally acts as a paracrine factor. However, high levels of PTHrP can be produced by neoplasms, thereby causing hypercalcemia (as in hyperparathyroidism).

4. Osteoprotegerin acts as a decoy inhibitor of RANKL, thereby inhibiting osteoclast-mediated bone resorption. Overexpression of osteoprotegerin would cause overly dense bone (osteopetrosis).

5. Vitamin D (i.e., 1,25-dihydroxyvitamin D) elevates Pi levels, which promotes the proper calcification of osteoid. Pi absorption by the GI tract occurs largely unregulated. However, Pi reabsorption by the proximal tubule in the kidney is enhanced by vitamin D. This is because the sodium-phosphate exchanger expressed in the kidney is NPT2a, which is under strong hormonal regulation.

6. PTH increases the filtered load because it increases serum calcium levels. Even though PTH increases the distal nephron calcium reabsorption and therefore the fractional reabsorption of calcium, the increase

in calcium filtered generally exceeds the increase in the quantity of calcium reabsorbed.

7. Paget's disease is characterized by high bone turnover. Calcitonin decreases bone resorption, which would decrease turnover rate.

8. Excess PTH increases serum calcium levels. The high calcium levels can increase intracellular calcium levels in cardiac cells, which can lead to cardiac arrest in systole.

9. Hyperparathyroidism increases renal excretion of calcium and phosphate, and the presence of the additional osmotically active electrolytes decreases renal water reabsorption.

10. PTH decreases HCO_3^- reabsorption in the kidney, which could produce metabolic acidosis. Because HCO_3^- reabsorption is inversely related to chloride (Cl^-) reabsorption, the decrease in HCO_3^- absorption would increase Cl^- reabsorption and produce hyperchloremia.

11. PTH acts on the distal nephron by increasing cAMP. The elevated urinary cAMP level reflects this mechanism of action of PTH.

12. The urinary calcium level is low because the low serum calcium levels result in a decreased filtered load for calcium even though fractional reabsorption of calcium is low in the absence of PTH.

13. Alkalosis increases protein binding of calcium, which decreases free calcium levels.

14. Cardiac contractility depends on the availability of intracellular calcium. Because much of the calcium involved in excitation-contraction coupling in cardiac cells comes from ECFs, when extracellular calcium drops, myocardial contractility decreases.

15. Alkaline phosphatase is produced by osteoblasts; elevated serum alkaline phosphatase levels indicate high bone turnover. Elevation of osteocalcin and hydroxyproline levels suggests that bone resorption has increased. Hydroxyproline is an amino acid that is a constituent of collagen.

CHAPTER 5

1. The neurohypophysis (pars nervosa, infundibular stalk, and median eminence) is derived from the infundibular down growth of the diencephalon. The adenohypophysis (pars distalis, pars tuberalis) is derived from Rathke's pouch, a carnial outgrowth of the oral ectoderm.

2. The median eminence is where releasing hormones are released and enter the hypothalamohypophyseal portal vessels, which run down the infundibular stalk.

3. Osmolality.

4. ADH is synthesized in the hypothalamus, specifically in the cell bodies or magnocellular neurons of the SON and PVN. ADH is synthesized as preprovasophysin, which is proteolytically processed during intra-axonal transport down the stalk. ADH is released from the axonal termini at the pars nervosa.

5. ADH secretion is no longer regulated according to normal servomechanisms. The unregulated, inappropriately high ADH levels lead to excess volume and decrease osmolality. The increased volume stimulates ANP, promoting sodium loss. The decreased osmolality further contributes to hyponatremia.

6. If you withhold water from a person with psychogenic diabetes insipidus, urine volume and osmolality will return to normal and ADH can be measured in serum. However, in a person with neurogenic diabetes insipidus, ADH secretion does not increase when water is withheld, urine volume continues to remain higher than normal, and osmolality is lower than normal.

7. Aquaporin 2 and the vasopressin 2 receptor.

8. The prooxyphysin and provasophysin genes evolved from a common ancestral gene through gene duplication. Oxytocin and ADH (vasopressin) are both 9 amino acids peptides produced by magnocellular neurons and released at the pars nervosa.

9. A primary endocrine deficiency usually means the loss (or drastic reduction) of the peripheral hormone that directly regulates physiology. Secondary or tertiary deficiencies mean loss of hormones that do not directly regulate physiology. Moreover, some basal level of primary hormone secretion may persist.

10. Secondary.

11. The GHRH receptor is coupled to a Gs-cAMP-PKA assay, and increases GH gene expression and somatotrope proliferation.

12. GH is a weak counter–regulatory hormone, and opposes insulin-dependent glucose uptake.

13. Cortisol and GH are both "stress hormones" that maintain blood glucose during stress. As expected, stress increases CRH and GHRH. TRH is inhibited by cortisol, and thus is decreased by stress—this would decrease metabolic demands during stress. Similarly, the reproductive system imposes significant metabolic demands, and its activity is decreased during stress. Thus, GnRH is decreased by stress.

14. ACTH binds to the MC1R on melanocytes with low affinity. However, primary hypercortisolism leads to high ACTH levels, sufficient to activate the MC1R.

CHAPTER 6

1. In hypothyroidism, cholesterol synthesis decreases. However, the LDL receptor levels also decrease. These receptors play a crucial role in cellular uptake and hence use of the cholesterol-rich LDLs. Consequently, serum cholesterol levels rise, not because more cholesterol is synthesized, but because cholesterol cannot be cleared effectively from the circulation.

2. The metabolism of administered drugs decreases in hypothyroidism. Therefore medication dosages frequently need to be decreased to prevent overmedication.

3. As the binding affinity decreases, serum free T_4 rises, which results in lower levels of TSH released. T_4 secretion drops until total serum T_4 drops to a point at which free T_4 is returned to normal. Total serum T_4 remains low as long as the binding affinity is low.

4. The increased estrogen production resulting from the pregnancy increases liver TBG production.

As TBG levels increase, serum hormone binding increases. To maintain normal serum free T_4 levels, more T_4 is secreted until a new equilibrium is established in which free hormone levels are close to normal and total levels (bound plus free) are high. Normal pregnant women have significant thyroidal changes during pregnancy, but they are not considered to be hyperthyroid.

5. The size of the thyroid decreases because TSH is suppressed, and TSH stimulates growth of the gland. Because TSH secretion decreases, T_4 synthesis and secretion decrease.

CHAPTER 7

1. Norepinephrine is synthesized in the secretion granule, and then moves into the cytoplasm, where almost all is converted to epinephrine by the cytoplasmic enzyme, phenylethanolamine-N-methyltransferase (PNMT). Epinephrine is actively transported back into the granule for secretion.

2. Epinephrine acts as a counter–regulatory hormone at the liver—it stimulates glycogenolysis, gluconeogenesis, and ketogenesis. At the adipocyte, epinephrine has a strong lipolytic action, through the activation of hormone-sensitive lipase (HSL).

3. Catecholamines act through binding to adrenergic receptors. The primary action on a given organ will be determined by the relative density of the different adrenergic isotypes. The $\beta2$ adrenergic receptor is coupled to the Gs/cAMP/PKA pathway, which promotes vascular smooth muscle relaxation (through phosphorylation of myosin light chain kinase), and thus, vasodilation. Other vessels have a high density of $\alpha1$ receptors, which are coupled to a Gq/PLC/IP$_3$/Ca^{2+} signaling pathway that promotes vasoconstriction.

4. See table below.

	3β HSD	CYP17 (17 HYDROXYLASE FUNCTION)	CYP17 (17/20 LYASE FUNCTION)	CYP21B	CYP11B1	CYP11B2
zona glomerulosa	(+)	(−)	(−)	(+)	(−)	(+)
zona fasciculata	(+)	(+)	(−)	(+)	(+)	(−)
zona reticularis	(−/+)	(+)	(+)	(−)	(−)	(−)

5. Exogenous glucocorticoids inhibit ACTH, which normally is tropic to the adrenal cortex.

6. Excessive ACTH will drive adrenal androgen synthesis in the zona reticularis. The high levels of weak androgens lead to higher levels of testosterone and DHT being produced peripherally in such cells as hair follicle cells.

7. Aldosterone increases the synthesis of ENaC (α-subunit). Aldosterone also increases Sgk–1 gene expression. Sgk–1 prevents the ability of a protein, called Nedd 4-2, from targeting ENaC for degradation. Thus, aldosterone promotes Na+ reabsorption by increasing the synthesis and stability of ENaC in the apical membrane of the distal tubule.

8. Orthostatic hypotension is due to loss of sympathetic tone to adjust for the pull of gravity on the blood. A pheochromocytoma produces chronic high levels of catecholamines, which down-regulate all adrenergic receptors. In Addison's disease, very low levels of aldosterone deplete the intravascular volume, reducing blood pressure. Low cortisol will decrease angiotensinogen production by the liver, and decreases adrenergic receptor expression (especially $\alpha 1$) and signaling in blood vessels. Further, very low levels of cortisol decrease PNMT levels, and thus, adrenomedullary production of epinephrine.

9. Primary adrenal insufficiency involves aldosterone and glucocorticoid production, whereas secondary insufficiency involves only glucocorticoid production.

CHAPTER 8

1. The Sertoli cells form occluding junctions just apical to the spermatogonia—it is these junctions between adjacent Sertoli cells that create the basal and adluminal compartments of the seminiferous epithelium.

2. Loss of 17β–HSD (type 3) would result in no testicular production of bioactive androgens (T or DHT). This would result in minimal spermatogenesis and development of male genitalia. In fact, the external genitalia would likely form as female. The excessive androstenedione produced by the Leydig cell due to elevated LH (think "reduced negative feedback") would be converted to estrone and estradiol 17β, as well as some conversion to testosterone and DHT. However, estrogen production prevails in these individuals, so that "female" breast development occurs.

3. The testis develop normally and independently of DHT. Normal fetal production of T causes development of the mesonephric (male) tract, and normal fetal production of antimüllerian hormone causes the paramesonephric (female) tract to regress. DHT is required for normal development of the prostate and external genitalia. 5α-reductase type 2 is required for male development of the external genitalia in utero. Thus, loss of this enzyme will give rise to "default" female genitalia.

4. Normal spermatogenesis is absolutely dependent on LH-driven intratesticular production of T, which leads to extremely high levels of T within the seminiferous tubules. Exogenous androgens will increase blood T levels enough to inhibit LH, which will actually result in decreased intratesticular levels of T.

5. 1, mitosis of spermatogonia; 2, loss of most cytoplasm; 3, incapacitation; 4, mixing of sperm with secretions from seminal vesicles and prostate.

CHAPTER 9

1. Meiotic maturation of the primary oocyte to an egg (secondary oocyte at metaphase II). Only this cell can be fertilized.

2. LH receptor is always expressed on thecal cells. LH receptor is not expressed in granulosa cells until in a large preovulatory follicle. LH receptor is expressed on luteinized theca and granulosa cells. LH expression is induced by FSH during the late follicular phase of the ovary. Lack of LH receptors would make the follicle insensitive to the LH surge—there would be no meiotic maturation of the oocyte, nor ovulation, nor luteinization.

3. The LH surge induces the following during the periovulatory period: 1, meiotic maturation of the oocyte; 2, cumulus expansion and breakdown of contact between cumulus and mural granulosa cells; 3, secretion of hydrolytic enzymes which

erode the follicular and ovarian wall, and the basal lamina of the mural granulosa, allowing for direct vascularization; 4, luteinization of the follicle cells, leading to the onset of progesterone secretion.

4. The theca cells convert cholesterol to androstenedione. However, theca express little 17β–HSD and essentially no CYP19 aromatase, and, thus, cannot produce estradiol. The androstenedione must enter the granulosa cells, which convert it to estradiol.

5. For example, estrogen has a negative and positive feedback on pituitary gonadotropes, stimulates growth of the uterine endometrium, stimulates ductal growth in the breasts, stimulates ciliogenesis in the oviduct, and stimulates secretion of a thin, watery mucus by the cervix. Non-reproductive actions of estrogen include bone mineralization, growth and epiphysial plate closure, increased HDL and decreased VLDL and LDL production, increased vasodilation in general, maintenance of healthy skin, and increased lipolysis.

6. The endometrium would not fully develop secretory activity, would not fully express surface proteins involved in implantation, and would undergo early menses.

7. The ovarian reserve indicates the number of primordial follicles in the ovary at any given time. The ovulatory quota is the number of eggs ovulated per month, which is one in humans. The ovarian reserve declines continually to meet the ovulatory quota. During menopause, the ovarian reserve becomes insufficient to support the ovulation of one follicle per month.

8. The oviducts, uterus, and upper third of the vagina.

9. There is a selective rebound in FSH secretion.

10. Selection of recruited follicles.

CHAPTER 10

1. Implantation is associated with the following events: 1, differentiation of the trophoblast into cytotrophoblasts and syncytiotrophoblasts. Syncytiotrophoblasts express adhesion molecules and hydrolytic enzymes that allow for invasion, and hCG that rescues the corpus luteum; 2, the appearance of uterine receptivity, which occurs in a window of time corresponding to the midluteal phase of the ovary, and involves upregulation of adhesive molecules and downregulation of anti-adhesive molecules on the apical surface of the uterine epithelium; 3, the stromal cells of the uterine endometrium undergo decidualization, involving the production of glycogen, as well as expressing adhesive proteins, forming cell-cell contacts to wall off the site of implantation, and the release of growth factors and molecules that keep the invading syncytiotrophoblasts in check.

2. Placental progesterone is completed solely by the syncytiotrophoblast—and is independent of fetal viability. Estriol requires the fetal hypothalamus, pituitary, adrenal and liver, as well as the syncytiotrophoblast of the placenta. Thus, fetal and placental health impacts estriol synthesis.

3. Estrogen is not needed for a normal pregnancy, except for the development of the breasts for nursing, and for sufficiently responsive myometrium for labor to occur.

4. Complete loss of CYP17 would stop DHEAS synthesis, and thus, estrogen production by the placenta. The fetal adrenal definitive zone also produces cortisol, which would not be made in the absence of CYP17. Thus, fetal ACTH would be increased.

5. hCG increases rapidly during the first trimester, and cross-reacts with the TSH receptor on the maternal thyroid. hCG production declines to a lower steady level after the first trimester, thereby terminating the hyperthyroidism.

6. Respiratory changes in response to progesterone include increased minute volume and increased tidal volume.

7. Prolactin inhibits GnRH and thus promotes infertility. During very regular nursing, high prolactin levels cause lactational amenorrhea, which inhibits pregnancy while a newborn is being nursed. The most common type of pituitary tumor is the prolactinoma. This is associated with pathologically elevated prolactin, amenorrhea, and infertility.

8. To induce meiotic maturation of the primary oocyte to an egg at metaphase II.

APPENDIX C

Comprehensive Multiple-Choice Examination

1. Which hormone has a receptor that is structurally similar to the estrogen receptor?
   a. Insulin
   b. Epinephrine
   c. FSH
   d. Thyroid hormone

2. According to the second-messenger hypothesis, the second messenger is the:
   a. Hormone carrying the signal to the target organ
   b. Receptor located on the cell membrane
   c. Intracellular chemical messenger
   d. Receptor located in the cell nucleus

3. Which hormone would have an N-signal peptide as a portion of the original gene transcript?
   a. GH
   b. Cortisol
   c. Epinephrine (catecholamine)
   d. T_4 (thyroid hormone)

4. G_s proteins serve as transducers in the actions of:
   a. Testosterone
   b. PRL
   c. GH
   d. TSH

5. Which one of the following hormones does not have intracellular receptors?
   a. T_3
   b. Estrogens
   c. Cortisol
   d. Epinephrine

6. Transcription factors include:
   a. Estrogen receptors
   b. The hormone response element
   c. Heat shock proteins
   d. Phosphodiesterase

7. Which hormone is *not* biologically effective if administered orally?
   a. T_4 (thyroid hormone)
   b. Estradiol (an estrogen)
   c. GH
   d. Cortisol

8. You have discovered a "new" hormone that is a protein with a molecular size of 180 amino acids. Which statement is most likely to be correct about this hypothetical hormone?
   a. It will probably have its action by entering the cell and binding to a nuclear receptor.
   b. It will probably need to be relatively tightly associated with plasma proteins to be carried in any appreciable quantities in blood.
   c. It can be effectively administered orally.
   d. It will be stored in the cell in membrane-bound secretory vesicles.

9. You learn that the new hormone discussed in question 8 activates phospholipase C. Given that information, which one of the following changes is most likely to occur following hormone administration?
   a. Intracellular DAG levels will increase.
   b. Cytosolic calcium concentrations will decrease.
   c. Calcium association with calmodulin will decrease.
   d. Phosphorylation of protein tyrosine residues will increase.

10. Factors known to increase ACTH secretion include all of the following *except:*
    a. Stress
    b. ADH
    c. Hyperglycemia
    d. CRH

11. Ketosis is not likely to occur in acromegaly because:
    a. GH is not a lipolytic hormone
    b. GH inhibits beta oxidation
    c. GH stimulates lipoprotein lipase
    d. Most individuals with acromegaly have suffi-cient insulin production to suppress ketosis

12. Adults with gigantism characteristically have dis-proportionately long arms and legs relative to their height. This occurs because:
    a. They frequently have delayed puberty because of decreased gonadotropin secretion.
    b. GH stimulates long bone growth but not membranous or appositional bone growth.
    c. GH acts on bone by stimulating IGF produc-tion, and IGFs act only on long bones.
    d. GH acts preferentially on distal appendages, and hence the term *acromegaly* is applied to adults with hypersecretion of GH.

13. A patient had a difficult delivery 6 months ago with excessive blood loss. When she returns to her obstetrician for her 6-month follow-up visit, she mentions that her menstrual cycles have not resumed even though she is not nursing her infant. Her physician suspects postpartum pituitary necrosis. If correct, all of the following would be present *except:*
    a. Thyroid atrophy
    b. Low serum cortisol levels
    c. Diabetes insipidus
    d. Low serum LH levels

14. Correct statements about POMC include all of the following *except:*
    a. It is a prohormone for β-LPH
    b. It contains the amino acid sequences of MSH
    c. Its synthesis is regulated by CRH in the adult human pituitary
    d. It is synthesized from ACTH

15. In a normal individual with a typical sleep/wake cycle, the highest cortisol levels occur at:
    a. 6 AM
    b. 11 AM
    c. 5 PM
    d. 11 PM

16. Which statement best describes the relationship between GH and IGF-I?
    a. There is always a direct relationship between serum concentrations of GH and IGF-I.
    b. IGF-I mediates most, if not all, of the growth-promoting actions of GH.
    c. GH is protein anabolic, whereas IGF-I is not.
    d. GH is produced only in the pituitary, whereas IGF-I is produced only in the liver.

17. A 40-year-old man presents with severe joint pain. His teeth are widely spaced, and his hands, nose, and feet are unusually large. He comments that over the last 10 years, his shoe size has grown from a 10 to a 16. You order a detailed serum profile. Which of the following results would you expect from the blood analyses, and what is the correct reason?
    a. Serum IGF-I levels are high secondary to high GH levels.
    b. Serum TSH levels are high, and excessive thy-roid function is responsible for the bone pain.
    c. Serum IGF-I levels are low because of an insulin deficiency.
    d. Serum glucose levels are low because of increased insulin sensitivity.

18. Increased insulin sensitivity in panhypopitu-itarism is caused by:
    a. High serum insulin-induced receptor down regulation
    b. Low serum thyroid hormone levels
    c. High serum cortisol levels
    d. Low serum GH levels

19. IGF-I acts to:
    a. Increase blood glucose
    b. Stimulate lipolysis
    c. Stimulate cellular division (hyperplasia)
    d. Inhibit cartilage growth

20. ADH is:
    a. Produced in the posterior pituitary
    b. A neural hormone
    c. Carried in the blood bound to the protein neurophysin
    d. A large protein that must be administered by injection

21. Actions of ADH include:
    a. Stimulation of ACTH synthesis and secretion
    b. Inhibition of renal cAMP production
    c. Antagonism of the actions of oxytocin
    d. Inhibition of the sensation of thirst

22. Your patient has an ADH-secreting pulmonary carcinoma (syndrome of inappropriate ADH secretion—SIADH). As a result of unregulated ADH secretion, you would expect to find:
    a. Retention of water resulting in volume expansion
    b. A low urinary osmolality
    c. Increased renal sodium reabsorption
    d. A high serum sodium concentration

23. A 25-year-old woman develops a nonfunctional hypothalamic tumor that results in a complete inability to produce oxytocin. The most likely pathological response to this deficiency is:
    a. Inability to ovulate
    b. Amenorrhea
    c. Hypertension
    d. Inability to lactate normally
    e. Inability to deliver a child vaginally

24. T_4 rather than T_3 is generally thought to be the most appropriate treatment for hypothyroidism. T_4 normally is the most appropriate hormone to use because it:
    a. Is the more potent hormone
    b. Has a higher binding affinity for the thyroid hormone receptor
    c. Has a larger extrathyroidal pool with a slower turnover rate
    d. Is the only form of thyroid hormones that can be transported into cells

25. Which pathologic condition would most likely cause increased thyroidal radioactive iodide uptake?
    a. Primary hypothyroidism
    b. Secondary hypothyroidism
    c. Graves' disease

26. All but one of the answers below list common symptoms of hyperthyroidism and the correct physiological basis for the symptom. For an answer to be correct, both the symptom and the explanation must be correct. Which answer is *incorrect*?
    a. The resting heart rate increases because circulating levels of catecholamines increase. Excess

thyroid hormones stimulate the release of more adrenal catecholamines.
    b. Myocardial contractility increases because thyroid hormones act directly on the heart and act indirectly by potentiating the effect of catecholamines on the myocardium.
    c. Peripheral resistance decreases because of cutaneous vasodilation as a thermoregulatory response.
    d. The circulating half-lives of most exogenously administered drugs decrease because the rate of metabolism increases and drug inactivation is more rapid.

27. Mrs. J is a 58-year-old postmenopausal woman weighing 186 pounds. The serum T_4 is 8 μg/dl (normal is 6 to 12 μg/dl), TSH is 4 μU/ml (normal is 2 to 10 μU/ml), and she complains of depression. Her doctor prescribes a low dosage of T_4 to "pep her up." What changes would you expect to see 4 weeks after the initiation of treatment?
    a. The size of the thyroid will be reduced.
    b. Serum TSH will be greater than 4 μU/ml.
    c. Serum T_4 will be less than 8 μg/dl.
    d. The basal metabolic rate will be elevated.

28. If a person with normal thyroid function is treated with T_3, which of the following changes will become apparent within 48 hours?
    a. Serum T_4 will drop.
    b. TG synthesis will increase.
    c. Iodide uptake by the thyroid will increase.
    d. Serum TG levels will rise.

29. Mr. Z is a 27-year-old man with a readily apparent thyroid goiter. He comments that he has gained 3 pounds in the last year, and you notice that his weight is approximately 15 pounds greater than normal for his age and frame. What can you conclude about this patient's thyroid function?
    a. The goiter indicates that he is hyperthyroid.
    b. The combination of the excessive weight and the goiter indicates that he is hypothyroid.
    c. He is probably euthyroid because, although a goiter can occur in both euthyroid and hyperthyroid individuals, the weight gain eliminates the possibility of hyperthyroidism.
    d. It is not possible to draw any conclusions about his thyroid status from the information provided.

30. Which of the following relationships between the disorder indicated below and the probable clinical observations is the most appropriate?
    a. Primary (thyroidal) hypothyroidism: ↓ serum T_4; ↓ serum TSH; ↓ radioactive iodide uptake (RAIU); ↓ response of TSH to TRH following a TRH challenge
    b. Secondary (pituitary) hypothyroidism: ↓ serum T_4; ↓ serum TSH; ↓ RAIU; little or no change in TSH secretion following a TRH challenge
    c. Primary (thyroidal) hypothyroidism: ↓ serum T_4; ↑ serum TSH; ↓ RAIU; ↓ TSH secretion following a TRH challenge
    d. Tertiary (hypothalamic) hypothyroidism: ↓ serum T_4; ↑ serum TSH; ↓ RAIU; ↓ TSH secretion following a TRH challenge

31. Biologic actions of thyroid hormones include all of the following *except:*
    a. Stimulate protein synthesis and proteolysis
    b. Increase Na-KATPase activity
    c. Stimulate glycogenesis
    d. Increase oxidative phosphorylation
    e. Stimulate growth and vascularity of the thyroid gland

32. Which pair of symptoms and causes is most appropriate for hypothyroidism?
    a. The skin is warm and moist because of peripheral vasodilation.
    b. Diarrhea occurs because of increased GI secretion and motility.
    c. Puberty is delayed or absent because TSH reacts with LH and FSH receptors.
    d. Myxedema occurs because mucopolysaccharides accumulate in the extracellular spaces.
    e. There is a tendency to gain weight because appetite increases.

33. If you withdraw insulin from an insulin-dependent diabetic patient, you would expect to see all of the following *except:*
    a. A decrease in urinary bicarbonate levels
    b. An increase in renal ammonium production
    c. An increase in the release of alanine and glutamate from skeletal muscle
    d. A decrease in BUN (blood urea nitrogen)
    e. A decrease in $PaCO_2$

34. Correct cause-and-effect relationships following insulin withdrawal in a person with diabetes mellitus include:
    a. The ratio of potassium concentration inside the cell to potassium concentration outside the cell decreases in untreated diabetes for multiple reasons, including decreasing secondary to intracellular H{ΣY}+{/ΣY} buffering, which results in a shift of potassium to the extracellular compartment.
    b. Ketonemia (excess ketone bodies in serum) per se does not increase urine flow because it is entirely reabsorbed in the renal tubule.
    c. Urinary phosphate decreases because renal excretion of H{ΣY}+{/ΣY} results in increased phosphate reabsorption.
    d. Serum sodium rises because of hemoconcentration that results from a net fluid shift from the extracellular compartment to the intracellular compartment.
    e. Glomerular filtration rate increases as a result of increased serum glucose concentration.

35. The most effective direct stimulus for the release of glucagon is:
    a. A decrease in serum alanine
    b. An increase in serum glucose
    c. Somatostatin
    d. Insulin (direct action on the alpha cell)

36. People with non-insulin–dependent diabetes mellitus are generally not ketosis prone. This is thought to be a result of:
    a. The lack of an increase in glucagon in these individuals
    b. The presence of insulin in these individuals
    c. Their obesity
    d. The fact that, unlike insulin-dependent diabetic patients, their blood glucose levels do not tend to rise significantly

37. Metabolic actions of insulin include all of the following *except:*
    a. Increased glycogenesis
    b. Decreased gluconeogenesis
    c. Increased basal metabolic rate
    d. Increased skeletal muscle amino acid uptake (especially branched-chain amino acids)

38. The hormone *least* likely to be diabetogenic in excess is:
    a. Cortisol
    b. GH
    c. hCG
    d. hPL

39. Which of the following relationships about glucose transport into cells is correct?
    a. Glucose transport into the cells of the renal proximal tubule is via an insulin-sensitive transport system.
    b. Whereas the transport of glucose into skeletal muscle is regulated by insulin, the transport into adipocytes is independent of direct insulin actions.
    c. Exercise can increase the rate of glucose transport into skeletal muscle cells, even in the absence of insulin.
    d. Most areas of the brain have insulin-sensitive glucose transport systems.

40. In the statements below, which is the correct cause-and-effect relationship for diabetes mellitus?
    a. Ketoacidosis occurs when acetyl CoA entry into TCA cycle exceeds acetyl CoA production.
    b. Ketoacidosis occurs when beta oxidation depletes NAD.
    c. Osmotic diuresis occurs as a result of glucosuria, but not ketonuria, because ketone bodies are readily reabsorbed in the kidney.
    d. Hypertension occurs because ketone bodies are vasoconstrictors.

41. A decrease in the I/G ratio in serum will produce:
    a. A fall in blood glucose
    b. A rise in serum branched-chain amino acids
    c. A decrease in hormone-sensitive lipase activity
    d. An increase in lipoprotein lipase activity

42. An 8-year-old child with diabetes mellitus of 1 year's duration has had two severe episodes of diabetic ketoacidosis that have required hospitalization. Which of the following statements is most likely to be correct about his condition?
    a. He has increased frequency of certain HLA types.
    b. He would not be likely to have high titers of anti-islet cell antibodies.
    c. The serum fatty acid levels would have been low at the time of admission to the hospital.
    d. The pancreas would have fewer functioning alpha cells.

43. Secretion of PTH is increased by:
    a. An increase in serum magnesium concentration
    b. An increase in serum phosphate concentration
    c. An increase in dietary calcium
    d. A decrease in urinary calcium levels
    e. Treatment with thiazide diuretics

44. Hyperparathyroidism results in:
    a. Alkalosis
    b. Hyperchloremia
    c. Hyperphosphatemia
    d. Hypophosphaturia
    e. Hypocalcemia

45. Which cause-and-effect relationship is correct for a deficiency of active vitamin D (calcitriol)?
    a. Hypercalcemia occurs because of decreased intestinal calbindin levels.
    b. Hypophosphatemia occurs because of decreased intestinal phosphate absorption.
    c. Bone formation is increased because vitamin D blocks the action of PTH on bone resorption.
    d. Osteoporosis, but not osteomalacia, is associated with a calcitriol deficiency because calcitriol synergizes with PTH in its action on bone.

46. A 50-year-old man has low serum calcium and high serum phosphate levels. His urinary cAMP levels are low. He most likely suffers from:
    a. Hypoparathyroidism
    b. Hyperparathyroidism
    c. Vitamin D deficiency
    d. Cushing's syndrome

47. Renal osteodystrophy (bone problems associated with renal failure) is characterized by:
    a. A decrease in serum PTH levels
    b. An increase in urinary phosphate levels
    c. An increase in serum calcium levels
    d. A decrease in 1α-hydroxylase activity

48. Which set of serum values would be most typical of a patient with a calcium-mobilizing tumor?
    a. High serum phosphate, high serum calcium, and high serum PTH
    b. Low serum phosphate, high serum calcium, and high serum PTH

c. Low serum phosphate, high serum calcium, and low serum PTH

d. Low serum phosphate, low serum calcium, and high serum PTH

e. High serum phosphate, low serum calcium, and low serum PTH

49. Which set of serum values would be most typical of a patient with hyperparathyroidism?
    a. High serum phosphate, high serum calcium, and high serum PTH
    b. Low serum phosphate, high serum calcium, and high serum PTH
    c. Low serum phosphate, high serum calcium, and low serum PTH
    d. Low serum phosphate, low serum calcium, and high serum PTH
    e. High serum phosphate, low serum calcium, and low serum PTH

50. Which set of serum values would be most typical of a patient with a vitamin D deficiency?
    a. High serum phosphate, high serum calcium, and high serum PTH
    b. Low serum phosphate, high serum calcium, and high serum PTH
    c. Low serum phosphate, high serum calcium, and low serum PTH
    d. Low serum phosphate, low serum calcium, and high serum PTH
    e. High serum phosphate, low serum calcium, and low serum PTH

51. 1,25-dihydroxycholecalciferol:
    a. Increases bone mineralization by increasing serum calcium levels
    b. Decreases bone resorption by antagonizing the action of PTH on bone
    c. Decreases serum phosphate levels by decreasing renal phosphate reabsorption
    d. Decreases serum alkaline phosphatase levels by decreasing bone turnover

52. Bone loss associated with renal failure occurs because:
    a. The failing kidney is no longer capable of PTH production.
    b. Renal phosphate clearance decreases in renal failure.

c. The failing kidney increases activation of vitamin D.

d. Renal calcium clearance increases in renal failure.

53. A patient has hypercortisolism, and the MRI results indicate that there is hyperplasia of the right adrenal but the left adrenal appears smaller than normal. What does this generally indicate about the origin of the adrenal disorder?
    a. The adrenal hyperfunction most likely results from a secondary or tertiary disorder producing pituitary ACTH hypersecretion.
    b. The adrenal hyperfunction is most likely a result of an ACTH-secreting nonadrenal tumor.
    c. The adrenal hyperfunction is most likely a primary disorder resulting from malfunction of the adrenal gland.
    d. The hypercortisolism is probably not a result of an adrenal disorder but rather is the result of exogenous administration of glucocorticoids.

54. Mrs. Q is a 39-year-old woman complaining of polyuria and nocturia, and her fasting blood glucose level is high. Her hematocrit value is exceptionally high even though she is not dehydrated, and she has difficulty with deep knee bends. You notice that her face appears round and puffy, and, although her weight is slightly above normal for her frame, her arms and legs appear thin. Which one of the following conditions would be most likely to be correct about her condition?
    a. The liver glycogen levels would probably be low.
    b. Hypertension is a common occurrence in this disorder.
    c. Her cardiac output is likely to be lower than normal.
    d. She will probably have orthostatic hypotension.

55. Which of the following cause-and-effect relationships is correct?
    a. Weight gain in Cushing's syndrome is a result of the lipogenic action of cortisol.
    b. A person with adrenal insufficiency has difficulty excreting a water load in a normal period of time because of the actions of aldosterone on sodium and hence water reabsorption.

c. Anemia occurs in Addison's disease because of the action of cortisol on GI iron absorption and on erythropoietin release.

d. Skin darkening in Addison's disease indicates that the site of the disorder is in the pituitary rather than the adrenal.

e. Synthetic glucocorticoids are useful in the treatment of arthritis because they stimulate bone growth.

56. Mr. Jones is a 49-year-old brick mason who has come to you complaining of intermittent periods of cardiac palpitations accompanied by excessive sweating and headaches. You suspect he suffers from a pheochromocytoma. If you were to examine him shortly after one of these episodes, you would expect to find:

a. Postural hypotension

b. Hypoglycemia

c. Depressed serum FFAs

d. Low serum cortisol levels
The figure below shows the relationship between serum ACTH levels and serum cortisol levels under different conditions. The normal relationship is shown as a reference. Answer questions 57 to 59 using this figure.

57. A patient with an ACTH-secreting pulmonary tumor would most likely be represented by:

a. Point A

b. Point B

c. Point C

d. Point D

58. A patient with Cushing's disease and bilateral adrenal hyperplasia would most likely be represented by:

a. Point A

b. Point B

c. Point C

d. Point D

59. A patient with a functional adrenal cortical tumor would most likely be represented by:

a. Point A

b. Point B

c. Point C

d. Point D

60. In humans, total adrenalectomy is fatal without replacement therapy whereas hypophysectomy is not. This is because, after hypophysectomy:

a. The adrenal cortex undergoes compensatory hypertrophy.

b. The adrenal catecholamines compensate for the metabolic actions of cortisol.

c. The secretion of aldosterone is not markedly decreased.

d. Tissue requirements for corticosteroids decrease markedly.

61. Factors that increase serum cortisol concentrations include all of the following *except:*

a. Stress

b. Eating a high-carbohydrate meal

c. Pregnancy

d. Exercise

62. A 72-year-old man is suffering from nocturia. He also has difficulty with urination, decreased flow, and an inability to completely empty the bladder. The prostate is symmetrically enlarged, non-tender, and smooth. The predominant androgen associated with this enlargement is:

a. DHEA

b. Androstenedione

c. DHT

d. Testosterone

e. Androsterone

63. People with androgen insensitivity syndrome show developmental abnormalities. Which of the following primary or secondary sexual characteristics is most likely to be seen in these individuals? The presence of:

a. A prostate

b. A penis

c. Breast development at puberty

d. Descended testes

e. Pubic and axillary hair

64. Which serum patterns, relative to normal, are most likely to occur in androgen insensitivity syndrome?

a. ↑ LH, ↑ FSH, ↑ testosterone, ↑ estrogen

b. ↓ LH, ↓ FSH, ↑ testosterone, ↑ estrogen

c. ↓ LH, ↓ FSH, ↓ testosterone, ↑ estrogen

d. ↓ LH, ↓ FSH, ↓ testosterone, ↓ estrogen

e. ↑ LH, ↑ FSH, ↓ testosterone, ↓ estrogen

65. Characteristics of inhibin include that it:
    a. Is a steroid hormone
    b. Inhibits FSH secretion
    c. Is produced in the testis but not the ovary
    d. Contains two β chains

66. Which of the following is true regarding the determinants of sexual development?
    a. The presence of the gene for HY antigen on the Y chromosome determines whether a testis develops from the gonadal ridge.
    b. The presence of MIS determines whether the wolffian ducts develop.
    c. The presence of estrogen determines whether a vagina develops.
    d. The presence of DHT determines whether a prostate develops.

67. The anatomic site of the blood-testis barrier is the:
    a. Tight junction of the Sertoli cells
    b. Basal lamina (basement membrane) of the seminiferous tubules
    c. Testicular capsule
    d. Testicular interstitium
    e. Testicular capillary endothelium

68. Menopause results from:
    a. Ovarian failure
    b. Pituitary failure
    c. Hypothalamic failure
    d. All of the above

69. Which hormonal relationship most closely resembles that of inhibin and FSH?
    a. Estrogen and progesterone
    b. Estrogen and LH
    c. Somatostatin and estrogen
    d. GnRH and FSH

70. The most significant source of serum testosterone in the normal woman is:
    a. Liver production from ovarian estradiol
    b. Peripheral production from adrenal DHEA
    c. Ovarian granulosa cell production
    d. Luteal cell production

71. Cessation of growth after adolescence is a result primarily of:
    a. A decrease in GH secretion
    b. An increase in androgen and estrogen secretion
    c. An increase in cortisol secretion

d. A decrease in thyroxine secretion
    The figure at the top of the page represents serum levels of a hormone during the menstrual cycle. This is a typical 28-day cycle, and the graph begins on day 1 of the cycle. Answer questions 72 to 74 using this graph.

72. Ovulation will most likely occur 12 to 36 hours after this time:
    a. Point A
    b. Point B
    c. Point C

73. There should be an optimally developed secretory endometrium at this time:
    a. Point A
    b. Point B
    c. Point C

74. Both estrogen and progesterone levels in serum are high at this time:
    a. Point A
    b. Point B
    c. Point C

75. Progesterone acts to stimulate:
    a. Uterine contraction
    b. Endometrial proliferation
    c. Mammary gland lobular-alveolar development
    d. Production of thin, watery, slightly alkaline cervical mucus
    e. Keratinization (cornification) of the vaginal epithelium

76. Which of the following observations would be the most effective indicator that ovulation has occurred?
    a. A drop in body temperature
    b. A rise in serum progesterone levels
    c. A rise in serum estrogen levels
    d. A surge in serum LH levels
    e. A surge in serum FSH levels

77. The most effective early test for pregnancy involves measuring serum or urinary levels of which hormone?
    a. Estradiol
    b. Progesterone
    c. hPL
    d. hCG
    e. Estriol

78. Which maternal serum hormonal changes would most effectively indicate death or impairment of the fetus?
    a. Decreased estradiol levels
    b. Decreased estriol levels
    c. Decreased progesterone levels
    d. Decreased hCG levels
    e. Decreased hPL levels

79. What is the predominant cause of the diabetogenicity of pregnancy?
    a. Increased pancreatic insulin secretion
    b. Increased placental hPL secretion
    c. Increased pancreatic glucagon secretion
    d. Increased maternal GH secretion
    e. Increased placental ACTH secretion

80. Amnionic fluid is best described as:
    a. More closely approximating the constituency of maternal extracellular fluids than that of fetal extracellular fluids
    b. Being formed primarily as an excretory product of the amnionic membrane
    c. Containing fetal urine
    d. Having production regulated by hCG levels

APPENDIX D

HORMONE	NORMAL RANGE – CONVENTIONAL UNITS
Adrenal Steroids, plasma	
Aldosterone, supine, saline suppression	<8.5 ng/dL
Aldosterone, upright, normal diet	5-20 ng/dL
Cortisol	
8 AM	5-25 µg/dL
4 PM	3-12 µg/dL
Overnight dexamethasone suppression	<5 µg/dL
Dehydroepiandrosterone (DHEA)	2-9 µg/dL
DHEAS	50-250 µg/dL
Adrenal Steroids, urine	
Aldosterone	5-19 µg/day
Cortisol, free	20-100 µg/day
17-Hydroxycorticosteroids	2-10 mg/day
17-Ketosteroids	
Men	7-25 mg/day
Women	4-16 mg/day
Angiotensin II, plasma	10-60 pg/mL
Antidiuretic Hormone (ADH; vasopressin)	
Random fluid intake	1-3 pg/mL
Dehydration 18-24 h	4-14 pg/mL
Calciferols (Vitamin D_3), plasma	
1,25-dihydroxyvitamin D_3	15-60 pg/mL
25-hydroxyvitamin D_3	8-40 ng/mL
Calcitonin, plasma	
Normal	<19 pg/mL
Medullary thyroid cancer	>100 pg/mL
Calcium, ionized serum	4-5.6 mg/dL
Catecholamines, urine	
Free catecholamines	<100 µg/day
Epinephrine	<50 µg/day
Metanephrine	<1.3 ng/day
Norepinephrine	15-89 µg/day
Vanillylmandelic acid (VMA)	<8 mg/day

Continued

HORMONE	NORMAL RANGE – CONVENTIONAL UNITS
Cholesterol, total plasma	
Desirable	<200 mg/dL
HDL Cholesterol	
Desirable	>69 mg/dL
LDL Cholesterol	
Desirable	<130 mg/dL
Corticotropin (ACTH), plasma, 8 AM	9-52 pg/mL
Electrolytes	
Chloride, serum	98-106mEq/L
Sodium, serum	136-145 mEq/L
Free Fatty Acids, plasma	10.6-18 mg/dL
Gastrin, plasma	<120 pg/mL
Glucagon, plasma	50-100 pg/mL
Glucose, plasma	
Overnight fast, normal	75-115 mg/dL
Glucose Tolerance Test	
2 hr plasma glucose, normal	<140 mg/dL
2 hr plasma glucose, diabetes mellitus	>200 mg/dL
Gonadal Steroids	
Dihydrotestosterone	
Women	0.05-0.3 ng/mL
Men	0.25-0.75 ng/mL
Estradiol	
Women, basal	20-60 pg/mL
Women, ovulatory surge	>200 pg/mL
Men	<50 pg/mL
Progesterone	
Women, luteal phase	2-20 ng/mL
Women, follicular phase	< 2 ng/mL
Men	< 2 ng/mL
Testosterone	
Women	<1 ng/mL
Men	3-10 ng/mL
Gonadotropins, plasma	
Follicle-stimulating hormone (FSH)	
Women, basal	1.4-9.6 mIU/mL
Women, ovulatory surge	2.3-21 mIU/mL
Women, postmenopausal	34-96 mIU/mL
Men	0.9-15 mIU/mL
Luteinizing hormone (LH)	
Women, basal	0.8-26 mIU/mL
Women, ovulatory surge	25-57 mIU/mL
Women, postmenopausal	40-104 mIU/mL
Men	1.3-13 mIU/mL

HORMONE	NORMAL RANGE – CONVENTIONAL UNITS
Growth hormone, plasma	
After 100 g glucose orally	<2 mg/mL
After insulin-induced hypoglycemia	>9 ng/mL
Human chorionic gonadotropin (hCG)	
Men and nonpregnant women	<3 mIU/mL
Insulin, plasma, fasting	5-20 µU/ml
Insulin-like Growth Factor (IGF-I)	0.35-2.2 U/mL
Ketone bodies	
Acetoacetate	<1 mg/dL
β-Hydroxybutyrate	<3 mg/dL
Lactate, plasma	5-20 mg/dL
Magnesium, serum	1.8-3.0 mg/dL
Osmolality, plasma	285-295 mOsmol/L
Oxytocin, plasma	
Random	1.25-5 ng/mL
Women, ovulatory surge	5-10 ng/ml
Parathyroid hormone, serum (Intact PTH)	10-65 pg/mL
Phosphorus, inorganic, serum	3.0-4.5 mg/dL
Prolactin, serum	
Nonpregnant women and men	2-15 ng/ml
Pyruvate, plasma	0.3-0.9 mg/dL
Renin activity, plasma, normal sodium intake	
Standing	9.3 +/− 4.3 ng/mL/h
Supine	3.2 +/− 1 ng/mL/h
Thyroid function tests	
Free thyroxine estimate	0.7-2.0 ng/dL
Radioactive iodine uptake, 24 h	5-30%
Resin T_3 uptake, serum	25-35%
Reverse T_3 (rT_3), serum	10-40 ng/dL
Thyrotropin (TSH), serum	0.5-5 µU/mL
Thyroxine (T_4), serum	5-12 µg/dL
Triiodothyronine (T_3), serum	70-190 ng/dL
Triglycerides, plasma	<160 mg/dL

INDEX

[Page numbers followed by f indicate figures; t, tables; b, boxes.]

A

AA. *See* Amino acids
Abortion, 286
Acetoacetate, 46
Acetyl CoA carboxylase, 61
Acetylcholine, 30, 166
Acid labile subunit (ALS), 130
Acidophils, 117
Acinar cells, pancreatic, 35-36, 37f
Acne, 252
Acromegaly, 132-133, 134f
Acrosome reaction, 262, 262f
ACTH. *See* Adrenocorticotropic hormone
Addison's disease, 188, 188f
Adenohypophysis, 107, 117-137, 118t,
    119f-126f, 128f-129f, 132f-136f
    endocrine cell types of, 118t
    endocrine function of, 121
Adenosine triphosphate (ATP)
    amino acid production of, 46, 46f
    carbohydrate production of, 44-45
    for cells, 43-44, 44f
    FFA production of, 45-46, 46f
    ketone body production of, 46, 47f
    sensitive K⁺, 54, 55f
Adenylyl cyclase, 10
ADH. *See* Antidiuretic hormone
Adipocytokine, 74
Adiponectin, 73b, 74
    receptor, 75
AdipoR1, 75
AdipoR2, 75
Adipose cells, 51
Adipose tissue, 43
    as endocrine organ, 73-76, 73b
    energy storage and, 47
    glucose storage in, by insulin, 62,
        62b, 63f
    hepatic metabolism and, during fast,
        64-65, 64f
    hormones, 73b
    ingested lipid storage in, by insulin,
        62, 63f
    TG release in, 51
Adiposity, 74
    truncal, 177
Adrenal androgens
    psychologic actions of, 180, 182
    zona reticularis makes, 179-180, 180f

Adrenal cortex, 4, 4b, 120, 163-164, 170
    fetal, 273f
    pathologic conditions involving, 188-191,
        188f, 189b, 189t-190t, 190f
    steroidogenic pathways for, 171f
Adrenal glands
    anatomy, 163-164, 165f-166f
    fetal, 278, 278b
    key words, 192-194
    maternal, 279
    self-study, 194
    structure, 163, 164b
    summary, 191-192
Adrenal glucocorticoids, 97
Adrenal hormone epinephrine, 43
Adrenal medulla, 164
    pathologic conditions involving, 170,
        170b
Adrenal steroid hormones, 97
Adrenocortical excess, 188-191,
        189t, 190f
Adrenocortical insufficiency, 188,
        188f, 189b
Adrenocorticotropic hormone (ACTH),
        121, 123f
Adrenomedullary catecholamines, 167-168
African pigmy, 131
Albumin-uria, 71
Aldosterone, 163, 182-183, 184f
    actions, 183, 185f
    metabolism, 183-187, 186f
    secretion, 187-188, 187b, 187f
Alpha adrenergic receptors, 167-168, 168t
α Cells, in islets, 52
ALS. *See* Acid labile subunit
Amenorrhea, lactational, 135, 284f, 284f
Amidated gastrins, 31
Amino acids (AA)
    aromatic, decarboxylase, 164, 166
    ATP production by, 46, 46f
    G-17, 31, 31f
    oxidation of, 44
AMP kinase, 67
Anabolic pathways, storing energy, 58-62,
        58b, 59f-60f
Androgen, 4, 5t, 97. *See also* Adrenal
        androgens
    actions, 204-207, 205f-207f, 206b, 206t
    insensitivity syndrome, 218, 218f

Androgen—cont'd
    intratesticular, 204, 205f
    mechanisms of, 206-207
    metabolism of, 207, 207f
Androgen receptor (AR), 5, 202
Androgen-response-element (ARE),
        20, 207
Android adiposity, 74
Andropause, 217
Anemia, 177
Angiogenic factors, 233
ANP. *See* Atrial natriuretic peptide
ANS. *See* Autonomic nervous system
Antagonists, 1
Anterior pituitary, 108
Antidiuresis, 112
Antidiuretic hormone (ADH)
    actions, 112-117, 112f-114f
    degradation, 115
    plasma, blood volume and, 114f
    plasma, plasma osmolality and,
        113f, 116f
    structure, 110-111, 110f
Antral follicle, 228-230, 229f-230f
Apo B48, 48
apoE, 49
Apoproteins (Apos), 47-48, 49f
Apoproteins B100, 49, 50f
Apos. *See* Apoproteins
Appetite, increased, 177
APS protein, 57
Aquaporin 2, 112
AR. *See* Androgen receptor
ARE. *See* Androgen-response-element
Aromatic amino acid decarboxylase,
        164, 166
β-Arrestins, 14
Atherogenic change, 50
ATP. *See* Adenosine triphosphate
Atrial natriuretic peptide (ANP), 116
Autocrine signal, 24
Autonomic nervous system (ANS), 27, 27f
Autosomal-recessive hypophosphatemic
        rickets, 96
Autosomes, 211

B

Basal metabolic rate (BMR), 152-153
Basic multicellular units, 90

Basophils, 117
Beta adrenergic receptors, 167, 168t
β cells
    GLP and, 37-39
    in islets, 52-53
Bidirectional facilitative glucose
        transporters, 45, 45t
Bile duct, anatomy, 36f
Bioactive 17 amino acid gastrin (G-17),
        31, 31f
6-Bisphosphatase, 51
Bitemporal hemianopia, 135
Blastocyst, 264, 265f
    "hatched," 266f
Blood volume, plasma ADH and, 114f
Blood-epididymis barrier, 210
BMR. See Basal metabolic rate
Bone
    adult, histophysiology of, 90-93, 91f
    Ca²⁺ handling by, 90
    cancellous, 90, 91f
    compact, 90, 91f
    cortisol and, 177
    loss, in renal failure, 102f
    Pi handling by, 90
    problems, of renal failure, 101-102,
        101f-102f
    shaft, 91f
Bone accretion, 90
Bone resorption, 90, 91f, 177
Brain, 43
Breasts, 225
    anatomy of, 283f
Broad ligament, 225
Bronchiolar smooth muscle, 168
Bruit, 141
Buffalo hump, 189t, 190

C
Ca²⁺. See Calcium
Calbindin-Ds, 90
Calcifediol, 85f, 87
Calcitonin
    hormonal regulation of, 95
    receptor, 96
Calcitonin gene-related peptide
        (CGRP), 95
Calcitrol, 81
Calcium (Ca²⁺), 81
    ATPases, 12
    balance, pathologic disorders of, 97-102,
        98b-99b, 98f-102f
    channels
        epithelial, 89-90
        in signal transduction pathway,
            12, 12f
        voltage-gated, 55
    as dietary element, 81-82, 82f, 82t
    forms of, 81-82, 82f
    handling, 88-90, 89f
        by kidneys, 93, 94f
    homeostasis, summary, 102-103

Calcium (Ca²⁺)—cont'd
    inflammatory cell regulation and, 97
    intestinal absorption of, 89f
    levels, 55, 55f
    metabolism regulation of, 97
    NCX, 90
    physiologic regulation of, 93, 95
    PMCA, 90
    secretion dose-response curve, 84f
    sensing receptor, 83
Calcium-calmodulin system,
        activation of, 18f
Calcium-response element, 84
cAMP. See Nephrogenous cyclic adenosine
        monophosphate
cAMP response element-binding protein
        (CREB protein), 13
Cancer
    ovarian, 226
    regulators overexpressed by, hormonal
        regulation of, 96-97
Carbohydrate, 117b
    ATP production, 44-45
Carboxyl terminal ligand-binding domain,
        subdomains of, 18, 20
Cardiac output, 168
Cardiovascular dysmetabolic syndrome, 71
Cardiovascular system
    changes, during pregnancy,
        279-280, 279b
    cortisol and, 177
    thyroid hormone actions on, 154
Carnitine palmityl-transferase (CPT),
        45, 46f
Carpal-pedal spasms, 100
Catecholamines
    action mechanism of, 166-167, 167f
    adrenomedullary, 167-168
    characteristics of, 4b
    metabolism of, 168-169, 169f
    structure based classes of, 8b
    structure of, 4f
    synthesis of, 4
Catechol-O-methyltransferase (COMT),
        168-169, 169f
CBG. See Corticosteroid-binding
        globulin
CCK. See Cholecystokinin family
Cells
    α, 52
    acinar, 35-36, 37f
    adipose, 51
    ATP role for, 43-44, 44f
    β, 37-39, 52-53
    chief, 29
    chromaffin, 164
    ciliated, 242f
    ECL, 30-31
    endocrine, 25, 118t
    endothelial dysfunction, 71, 72f
    enteroendocrine, 25-26, 26f, 26t
    follicle, 226, 226f

Cells—cont'd
    follicular, 141, 142f
    inflammatory, 97, 177
    Leydig, 198, 205f-206f, 207
    ovarian surface epithelial, 225
    paracrine factor-producing, 27, 27f
    parafollicular C, 95
    principal, 83
    secretory, 242f
    Sertoli, 199-204, 201b, 203f,
        207-208, 209f
    specificity, 44
    sperm, 199, 200f
    steroidogenic, 5-6, 6f
    target, 1
Cellular responses
    events for, 15f
    to hormones, 9-21, 10f-19f
Centrosome, 263, 264f
Cephalic phase, 30, 32f
Cervical mucus, hormonal regulation of,
        245-246, 245b
Cervix, structure of, 240f, 245
CETP. See Cholesterol ester transfer
        protein
c-Fms, 92
CGRP. See Calcitonin gene-related peptide
Chemical nature, of hormones, 2-8, 2b,
        3f-8f, 4b, 5t, 7b-8b
Chemical signaling, different modes of, 24
Chief cells, 29
Cholecalciferol, 86
Cholecystokinin family (CCK), 28, 28t,
        31-32
    enterotropic actions of, 39
    during intestinal phase, 34
    primary stimulus of, 35-36, 37f
    production of, 35
    receptors of, 28, 35
Cholesterol, side-chain of, 171
Cholesterol ester hydrolyase, 170
Cholesterol ester transfer protein
        (CETP), 50
Cholesterol-rich low-density
        lipoprotein, 50
Chorion frondosum, 269, 269f
Chorion laeve, 269, 269f
Chromaffin cells, 164
Chromaffin granule, 166
Chromogranins, 166
Chvostek's sign, 100
Chylomicron, 47, 49f
    remnants, 49
Chyme, 30
Ciliated cells, 242f
Circadian rhythms, 21, 21f
Circulation, hormone transport in, 8-9
Cleavage stages, early
    in eggs in vitro fertilization, 266f
    in embryos, 265f
Cleidocranial dysplasia, 90
Closing cone, 92

Colloid, 141
COMT. *See* Catechol-*O*-methyltransferase
Congenital adrenal hyperplasia, 191
Connecting peptide, 53
Connective tissue, cortisol and, 177-178
Conn's syndrome, 191
Contiguous lumen, 208
Contraception, 285-286
Co-repressors, 20
Corpus luteum, 224
  endocrine function of, 235-236, 235f
  growth, 234-235, 236f
  histologic features of, 236f
Corticosteroid-binding globulin (CBG),
    6, 175
Corticosteroids, relative potencies of, 190t
Corticosterone, 173, 174f, 175
Corticotropes, 121
Corticotropin-releasing hormone (CRH),
    placental, fetal adrenal axis and,
    281-282
Cortisol, 120, 163
  actions, 175-178, 175b, 176f
  bone and, 177
  cardiovascular system and, 177
  connective tissue and, 177-178
  fetal development and, 178
  gastrointestinal actions and, 178
  kidney and, 178
  metabolic actions of, 175-176, 176f
  muscles and, 178
  production, 178-179, 178b, 179f
  reproductive system and, 177
  synthesis, 171-175, 171f-174f
  zona fasciculata and, 170-175,
    171f-174f
Cortisone, 175
Coupling, 145, 145f
  stimulus-secretion, 2-3
CPT. *See* Carnitine palmityl-transferase
Craniopharyngiomas, 107
CREB protein. *See* cAMP response
    element-binding protein
Cushing's disease, 188-191, 190f
Cutting cone, 92
Cyclic AMP, 10-11
  in signal transduction pathway, 11f
Cyclic GMP, 11-12
Cyclic nucleotide monophosphates,
    noncovalent binding of, 10, 11f
Cyclopentanoperhydrophenathrene
    ring, 4, 5f
Cyp1α gene, 87, 88f
CYP11A1, 171
CYP11B1, 173, 174f, 183
CYP21β, 173, 174f
Cytochrome p450 mono-oxidase gene
    family, 171
Cytoplasmic events, by PKA, to produce
    cellular response, 15f
Cytoplasmic tyrosine kinases, receptors
    associated with, 17, 17f

D
D$_2$ receptor, 134
DAG. *See* Diacylglycerol
Dawn phenomenon, 72-73
DBP. *See* Vitamin D-binding protein
Decapacitation, 210
Decidua, 269-270, 269f-270f
Decidualization, 265
Decondensation, 263
Degradation, of ADH, 115
Dehydroepiandrosterone sulfate
    (DHEAS), 163, 180
Deiodinases, 147f
Deoxycorticosterone (DOC), 173,
    174f, 175
Dephosphorylation, 10f
DHEAS. *See* Dehydroepiandrosterone
    sulfate
DHEA-sulfotransferase, 180, 181f
DHT. *See* 5α-Dihydrotestosterone
DI. *See* Diabetes insipidus
Diabetes insipidus (DI), 115-116,
    115t, 116f
Diabetes mellitus (DM). *See also* Type 1
    diabetes mellitus; Type 2
    diabetes mellitus
  acute complications of, 69-70, 70f
  classifications of, 65-66
  long-term sequelae of, 70-71, 72f
  management, 72-73
  non-insulin-dependent, 67
  overview, 65
  symptoms of, 68-69, 68b, 68f
  underlying causes of, 66f, 67-68
Diabetic ketoacidosis, 69, 70f
Diabetic retinopathy flow chart, 72f
Diabetogenic hormone, 130
Diabetogenicity, of pregnancy, 281
Diacylglycerol (DAG), 12, 70
  in signal transduction pathway, 13f
Diaphragma sellae, 109
Dietary TG, 47-49, 49f
Diet-induced obesity, 43
Digestion
  partial, of VLDLs, 50
  of protein, 4
Digestive period, glucose partitioning
    during, 63f
5α-Dihydrotestosterone (DHT), 204,
    205f-206f, 206
Dihydroxyphenylalanine
    (DOPA), 164
1,25-Dihydroxyvitamin D, 81, 87, 89t
  biosynthesis, 85f
  psychological importance of, 82
  response, to hypercalcemic challenge,
    93, 95, 95f
Diiodotyrosine (DIT), 142, 143f
DIT. *See* Diiodotyrosine
Diuresis, 112
DOC. *See* Deoxycorticosterone
Docking protein, 2

Dominant follicle, 230-231
  during preovulatory period, 231-234,
    232f-233f
DOPA. *See* Dihydroxyphenylalanine
Dopamine, 133-134, 164
Duodenum, 34, 36f
Dwarfism, 131-132, 132f

E
Early phase, of insulin release, 54, 54f
ECL. *See* Enterochromaffin-like cells
ED. *See* Erectile dysfunction
Effector proteins, 9
Egg activation, 261
Eicosanoids, 8
Ejaculatory duct, 208
Electrolyte depletion, 69
Electron transport chain, 45
Embryogenesis, early, 264-266, 265f-266f
Embryotroph, 267, 268f
Emergency contraception, 286
Emission, 210
Empty sella syndrome, 109
Empty shell syndrome, 136, 136f
Endemic cretinism, 154, 155f
Endemic system, fetal, 277-278, 278f
Endocrine axes, 117-121, 117t, 119f-120f
Endocrine cell mass, largest bodily, 25
Endocrine cell types,
    of adenohypophysis, 118t
Endocrine disorders, 119f, 120-121
Endocrine function
  of adenohypophysis, 121
  of corpus luteum, 235-236, 235f
  of ovarian follicle, 227
  of placenta, 271-272
Endocrine glands
  outside GI tract, 27
  secretions of, 1
Endocrine organ
  adipose tissue as, 73-76, 73b
  peripheral, 120
Endocrine pancreas, 52-53
Endocrine secretion, hormonal
    rhythms of, 21, 21f
Endocrine signal, 24
Endocrine system
  hormone context in, 1
  key words, 22-23
  self study, 23-24
  summary, 22-23
Endocytosis, 3
  GPCR inactivation and, 16f
  ligand-induced, 17
Endogenously-synthesized TG, 49-50, 50f
Endothelial cell dysfunction, 71, 72f
Energy
  homeostasis, 73-76, 73b
  protein and, 51
  release of
    during extended fast, 59f-60f,
      63-64, 64f

Energy—cont'd
        during interdigestive period, 59f-60f,
                63-64, 64f
        storage forms of, 47-50, 48f-50f
                adipose tissue and, 47
                anabolic pathways, 58-62, 58b,
                        59f-60f
Energy metabolism
        key words, 77-79
        overview of, 43-52, 44f, 45t,
                46f-50f, 52f
        self-study problems, 79
        summary, 51-52, 76-77
ENS. See Enteric nervous system
Enteric nervous system (ENS), 27, 27f
        gastric function and, 30
Enterochromaffin-like cells (ECL), 30-31
Enteroendocrine cells
        closed/open, 26f
        along GI tract, 25-26, 26t
Enteroendocrine hormone families,
        receptors of, 27-29, 28t
Enteroendocrine regulation, of exocrine
                pancreas, gallbladder and,
                33-37, 36f-37f
Enterogastrones, 33
Enterotropic action, of GI hormones,
                39-40
Epididymis, 198, 198f, 208, 210
Epinephrine, 4, 4f, 58, 163
        rising levels of, 59f-60f, 63-64
        synthesis, 164, 166, 167f
Epithelial calcium channels, 89-90
ER. See Estrogen receptor
ERE. See Estrogen receptor element
Erectile dysfunction (ED), 211
Erythromycin, 37
Erythropoietin, 177
Estradiol 17β, 97
        biology of, 247-249, 247f
Estrogen, 4, 5t, 120
        biological effects of, 248
        deficiency, 251
        feedback loops, 224
        mechanisms of, 247, 247f
        in parturition, 282
        peripheral conversion to, 204, 205f
        during pregnancy, 273f, 274, 275f
Estrogen receptor (ER), mechanisms of,
                5, 247, 247f
Estrogen receptor element (ERE), 20
Euthyroid, 149, 149b
Exendins, 39
Exocrine glands, secretions of, 1
Exocrine pancreas. See also Pancreas
        anatomy, 36f
        enteroendocrine regulation and,
                gallbladder and, 33-37, 36f-37f
        gland, 33, 36f
        hormonal regulation of, 37f
Exocytosis, 2-3
Exophthalmos, 158, 158f-159f

Extended fast, energy release during,
                59f-60f, 63-64, 64f
Extracellular K+, 188
Extrathyroidal pools, 145
Extrinsic regulators, 27, 27f

F
Familial benign hypocalciuric
                hypercalcemia (FBHH), 84
FAS. See Fatty acid synthase complex
Fast. See also Extended fast
        hepatic metabolism during,
                64-65, 64f
Fasting-to-fed state transition, 58-62,
                58b, 59f-60f
Fatty acid synthase complex (FAS), 61
Fatty liver, 67
FBHH. See Familial benign hypocalciuric
                hypercalcemia
Feedback loops
        estrogen, 224
        negative
                on gastric secretion, 34f
                in stomach, 32-33, 34f
        passive, on gastric secretion, 34f
        positive, 116-117
Female reproductive system. See also
                Reproductive tract function
        anatomy of, 225f
        key words, 254-256
        male v., 223-225, 224f
        ontogeny of, 249-251, 249f-251f, 250t
        self-study problems, 256-257
        summary, 253-254
        tract, 224, 239-247, 240f-246f
                development of, 249, 249f
Fertilization, 225
        changes during, 261-264, 262f, 264f
        events, 262f
        during first week, 265f
        human menstrual cycle synchronization
                with, 260f
        implantation and, 259-261, 260f
        key words, 288-290
        summary, 287-288
Fetal adrenal axis, placental CRH and,
                281-282
Fetal development
        cortisol and, 178
        of glands, 273f, 277-278, 278b
        of male reproductive system, 215t
        of membranes, 269f
Fetal endocrine system, 277-278, 278f
FFAs. See Non-esterified fatty acids
FGF23. See Fibroblast growth factor 23
Fibrate family, 75
Fibroblast growth factor 23
                (FGF23), 96
"Fight or flight" response, 168
First embryonic cleavage, 264
Flaccid state, 211
Follicle cells, 226, 226f

Follicle stimulating hormone (FSH),
                3, 208f, 233f
        relative serum, in women, 250f
        rhythms of, 21f
Follicular atresia, 227, 236
Follicular cells, 141, 142f
Follicular development
        late, regulation of, 236-239, 238f
        monthly menstrual cycle and, 236, 237f
Follicular growth, phases of, 237f
Follicular phase, 223
Food-induced hypercortisolism, 38
Fructose, 211
Fructose-1, 51
Fructose-1,6-bisphosphatase, 61
FSH. See Follicle stimulating hormone
Fundus, 29, 29f

G
G protein-coupled receptor (GPCR), 13
        endocytosis and, 16f
        GI hormones binding to, 27-28
        receptors, 13, 14f, 27-28
        in signal transduction pathway, 14f
G proteins, 10, 11f
        in signal transduction pathways, 11f
        signaling using, 13-14, 14f
G-6-P. See Glucose-6-phosphate
G-17. See Bioactive 17 amino acid gastrin
Gα. See α subunit
Ga protein, 13-14
GAGs. See Glycosaminoglycans
Gallbladder
        anatomy, 36f
        enteroendocrine regulation and,
                exocrine pancreas and,
                33-37, 36f-37f
        function, 34
Gamete, 227-231, 234-235
Gametogenesis, 197
Gametogenic function, 223
Gastric acid, 39
Gastric function
        emptying, 33, 34f
        ENS and, 30
        inhibition of, 32-33, 34f-35f
        interdigestive phase of, 36-37
        key words, 41
        regulation of, overview of, 29-30, 29f
        release, 33
        self-study, 41
        stimulation of, gastrin and, 30-32,
                31f-32f
        summary, 40
Gastric inhibitory peptide (GIP), 38
Gastric motility, regulation of, 29-30
Gastric phase, 30, 32f
Gastric secretion
        feedback loops of, 34f
        regulation of, 29-30
                during gastric phase, 33f
                during intestinal phase, 35f

Gastrin family, 28, 28t
  gastric function stimulation by, 30-32,
      31f-32f
  other effects of, 39
  production of, 30-31, 31f
  in stomach, 30
Gastrin intermediates, 31f
Gastrin-releasing peptide (GRP), 30
Gastrointestinal changes, during
      pregnancy, 281
Gastrointestinal tract
  cortisol and, 178
  endocrine glands outside of, 27
  enteroendocrine cells along, 25-26, 26t
  hormones of
    enterotropic action of, 39-40
    GPCR binding to, 27-28
    models' of, 26-27
    peptides, 28-29
      insulinotropic actions of,
          37-39, 38f
Gastroparesis, 37
Gβ/γ. *See* β/γ subunit dimer
GEFs. *See* Guanine nucleotide
      exchange factors
Genitalia
  female
    external, 246f
    internal, 240f, 249f
  male
    external, 213, 214b, 215f
    internal, 212-213, 213b, 213f-214f
Germinal vesicle breakdown
      (GVBD), 238
GH. *See* Growth hormone
GH-binding protein, 127
Ghrelin, 28, 28t, 127
GHS. *See* Growth hormone secretagogue
Gi-α, 13
GIP. *See* Gastric inhibitory peptide
Gland. *See* Specific type, e.g., Endocrine
      glands
Glomerulosclerosis, 71
GLP. *See* Glucagon-like peptides
Glucagon, 28, 28t, 43
  actions of, 57, 57b
  prepro, 38, 38f
  receptor, 57
  rising levels of, 59f-60f, 63-64
  secretion, 57-58, 57t
  stimulation, secretion and, 168
  structure, 55f, 57
  synthesis, 57
Glucagon-like peptides (GLP), 28, 28t
  β cells and, 37-39
  enterotropic actions of, 39-40
  specific types, 38f, 39
Glucocorticoid, 4, 5t, 175
  adrenal, 97
Glucocorticoid receptor (GR), 5, 175
Glucocorticoid response element
      (GRE), 20

Glucogenesis, 51, 52f
Glucokinase, 45, 54, 59
Glucometabolic regulation, by insulin, 66
Gluconeogenesis, hepatic glycogenolysis
      and, 168
Glucose
  intolerance, 177
  metabolism, insulin steps in, 59f-60f
  oral, tolerance test, 68f
  oxidation of, 44
  partitioning of, during digestive
      period, 63f
  storage of
    in adipose tissue, 62, 62b, 63f
    as glycogen, 58-62, 58b, 59f-60f, 62b
    in skeletal muscle, 62, 62b
  transporters, 45, 45t
  trapping intracellular, 59-60, 59f-60f
Glucose-6-phosphate (G-6-P), 45, 47,
      48f, 51, 60
Glucose-6-phosphate dehydrogenase, 61
Glucose-dependent insulinotropic
      peptide, 28, 38
Glucose-sensor, 54
Glucose-sparing effect, 51, 65
Glucosuria, 68
Glucotoxicity, 70
Glucuronide, 6
GLUT 4-dependent uptake, 62, 63f, 65, 66
GLUT 4-mediated glucose uptake, 176
GLUTs, 45, 45t, 47, 51, 59
Glycerol kinase, 62
Glycogen, 47, 48f
  glucose storage as, insulin for, 58-62,
      58b, 59f-60f, 62b
  synthesis, 59f-60f, 60-61
Glycogen phosphorylase, 47, 48f, 61
Glycogen synthase, 47, 48f, 60
Glycogen synthase kinase 3, 60-61
Glycogenolysis, 168
Glycolysis, 45, 46f
Glycoproteins, structure based
      classes of, 8b
Glycosaminoglycans (GAGs), 156
GnRH, 238, 238f. *See* Gonadotropin-
      releasing hormone
Goiter, 124, 149
Goitrogens, 146
Gonadal hormones, 97
Gonadotropes, 121, 125-127, 126f
Gonadotropin-releasing hormone
      (GnRH), 125, 208f
Gonads, 197
GPCR. *See* G protein-coupled receptor
GPCR kinases (GRKs), 14
Gq-α, 13
GR. *See* Glucocorticoid receptor
Graves' disease, 150, 150f, 158f
Grb2, 15
GRE. *See* Glucocorticoid response element
GRKs. *See* GPCR kinases
Growth, 136-137

Growth factors (IGFs), 130
Growth hormone (GH), 3, 127
  actions of, 129-133, 132f-133f
  deficiency, in adults, 132
  excess, before puberty, 132, 133f
  metabolic actions of, 117b
  pathologic conditions involving,
      131-133, 132f-133f
  plasma, intravenous arginine infusion
      effect on, 129f
  serum, 129f
  in starvation, 131
Growth hormone secretagogue (GHS), 28
Growth hormone-releasing hormone, 127
GRP. *See* Gastrin-releasing peptide
Gs-α, 13
GTP. *See* Noncovalent guanosine
      nucleotide triphosphate
Guanine nucleotide exchange factors
      (GEFs), 10
  ligand-activated, 13
Guanylyl cyclase, 12
GVBD. *See* Germinal vesicle breakdown
Gynecoid adiposity, 74

H

Hashimoto's thyroiditis, 159
HAT. *See* Histone acetyltransferase
Haversian canal, 91f, 92
Haversian lacunae, 92
HbA$_{1c}$. *See* Hemoglobin A$_{1c}$
hCG. *See* Human chorionic gonadotropin
HCl. *See* Hydrochloric acid
HDAC. *See* Histone deacetylase
HDLs. *See* High-density lipoproteins
7 Helix transmembrane receptors, 13
Hemoglobin A$_{1c}$ (HbA$_{1c}$), 70-71
Hepatic gluconeogenic enzymes, 175
Hepatic glycogenolysis, gluconeogenesis
      and, 168
Hepatic ketogenesis, 168
Hepatic metabolism, during fast
  adipose tissue and, 64-65, 64f
  skeletal muscle and, 64-65, 64f
Hepatic steatosis, 67
Herring bodies, 111
Heterotrimeric G proteins, 13
Hexokinases, 45
Hexosamines, 70
High affinity, 9
High-density lipoproteins (HDLs),
      48, 49f
Hirsutism, 252
Histamine, 30
Histone acetyltransferase (HAT), 20
Histone deacetylase (HDAC), 20
Histotrophic nutrition, 260, 268f
Homeostasis
  Ca^{2+}, summary, 102-103
  energy, 73-76, 73b
  metabolic, 58-65, 58b, 59f-60f, 62b,
      63f-64f, 66f, 68b, 68f, 70f, 72f

Homeostasis—cont'd
    hormones in, 52-58, 53b, 54f-56f, 55t, 57b, 57t
    Pi, summary, 102-103
Hormonal desensitization, 14
Hormonal regulation
    of calcitonin, 95
    of cervical mucus, 245-246, 245f
    of mammary glands, 283-285, 284f
    during menstrual cycle, 236-247, 238f, 244f-245f
    of myometrium, 245
    of pancreatic secretion, 37f
    in regulators overexpressed, by cancer, 96-97
    of uterine endometrium, 242-245, 244f
Hormonal replacement therapy, 97
Hormonal resistance, 1
Hormonal rhythms, 21, 21f
Hormone response elements (HREs), 18, 19f, 20
Hormone sensitive lipase (HSL), 64f, 65
Hormones. See also Specific types, e.g., Thyroid hormone
    adipose tissue and, 73b
    cellular responses to, 9-21, 10f-19f
    characterization of, 25
    chemical nature of, 2-8, 2b, 3f-8f, 4b, 5t, 7b-8b
    circulatory transport of, 8-9
    classes of, structure based, 8b
    endocrine context of, 1
    GI tract and, 26-29, 39-40
    male production of, 206t
    as messengers, 1
    in metabolic homeostasis, 52-58, 53b, 54f-56f, 55t, 57b, 57t
    plasma levels of, 21f
    pre, 2, 3f
    prepro, 2, 3f
    pro, convertases, 2
    protein, 6, 6f-7f
    receptor and, 1
    releasing, 119, 120f
Hot flashes, 251
HPA. See Hypothalamus-pituitary-adrenal axis
HREs. See Hormone response elements
3β-HSD. See 3β-Hydroxysteroid dehydrogenase
HSL. See Hormone sensitive lipase
Human chorionic gonadotropin (hCG), 3, 265
    during pregnancy, 272, 272f
Human chorionic somatomammotropin. See Human placental lactogen
Human menstrual cycle, 223. See also Menstruation
    follicular development and, 236, 237f
    hormonal regulation in, 236-247, 238f, 244f-245f

Human menstrual cycle—cont'd
    synchronization of, with fertilization/implantation, 260f
Human placental lactogen, 127, 274-276, 275b, 276f
Hydrochloric acid (HCl), 29, 29f
    secretion, 31-32, 32f
β-Hydroxybutyrate, 46
3β-Hydroxysteroid dehydrogenase (3β-HSD), 171-172
25-Hydroxyvitamin D, 87
17-Hydroxyprogesterone, 172-173, 173f
Hydroxyapatite crystal, 92
Hyperactivation, 262
Hypercalcemia, 82
Hypercalcemic challenge
    1,25-Dihydroxyvitamin D response to, 93, 95, 95f
    PTH response to, 93, 95, 95f
Hypercalcemic tetany, 100f
Hyperchloremic acidosis, 98, 99f
Hypercortisolism, 189t
    food-induced, 38
    tertiary, 124
Hyperglycemia, 68, 68b, 68f
Hyperglycemic hormone, 129
Hyperinsulinemia, 177
Hyperlipemia, 69
Hyperparathyroidism, primary, 97-98, 98b, 98f-99f
    symptoms of, 98b
    x-ray, 98f
Hyperphosphatemia, 82
Hyperprolactinemia, 135
Hyperthyroid, 149, 149b, 157-159, 158b, 158f-159f
    x-ray, 152f
Hypocalcemia, 82
    parathormone-calciferol axis to, 96f
Hypocalciuria, 84
Hypoglycemia, 44, 44f
Hypoparathyroidism, 99-101, 99b
Hypophysectomy, 130
Hypophyseotropic hormones, 120f
Hypophysiotrophic, 119
Hypophysis, 107
Hypopituitarism, 135-136
Hypothalamic-hypophyseal-thyroid axis, 148f
Hypothalamic-pituitary-adrenal axis, 123f, 180f
Hypothalamic-pituitary-gonadal axis, 197
Hypothalamic-pituitary-ovarian axis, 224
Hypothalamic-pituitary-testis axis, 125, 126f, 207-208, 208f-209f
Hypothalamic-pituitary-thyroid axis, 125f
Hypothalamohypophyseal portal vessels, 118t, 119
Hypothalamohypophyseal tracts, 109, 110f

Hypothalamus, 109
    anatomy, 114f
    MRI, 108, 108f
    structure, 107, 108f
Hypothalamus/pituitary complex
    key words, 138-139
    overview, 107
    self-study problems, 138-139
    summary, 137-138
Hypothalamus-pituitary-adrenal axis (HPA), 121
Hypothalamus-pituitary-gonadal axis, 126f
Hypothalamus-pituitary-liver axis, 128f
Hypothalamus-pituitary-ovary axis, 125, 126f
Hypothyroid, 148-149
Hypothyroidism, 154-157, 155f, 156b, 157b, 157f

I
IDLs. See Intermediate-density lipoprotein particles
IGFBPs. See Insulin-like growth factor-binding proteins
IGFs. See Growth factors; Insulin-like growth factors
Immune response, 177
Immunosuppressants, 177
Impaired glucose tolerance, 38
Implantation, 225, 264-266, 265f-266f
    fertilization and, 259-261, 260f
    human menstrual cycle synchronization with, 260f
    interstitial, 264, 266f
    steps of, 267f
In vitro fertilization, 286-287
    cleavage stages in, 266f
Incretin action, 37-39, 38f
Incretins, 37
Infertility, 236
Inflammatory cells, 177
    metabolism regulation by
        of Ca^{2+}, 97
        of Pi, 97
Infundibulum, 107-108
Inhibin, 207-208
Inhibit insulin secretion, 168
Inorganic phosphate, 82, 82f
Inositol 1,4,5-triphosphate (IP_3), 12
    in signal transduction pathway, 13f
Insulin, 43
    actions of, 53, 53b
        on liver, 58b
    falling levels of, 59f-60f, 63-64
    glucometabolic regulation by, 66
    in glucose metabolism, 59f-60f
    ingested lipid storage promotion by, in adipose tissue, 62, 63f
    inhibit, secretion, 168
    pro, 53

Insulin—cont'd
  promotes glucose storage
    as glycogen, 58-62, 58b, 59f-60f, 62b
    by skeletal muscle/adipose, 62, 62b
  promotes protein synthesis, in many
    tissues, 62-63
  receptors, 16-17, 16f, 56-57, 56f
  release, phases of, 54, 54f
  secretion, 53-56, 55f, 55t
  serum levels of, 54f
  shock, 70
  in starvation, 131
  structure, 53, 54f
  synthesis, 53-54, 54f
Insulin insensitivity, 130
Insulin receptor (IR), 16-17, 16f, 56, 56f
Insulin receptor substrate (IRS), 16-17,
  16f, 57
Insulin resistance, 43
  causes of, 66
  other factors promoting, 67
  progression of, 66, 66f
  syndrome, 71
Insulin-like growth factor-binding
  proteins (IGFBPs), 130
Insulin-like growth factors (IGFs), 3, 117b,
  120, 127, 128f, 130-131
Insulinotropic actions, of GI peptides,
  37-39, 38f
Interdigestive period
  energy release during, 59f-60f,
    63-64, 64f
  motilin and, 36-37
Intermediate-density lipoprotein particles
  (IDLs), 50, 50f
Internal insemination, 197
Interstitial implantation, 264, 266f
Intervillous space, 270f, 271
Intestinal phase, 30
  CCK during, 34
  gastric secretion regulation during, 35f
  secretin during, 34
Intracellular messengers, 9
  lipid informational molecules as, 12
Intracellular responses, signaling from,
  18-21, 19f
Intracrine signal, 24
Intratesticular androgen, 204, 205f
Intrinsic factor, 29
Intrinsic GTPase activity, 10
Intrinsic regulators, 27, 27f
Iodide (I⁻), 144f
  oxidation, 144
Iodide transport, 142-144, 144f
Iodinated thyronines, 8f
Iodination, 144
Ion channels, receptors regulating, 18, 18f
IP₃. See Inositol 1,4,5-triphosphate
IR. See Insulin receptor
IRS. See Insulin receptor substrate
Islets of Langerhans, 52
Izumo, 262f, 263

J
JAK kinase, 17, 17f
Juvenile diabetes, 67
Juxtacrine signal, 24

K
KAL gene, 126
Kallmann syndrome, 126, 218-219
Ketoacidosis, 68-69
  diabetic, 69, 70f
Ketone body
  ATP production by, 46, 47f
  oxidation of, 44
  production, in liver, 47f
Key metabolic pathways, summary, 51-52
Kidneys
  Ca²⁺ handling by, 93, 94f
  cortisol and, 178
  excretion, of Pi, 101, 101f
  Pi handling by, 93, 94f
Kit ligand, 227
Klinefelter syndrome, 217-218, 217f

L
Lactation, mammogenesis and, 282-285,
  283f-284f
Lactational amenorrhea, 135, 284f
Lactotropes, 121, 133-135, 134f
Lamellae, 92
Laron dwarfs, 127
Late phase, of insulin release, 54, 54f
Leptin, 73b, 74
  resistance, 74
  structure, 74
Leptin receptor (LRb), 74
Let-down of milk, 117
Leukotrienes, 8
Leydig cells
  regulation of, 207
  steroidogenic pathways in, 198,
    205f-206f
LH. See Luteinizing hormone
Lid retraction, 158
Ligand-activated GEFs, 13
Ligand-induced endocytosis, 17
Ligands. See also Carboxyl terminal
    ligand-binding domain
  binding of, 1
  kit, 227
  RANKL, 92
Lipid, 117b
Lipid informational molecules, as
    intracellular messengers, 12
Lipid messengers, in signal transduction
    pathway, 13f
Lipogenesis, 177
Lipolysis, 168, 176
Lipolytic hormone, 129-130
Lipoprotein lipase (LPL), 48, 49f
Lipoprotein particle, 47, 49f
Liporegulation, 74
Lipotoxicity, 66, 66f

Liver, 43, 120. See also Hypothalamus-
    pituitary-liver axis
  fatty, 67
  insulin actions on, 58b
  ketone body production in, 47f
Lobules, 198, 200f
LPL. See Lipoprotein lipase
LRb. See Leptin receptor
Luteal phase, 235, 235f
  deficiency, 236
Luteinizing hormone (LH), 3, 208f, 216f
  relative serum, in women, 250f
  rhythms of, 21f

M
Macroangiopathies, 71
Magnetic resonance imaging (MRI),
    of hypothalamus/pituitary,
    108, 108f
Magnocellular, 109
Male oral contraceptive, 208
Male phenotype, 212f
Male reproductive system
  appropriate hormone production
    rates, 206t
  development of, 211-219, 212f-215f,
    213b-214b, 215t, 216f-218f, 217t
  diagram, 210f
  disorders involving, 217-219, 217f-218f
  female vs., 223-225, 224f
  fetal development of, 215t
  key words, 220-222
  overview, 197-198
  self-study, 220-222
  summary, 219-220
  tract, 198f, 208, 210-211, 210f
Mammary glands, 225
  hormonal regulation of, 283-285, 284f
  structure, 282-283, 283f
Mammogenesis, lactation and, 282-285,
    283f-284f
MAO. See Monoamine oxidase
MAP kinase. See Mitogen-activated
    protein kinase
Maternal endocrine changes, during
    pregnancy, 278-279
Maternal ovarian reproductive tract
    function, synchronization with,
    259-261, 260f
Maternal physiologic changes, during
    pregnancy, 279-281, 279b
Maturation-promoting factor (MPF), 263
MC2R. See Melanocortin 2 receptor
M-CSF. See Monocyte-colony stimulating
    factor
Median eminence, 108
Megalin, 87
MEK, 15
Melanocortin 2 receptor (MC2R), 121
Membrane receptors, signaling from
  using G proteins, 13-14, 14f
  using RTKs, 14-17, 15f-16f

Menopause, 223, 250-251
Menstrual phase, 244-245, 244f
Menstruation, 225. *See also* Human menstrual cycle
Mesonephric ducts, 212
Metabolic homeostasis, 58-65, 58b, 59f-60f, 62b, 63f-64f, 66f, 68b, 68f, 70f, 72f
Metabolic syndrome, 71
Metabolism, 117
Metanephrine, 169
Metformin, 67
Midcycle gonadotropin, 224
Migrating myoelectric complex (MMC), 37
Milk ejection, 117
Mineralocorticoid response element (MRE), 20
Mineralocorticoids, 4, 5t
MIT. *See* Monoiodotyrosine
Mitogen-activated protein kinase (MAP kinase), 15-16, 16f
MMC. *See* Migrating myoelectric complex
Monoamine oxidase (MAO), 168-169, 169f
Monocyte-colony stimulating factor (M-CSF), 92
Monoiodotyrosine (MIT), 142, 143f
"Morning sickness," 272
Motilin, 28, 28t
    gastric contractions and, 36-37
    interdigestive period and, 36-37
MPF. *See* Maturation-promoting factor
MRE. *See* Mineralocorticoid response element
MRI. *See* Magnetic resonance imaging
Mucigens, 29
Muscles. *See also* Skeletal muscle
    bronchiolar smooth, 168
    cortisol and, 178
    of stomach, 30
    vasodilation of, of arteriolar beds, 168
Myometrium, hormonal regulation of, 245
Myxedema madness, 152, 156

N

NCX. *See* Sodium/calcium exchanger
Negative feedback loop
    of gastric secretion, 34f
    in stomach, 32-33, 34f
Nephrogenous cyclic adenosine monophosphate (cAMP), 99f
    phosphodiesterases, 11
Nephropathies, 71
Neurocrine factor, 28
Neurocrine signal, 24
Neuroendocrine reflex, 116
    linking nipple suckling to, oxytocin/ prolactin release, 284f
Neuroendocrine signal, 24

Neurohypophysis, 107, 109-117, 110f-114f, 115t, 116f, 117b
Neuropathies, 71
Neurophysin, 110
Neurovascular structure, 109
Nicotinic receptors, 166
Nitric oxide (NO), 12
NO. *See* Nitric oxide
Noncovalent guanosine nucleotide triphosphate (GTP), 10, 11f
Nonenzymatic glycation, 70
Non-esterified fatty acids (FFAs), 44
    ATP production by, 45-46, 46f
    converted, to TGs, 45-46, 46f
Non-insulin-dependent diabetes mellitus, 67
Nonketotic hyperosmolar coma, 69-70
Nonretinal visual problems, 71
Norepinephrine, 4, 4f, 43, 58, 164
Nuclear events, by PKA, to produce cellular response, 15f
Nuclear receptor superfamily, 18
Nuclear receptor-hormone complexes, mechanisms of, 19f

O

Obesity, diet-induced, 43
OHSS. *See* Ovarian hyperstimulation syndrome
Oliguria, 68
Ontogeny, of female reproductive system, 249-251, 249f-251f, 250t
Oocytes, 223, 226
    development of, 230f
Oogonium, 223
Oral contraceptives, 285-286
Oral glucose tolerance test, 68f
Organification, 144, 145f
Osteitis fibrosa cystica, 98
Osteoblast, 90, 91f
    express factor, 91f, 92
Osteoclast, 90, 91f
Osteocyte, 92
Osteoid, 90
Osteomalacia, 93, 101
Osteon, 92
Osteopetrosis, 92
Osteoporosis, 92, 98
Ovarian cancer, 226
Ovarian follicle, 223, 225. *See also* Antral follicle; Dominant follicle; Preantral follicle
    endocrine function of, 227
    graafian, 230f
    growth of, 226-227, 226f-227f
Ovarian hyperstimulation syndrome (OHSS), 287
Ovarian pathophysiology, 251-252, 252f
Ovarian reserve, 227, 227f
Ovarian steroidogenesis, 232f-233f, 235f

Ovarian steroids
    metabolism of, 248-249
    transport of, 248-249
Ovarian surface epithelial cells, 225
Ovaries, 4, 4b, 120, 237-238
    anatomy of, 225-226, 225f
    fetal, 278
    histology of, 225-226, 226f
Oviduct, 239-241, 240f-241f
Ovulation, 233f
Oxidation, 44-45, 46f. *See also* β-oxidation I⁻, 144
Oxidative phosphorylation (OxPhos), 45
β-Oxidation, 45, 46f
Oxidized LDL, 50
OxPhos. *See* Oxidative phosphorylation
Oxyntic cells, 29
Oxytocin, 110-112, 110f-111f, 116-117, 117b
    in parturition, 282, 282f
    release, 284f

P

Paget's disease, 96, 100f, 101
Palmityl CoA desaturase, 61
Pancreas. *See also* Endocrine pancreas; Exocrine pancreas
    fetal, 277
Pancreatic acinar cells, 35-36, 37f
    secretin and, 35
Pancreatic islet, 43
Pancreatic polypeptide, 53
Pancreatic secretion, hormonal regulation of, 37f
Panhypopituitarism, 135-136
Panhypopituitary dwarfism, 131
Paracrine factor-producing cells, 27, 27f
Paracrine signal, 24
Parafollicular C cells, 95
Parathormone-calciferol axis, to hypocalcemia, 96f
Parathyroid glands
    anatomic position of, 83f
    fetal, 277
    psychological importance of, 82-83
Parathyroid hormone (PTH), 81
    actions of, 89t
    gene expression, 84f
    level, serum phosphate level and, in renal failure, 101f
    psychological importance of, 82
    receptor, 84-85
    response, to hypercalcemic challenge, 93, 95, 95f
    secretion, 83-84, 84f
    structure, 83-84
Parathyroid hormone-related peptide (PTHrP), 96
Parathyroid hormone-related protein (PTHrP), 276
Paraventricular nuclei (PVN), 109
Parietal cells, 29, 29f

Pars distalis, 108
Pars intermedia, 108
Pars nervosa, 108
Pars tuberalis, 108
Parturition, 225, 281-282, 282f
    estrogen in, 282
    oxytocin in, 282, 282f
    progesterone secretion in, 282
    prostaglandins in, 282
    uterine size in, 282
Parvicellular, 119
Passive feedback loop, on gastric
    secretion, 34f
Pathway 1, 20
Pathway 2, 20
PCOS. *See* Polycystic ovarian syndrome
Pentagastrin, 31
Pentose phosphate shunt, 61
Pep carboxykinase (PEPCK), 51
PEPCK. *See* Pep carboxykinase;
    Phosphoenolpyruvate
    carboxykinase
Peptides, 2-4, 2b, 3f. *See also* Glucagon-like
    peptides; Polypeptides
    ANP, 116
    CGRP, 95
    connecting, 53
    gastrointestinal tract, hormones of,
        28-29, 37-39, 38f
    GIP, 38
    glucose-dependent insulinotropic,
        28, 38
    GRP, 30
    PTHrP, 96
    signal, 2
    VIP, 28
    YY, 38
Perilipin proteins, 64f, 65
Peripheral conversion, of steroid
    hormone, 6, 6f
Peroxisome proliferator-activated receptor
    gamma (PPAR-γ), 73
PFK-1. *See* Phosphofructokinase-1
pH, 34
PH-20, 262
Phagosome, 145
Phenylethanolamine-*N*-methyl transferase
    (PNMT), 164
Pheochromocytoma, 170, 170b
PHEX. *See* Phosphate regulating gene with
    homologies to endopeptidases
    on the X chromosome
Phosphate (Pi), 81
    balance, pathologic disorders of, 97-102,
        98b-99b, 98f-102f
    fluxes, 82f
    handling
        by bone, 90
        by kidneys, 93
        by small intestine, 88-90, 89f
    homeostasis, summary, 102-103
    inorganic, 82, 82f

Phosphate (Pi)—cont'd
    kidney excretion of, 101, 101f
    metabolism regulation of
        by inflammatory cells, 97
        by steroid hormones, 97
    physiologic regulation of, 93, 95
    in plasma, 82, 82t
    sodium, co-transporter, 90
Phosphate regulating gene with
    homologies to endopeptidases
    on the X chromosome
    (PHEX), 96
Phosphatidylinositol-3-kinase (PI3K),
    12-13
    in signal transduction pathway, 13f
Phosphatidylinositol 3,4,5-triphosphate
    (PIP$_3$), 12
Phosphoenolpyruvate carboxykinase
    (PEPCK), 61, 175
Phosphofructokinase-1 (PFK-1), 61
Phosphofructokinase-2/fructose
    bisphosphatase 2, 61
Phospholipase A$_2$, 177
Phospholipase C, 13-14
Phosphorylase kinase, 61
Phosphorylation
    covalent, 10, 10f
    noncovalent, 10-12, 11f-12f
    OxPhos, 45
    in signal transduction pathway, 10f
Phosphotyrosine (pY), 15
Physiologic changes, during pregnancy,
    279-281, 279b
Physiologic regulation, of Ca^{2+}/Pi
    metabolism, 93, 95
Pi. *See* Phosphate
PI3K. *See* Phosphatidylinositol-3-kinase
PIP$_3$. *See* Phosphatidylinositol
    3,4,5-triphosphate
Pituicytes, 109
Pituitary apoplexy, 136
Pituitary gland
    anatomy, 114f
    anterior lobe of, 108
    development of, 109f
    fetal, 277
    maternal, 278-279
    posterior lobe of, 108
    structure, 107, 108f
Pituitary glycoprotein hormones, 124f
Pituitary gonadotrope, 237-238, 238f
PKA catalytic subunit, 11
    cytoplasmic events by, to produce
        cellular response, 15f
    nuclear events by, to produce cellular
        response, 15f
    in signal transduction pathway, 11f
PKG. *See* Protein kinase G
Placenta
    accreta, 266
    CRH, fetal adrenal axis and, 281-282
    endocrine function of, 271-272

Placenta—cont'd
    hormones, other types of, 276
    mature, 266-271, 267f-271f
    membrane, 271f
    steroid hormones and, 4, 4b
Placental lactogen, human, 127, 274-276,
    275b, 276f
Placental transport, 276-277, 277b
Placentation, 225
Plasma growth hormone, intravenous
    arginine infusion effect on, 129f
Plasma hormone levels, 21f
Plasma membrane calcium ATPase
    (PMCA), 90
Plasma osmolality, plasma ADH and,
    113f, 116f
PMCA. *See* Plasma membrane calcium
    ATPase
PNMT. *See* Phenylethanolamine-*N*-methyl
    transferase
Polycystic ovarian syndrome (PCOS),
    251-252, 252f
Polycythemia, 177
Polydipsia, 68
Polyols, 70
Polypeptides
    pancreatic, 53
    structure based classes of, 8b
Polyphagia, 68
Polyunsaturated fatty acids,
    eicosanoids and, 8
Polyuria, 68
POMC. *See* Pro-opiomelanocortin
Positive feedback loop, oxytocin/uterine
    motility, 116-117
Posterior pituitary, 108
Potassium ion (K$^+$), extracellular, 188
PPAR-α, 75
PPAR-γ. *See* Peroxisome proliferator-
    activated receptor gamma
PR. *See* Progesterone receptor
PRE. *See* Progesterone response element
Preantral follicle, 226f, 228
Preganglionic sympathetic neurons, 166
Pregnancy
    cardiovascular system changes during,
        279-280, 279b
    diabetogenicity of, 281
    estrogen during, 273f, 274, 275f
    gastrointestinal changes during, 281
    hCG during, 272, 272f
    maternal endocrine changes during,
        278-279
    maternal physiologic changes during,
        279-281, 279b
    progesterone during, 272-274, 273f
    renal changes during, 279b, 280-281
    respiratory system changes during,
        279b, 280
    summary, 287-288
Pregnenolone, 171-172
Prehormone, 2, 3f

Premature ovarian failure, 227
Preovulatory period, dominant follicle during, 231-234, 232f-233f
Preprogastrin, 30-31, 31f
Preproglucagon, 38, 38f
Preprohormone, 2, 3f
Preprooxyphysin, 110, 111f
Preprovasophysin, 110, 111f
Pretibial myxedema, 156
Primary villi, 267, 268f
Principal cells, 83
Pro-corticotropin releasing hormone (Pro-CRH), 122
Pro-CRH. See Pro-corticotropin releasing hormone
Progastrins, 31f
Progesterone, 120, 172
    biological effects of, 248
    biology of, 247-249, 247f
    biosynthesis, 273f
    during pregnancy, 272-274, 273f
    secretion, in parturition, 282
Progesterone receptor (PR), binding of, 5
Progesterone response element (PRE), 20
Progestins, 4, 5t
Prohormone convertases, 2
Proinsulin, 53
Prolactin, 127, 133, 134f-135f
    deficiency, 135
    pathologic disorders involving, 135
    release, 284f
Prolactin-releasing factor, 134
Proliferative phase, 224-225, 242-243, 244f
Pronuclear formation, 264f
Pro-opiomelanocortin (POMC), 121, 121f
Proprotein, 2
Propylthiouracil (PTU), 146
Prostacyclin, 8
Prostaglandins, 8
    in parturition, 282
Prostate gland, 210
Protein anabolic hormone, 129
Protein binding, 146-147, 146f
Protein hormones
    conversions of, 6, 6f
    pituitary glyco-, 124f
    ultrastructure of, 6, 7f
Protein kinase
    MAP, 15-16, 16f
    PKB, 13, 13f, 57
    PKG, 12, 12f
    regulatory subunit of, 10-11
Protein kinase B (PKB)
    dependent pathway, 57
    in signal transduction pathway, 13, 13f
Protein kinase G (PKG), activation of, 12, 12f
Protein phosphatase 1, 60
Protein synthesis, 3f
    insulin promotes, in many tissues, 62-63
Protein wasting, 69

Proteins, 117b. See also Apoproteins; G proteins; Glycoproteins; High-density lipoproteins; Very-low density lipoproteins
    CETP, 50
    chemical nature of, 2-4, 2b, 3f
    CREB, 13
    DBP, 87
    digestion of, 4
    docking, 2
    effector, 9
    energy and, 51
    Ga, 13-14
    IGFBP, 130
    perilipin, 64f, 65
    pro, 2
    shc, 57
    SREBP-1C, 73
    StAR, 170, 172f, 273
    sterol responsive element binding protein-1C, 59-60
    transport, 6
Proteolysis, 176
Pseudohypoparathyroidism, 99
Psychosocial dwarfism, 120
Psychosocial growth retardation, 137
PTH. See Parathyroid hormone
PTHrP. See Parathyroid hormone-related peptide; Parathyroid hormone-related protein
PTU. See Propylthiouracil
Puberty, 214-217, 215f-216f, 215t, 217t
    changes, in females, 249-250, 250f-251f, 250t
    GH excess, before, 132, 133f
Pulsatile rhythms, 120
    circadian rhythm relationship to, 21, 21f
PVN. See Paraventricular nuclei
pY. See Phosphotyrosine
Pyloric antrum, 29f, 30
Pyruvate carboxylase, 51, 52f
Pyruvate dehydrogenase (PDH), 60f, 61
Pyruvate kinase, increasing, 59f-60f, 61, 175

R
Radioactive iodide uptake (RAIU), 143-144, 144f, 162
RAIU. See Radioactive iodide uptake
RANKL, 97. See Receptor activator of NF-κB ligand
Ras, 15
Rathke's pouch, 107
Reactive oxygen species (ROS), 45
Receptor activator of NF-κB ligand (RANKL), 92
Receptor serine/threonine kinases, 17-18, 18f
Receptor tyrosine kinases (RTKs), 56, 56f
    signaling from, 14-17, 15f-16f

Receptors. See also Membrane receptors
    adiponectin, 75
    adrenergic, 167-168, 168t
    antagonist, 1
    AR, 5, 202
    calcitonin, 96
    CaSR, 83
    cck, 28
    cytoplasmic tyrosine kinases associated with, 17, 17f
    D_2, 134
    enteroendocrine hormone families and, 27-29, 28t
    ER, 5, 247, 247f
    ERE, 20
    glucagon, 68
    GPCR, 13, 14f, 27-28
    GR, 5, 175
    7 Helix transmembrane, 13
    high affinity of, 9
    hormones and, 1
    insulin, 16-17, 16f, 56-57, 56f
    leptin, 74
    MC2R, 121
    nicotinic, 166
    nuclear receptor-hormone complexes, 18, 19f
    PPAR-γ, 73
    PR, 5
    PTH, 84-85
    regulating ion channels, 18, 18f
    scavenger, 50
    TGF-β related, 17, 18f
    thyroid hormone, 8, 150-151, 151f
    TNF-α, 76
    vasopressin, 112, 112f
    VDR, 5
    vitamin D, 5, 87
5α-Reductase 2 deficiency, 218
Regulated secretory pathway, 2-3
Relative hypoinsulinemia, 66
Releasing hormones, 119, 120f
Renal changes, during pregnancy, 279b, 280-281
Renal failure
    bone loss in, 102f
    bone problems of, 101-102, 101f-102f
    PTH level, serum phosphate level and, 101f
Renin-angiotensinogen angiotensin system, 187f
Reproductive system. See also Female reproductive system; Male reproductive system
    cortisol and, 177
Reproductive tract function, 197
Respiratory system, changes, during pregnancy, 279b, 280
Rete testis, 198
Retinopathies, 71, 72f
Reverse T_3, 142

Rickets, 93, 96
  x-ray, 100f
ROS. *See* Reactive oxygen species
RTKs. *See* Receptor tyrosine kinases
Ruffled membrane, 92

S

Scanning electron micrograph, of surface
        ampullary endosalpinx, 242f
Scavenger receptors, 50
Scrotum, 198
Secretagogues, 25-26
Secretin
  discovery of, 25
  enterotropic actions of, 39
  family, 28, 28t
  during intestinal phase, 34
  pancreatic acinar cells and, 35
  primary short-term action of, 35
  primary stimulus for, 34
  -releasing factor, 34
Secretory cells, 242f
Secretory phase, 243-244, 244f
Sella turcica, 108f, 109
Semen, 210
Semenogelins, 211
Seminal vesicles, 210
Seminiferous tubules, 198, 200f
Senescence, 214-217, 215f-216f, 215t, 217t
Sertoli cells, 199-204, 201b, 203f,
        207-208, 209f
Serum growth hormone, 129f
Set-points, 1, 120
Sex chromosomes, 211
Sex-determining region Y (SRY), 212
Sex-hormone binding globulin (SHBG), 6
SHBG. *See* Sex-hormone binding globulin
Shc protein, 57
Sheehan's syndrome, 136
Signal peptidase, 2
Signal recognition complex, 2
Signal transducers and activators of
        transcription (STAT), 17
Signal transduction pathway
  Ca²⁺ channels in, 12, 12f
  characteristics of, 9-10
  cyclic AMP, 11f
  DAG in, 13f
  different modes of, 24
  G proteins in, 11f
  GPCR in, 14f
  intracellular responses and, 18-21, 19f
  IP₃ in, 13f
  IR in, 16-17, 16f
  lipid messengers in, 13f
  phosphorylation/dephosphorylation
        in, 10f
  PI3K in, 13f
  PKA catalytic subunit in, 11f
  PKB in, 13, 13f
  of steroid hormones, 19f
  of thyroid hormone, 19f

Skeletal muscle, 43
  glucose storage in, 62, 62b
  hepatic metabolism and, during fast,
        64-65, 64f
  thyroid hormone effects on, 154
Smads, 17
Small intestinal contractions, 36-37
Small intestine
  Ca²⁺ handling by, 88-90, 89f
  Pi handling by, 88-90, 89f
SOCS. *See* Suppressors of cytokine
        signaling
Sodium/calcium exchanger (NCX), 90
Sodium/Pi co-transporter, 90
Somatomedins, 130
Somatostatin, 30, 127
  action, 32
Somatotropes, 121, 127-129, 128f-129f
Somatotropin, 127
Somogyi effect, 72
SON. *See* Supraoptic nuclei
Sonogram, of polycystic ovary, 252f
Sperm, 197
  cells, 199, 200f
Spermatocyte, 202f
Spermatogenesis, 198, 201f
Spermatozoa, 198
Spinnbarkeit, 245f
Spiral arteries, 270f, 271
Sporadic congenital hypothyroidism, 152
SREBP-1C. *See* Sterol regulatory binding
        element protein 1C
SRY. *See* Sex-determining region Y
StAR protein. *See* Steroidogenic
        Acute Regulatory Protein
        (StAR Protein)
STAT. *See* Signal transducers and activators
        of transcription
Steroid hormones, 4-6, 4b, 5f-6f, 5t
  adrenal, 97
  Ca²⁺ metabolism regulation by, 97
  categories of, 4, 5t
  ovarian, 248-249
  peripheral conversion of, 6, 6f
  Pi metabolism regulation by, 97
  placenta and, 4, 4b
  signal transduction pathway of, 19f
  steroidogenesis of, 5-6, 6f
  structure based classes of, 8b
Steroidogenic Acute Regulatory
        Protein (StAR Protein), 170,
        172f, 273
Steroidogenic cell, 5-6, 6f
Steroidogenic pathways
  for adrenal cortex, 171f
  in Leydig cells, 198, 205f-206f
Sterol regulatory binding element protein
        1C (SREBP-1C), 73
Sterol responsive element binding
        protein-1C, 59-60
Stimulus-secretion coupling, 2-3

Stomach
  anatomy, 29f
  function, 29
  gastrin in, 30
  muscles of, 30
  negative feedback loop in, 32-33, 34f
Storage, 145
Stress hormones, 129
Subacute thyroiditis, 159
α Subunit (Gα), 13
β/γ Subunit dimer (Gβ/γ), 13
Sulfate conjunction, 6
Sulfonylurea drugs, 55
Suppressors of cytokine signaling
        (SOCS), 17, 57
  role of, 17f
Supraoptic nuclei (SON), 109
Suprarenal gland, 163
Surface ampullary endosalpinx, scanning
        electron micrograph of, 242f
Sympathetic neurotransmitter, 43
Syncytiotrophoblasts, 264, 266f
Syndrome X, 71

T

T1DM. *See* Type 1 diabetes mellitus
T2DM. *See* Type 2 diabetes mellitus
T₃. *See* Triiodothyronine
T₄. *See* Thyroxine
Tanner stages, 216f, 217t
  in female puberty, 250t, 251f
Target cell, 1
Target organ, 1
TBG. *See* Thyroid hormone-binding
        globulin
Tertiary hypogonadotropic hypogonadism,
        126
Testis, 4, 4b, 120. *See also* Hypothalamic-
        pituitary-testis axis
  fetal, 278
  histophysiology of, 198-204, 200f-203f,
        201b
  intratubular compartment of, 199-204,
        200f-203f, 201b
  peritubular compartment of, 204
  rete, 198
Testosterone, 120, 198, 205f-206f, 213
  DHT, 204, 205f-206f, 206
  intratesticular, circulating vs., 209f
  peripheral actions, 206
  plasma, levels, 216f
Tetrac, 148
TGF-β related receptors, 17, 18f
TGs. *See* Triglycerides
Thiophorase, 46, 47f
Thioureas, 146
Thirst, regulation of, 115
Thromboxanes, 8
Thyroglobulin, 141, 142f
  synthesis, 144, 144f
Thyroid antibodies, 162
Thyroid deiodinase, 145

Thyroid function, tests of, 161-162, 161t-162t
Thyroid gland, 120
  anatomy, 141, 142f
  fetal, 277-278
  histology, 141, 142f
  key words, 159-160
  maternal, 279
  pathologic conditions involving, 154-159, 155f, 155t, 156b-158b, 157f-159f
  self-study, 160
  summary, 159-160
Thyroid hormone, 7-8, 7b, 8f, 120
  action mechanisms, 150-154, 151b, 151f-152f
  actions, on cardiovascular system, 154
  actions, on skeletal muscle, 154
  evaluation, serum tests for, 161t
  growth and, 152
  metabolic actions of, 152-153
  metabolism of, 147-148
  mimicking sympathetic nervous system activity, 153-154
  physiologic action of, 155t
  receptors, 8, 150-151, 151f
  secretion, 145, 145f
  signal transduction pathway of, 19f
  synthesis, 142-145, 143b, 144f-145f
    compounds altering, 156
  transport, 146-147, 146b
  tyrosine and, 7b
Thyroid hormone response elements (TREs), 20
Thyroid hormone-binding globulin (TBG), 7-8
Thyroid peroxidase (TPO), 144
Thyroid stimulating hormone (TSH), 149-150, 149f
Thyroiditis, 159
Thyroid-responsive element, 150
Thyroid-stimulating hormone receptor, 150-151
Thyronines, iodinated, 8f
Thyrotoxicosis, 157
Thyrotropes, 121, 124-125, 125f
Thyrotropin, 143
Thyrotropin-releasing hormone (TRH), 124-125, 125f, 148-149, 149f
  responses to, 162t
Thyroxine (T$_4$), 141, 146f, 147-148, 161-162, 161t
Thyroxine-binding globulin, 146
TNF-α. See Tumor necrosis factor-α
TNF/nerve growth factor family, 76
TPO. See Thyroid peroxidase
Transamination, 51
Transcription factors, general, 19f

Transduced signal, 9
Transforming growth factor (TGF)-β family, 17, 18f
Transport proteins, 6
Transthyretin, 146
Trapping intracellular glucose, 59-60, 59f-60f
TREs. See Thyroid hormone response elements
TRH. See Thyrotropin-releasing hormone
Triac, 148
Tricarboxylic acid cycle, 45
Triglycerides (TGs), 47-50, 49f-50f
  dietary, 47-49, 49f
  endogenously-synthesized, 49-50, 50f
  FFAs converted to, 62
  partitioning of, during digestive period, 63f
  release of, in adipose cells, 51
  synthesis, 59f-60f, 61
Triiodothyronine (T$_3$), 142, 147-148, 161-162, 161t
Tropic hormones, 118t, 119
Trousseau's sign, 100, 100f
TrpV5, 89-90
TrpV6, 89-90
Truncal adiposity, 177
TSH. See Thyroid stimulating hormone
Tumor necrosis factor-α (TNF-α), 67, 73b, 74, 92
  receptor, 76
  structure, 75-76
Tumor-induced rickets/osteomalacia, 96
Turner syndrome, 251, 252f
Type 1 diabetes mellitus (T1DM), 43, 65
  characteristics of, 67-68
Type 2 diabetes mellitus (T2DM), 43
  diagnosis, 66
Tyrosine, 4b, 4f, 164, 167f
  thyroid hormone and, 7b
Tyrosine hydroxylase, 164

U
Ultradian rhythms, 21, 21f
Urea cycle, 51
Uterine endometrium, 224
  hormonal regulation of, 242-245, 244f
  structure of, 243f
Uterine size, in parturition, 282
Uterus, structure of, 241-242, 243f

V
Vagal parasympathetic nervous system, stimulation of, 30
Vagina, 246
Vagovagal reflex, 31
Vanillylmandelic acid (VMA), 169

Vas deferens, 208
Vasculosyncytial membrane, 271, 271f
Vasoactive intestinal peptide (VIP), 28
Vasoconstriction
  through alpha adrenergic receptors, of high capacity vessels, 168
  of splanchnic arterioles, 168
Vasodilation, of muscle arteriolar beds, 168
Vasopressin, 110-112, 110f-111f
  receptors, 112, 112f
VDR. See Vitamin D receptor
Very-low density lipoproteins (VLDLs), 49-50, 50f
  partial digestion of, 50
  remnants, 50
Villar lymphatics, 47, 49f
Villi
  development of, 267, 268f, 269-271, 271f
  primary, 267, 268f
VIP. See Vasoactive intestinal peptide
Vitamin B$_{12}$, efficient absorption of, 29
Vitamin D, 4, 85-86, 85f
  deficiency, 87, 100f, 101
  response elements, 87
  structure, 86
  synthesis, 86, 86f
Vitamin D receptor (VDR), 5, 87
Vitamin D$_2$, 86, 86f
Vitamin D$_3$, 86, 86f
Vitamin D-binding protein (DBP), 87
VLDLs. See Very-low density lipoproteins
VMA. See Vanillylmandelic acid
Voltage-gated Ca^{2+} channels, 55

W
"Window of receptivity," 260
Wolff-Chaikoff effect, 145

X
X-linked hypophosphatemia, 96
X-ray
  hyperparathyroidism, 98f
  hyperthyroid, 152f
  rickets, 100f

Z
Zollinger-Ellison syndrome, 30, 39
Zona fasciculata, 166f, 170-179, 171f-174f, 175b, 176f, 178b, 179f
  cortisol and, 170-175, 171f-174f
Zona glomerulosa, 182-188, 184f-186f, 187b, 187f
Zona reticularis, 166f, 170, 179-182, 180f-181f
  makes adrenal androgens, 179-180, 180f
  regulation of, 182, 182f